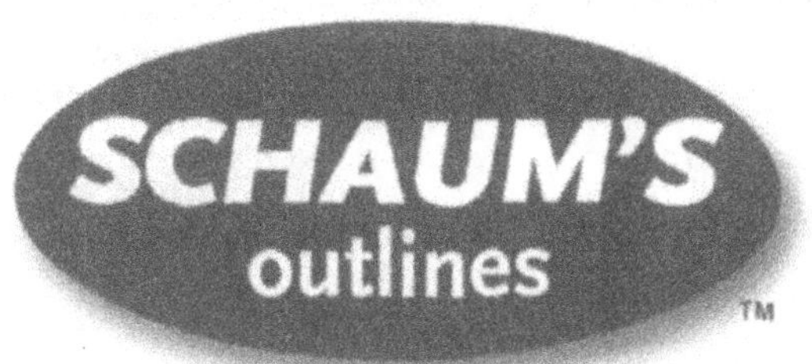

Pathophysiology

Thomas Betsy
Professor,
Bergen County Community College

Schaum's Outline Series

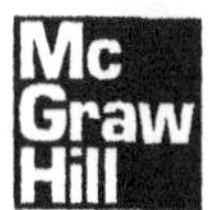

New York Chicago San Francisco Lisbon London Madrid
Mexico City Milan New Delhi San Juan Seoul
Singapore Sydney Toronto

The **McGraw-Hill** *Companies*

2 3 4 5 6 7 8 9 10 QVS/QVS 1 9 8 7 6 5 4

ISBN: 978-0-07-162369-8
MHID: 0-07-162369-8

Schaum's Outline of
PATHOPHYSIOLOGY

Library of Congress Cataloging-in-Publication Data

Betsy, Tom.
Schaum's outline of pathophysiology / Thomas Betsy.
p.; cm. – (Schaum's outline series)
Other title: Outline of pathophysiology
Summary: "This book provides a review for the undergraduate course in Pathophysiology for nursing students"—Provided by publisher.
ISBN-13: 978-0-07-162369-8
ISBN-10: 0-07-162369-8
1. Physiology, Pathological—Outlines, syllabi, etc. I. Title. II. Title: Outline of pathophysiology.
III. Series: Schaum's outline series.
[DNLM: 1. Pathology—Examination Questions. 2. Pathology—Nurses' Instruction. 3. Pathology—Outlines.
4. Physiology—Examination Questions. 5. Physiology—Nurses' Instruction. 6. Physiology—Outlines.
QZ 18.2 B564s 2010]
RB113.B456 2010
616.07—dc22 2010010397

This book is dedicated to my wife, Shelley, and my babies, Juliana and Thomas, for their love, laughter, and smiles and for tolerating the nights and weekends when Daddy was away working on the manuscript. And to my students, whose love of education inspires me and makes teaching the best job in the world.

Contents

To the Student

Thank you for reading *Schaum's Outline of Pathophysiology.* This book is designed to help guide you through the subjects of pathology and pathophysiology, as well as provide a review of anatomy and physiology.

The information used in preparing this outline came from what I believe to be reliable and accurate sources. This outline is intended to be a study guide, and in no way, shape, or form is a substitute for your textbooks or your professors' notes.

This outline is informational and is in no way intended to be used in the diagnosis or treatment of any condition, pathology, or disease. If you feel that you have a condition, pathology, or disease, it is highly recommended that you seek the evaluation or advice of a health-care professional.

I wish you the best of luck in all your endeavors in the fields of science and health.

Tom Betsy

Acknowledgments

I would like to acknowledge and thank Mrs. Joan Sisto for her countless hours on the computer. Joan has assisted me for most of my professional career. I cannot thank her and her husband, Ronnie, enough.

I would like to thank my colleagues and friends, professors John Smalley, Fred Benedict, and Daniel Donatacci for all their technical help and advice.

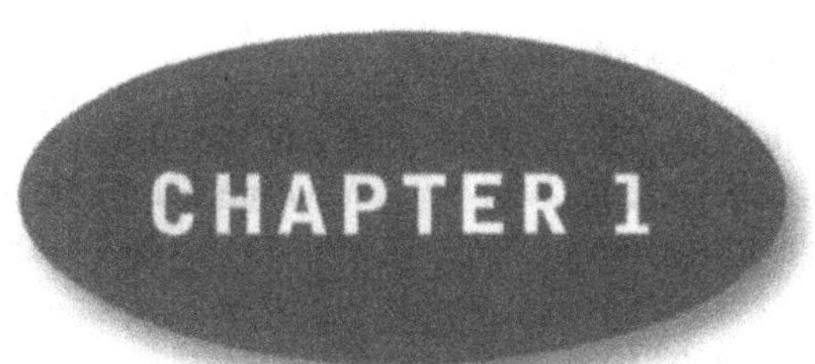

Pathology, Pathophysiology, and the Different Types of Disease-Causing Agents

The study of pathology and the agents that cause disease are essential to anyone who is pursuing a career in health care. In this book, we will make it easy to understand many of these disease-causing agents, their routes of infection, infection control, immunity, and the pathologies that affect the various systems of the human body.

Objectives

This chapter will introduce various terms and definitions associated with the field of pathophysiology and common medical terminology used in health-care settings.

Keywords:

Anatomy	Local Disease	Clinical Disease	Syndrome	
Physiology	Systemic Disease	Subclinical Disease	Congenital Disorder	
Homeostasis			Pathogen	
Disease				
Symptom				
Sign	Acute Disease			
	Subacute Diseasc			
	Autoimmune Disease			
	Cancerous Diseases		Diagnosis	Pathology
	Chronic Disease		Pathologist	

1.1 Overview

What Is Anatomy?

Anatomy is the study of body structures. An example would be the heart. The heart is an organ that has a specific task.

What Is Physiology?

Physiology is the study of the functions or tasks of those body structures. An example would be the heart pumping blood filled with oxygen and nutrients to the cells and tissues of the body, as well as pumping deoxygenated blood and wastes away from these cells and tissues.

What Is Homeostasis?

Homeostasis is the "steady state" or equilibrium of the body. This is a condition in which all the chemical reactions occurring in the body (metabolism) are being maintained properly despite any external fluctuations in the external environment and in which all the cells (that make up tissues), all the tissues (that make up organs), all the organs (that make up organ systems), and all the 11 organ systems that make up the organism (in this case humans) are working at their optimal levels or peak performances. This is what we call "health."

What Two Systems Maintain Homeostasis?

The two systems of the body that primarily maintain homeostasis are the ***nervous system*** (which we will review in Chapter 18) and the ***endocrine system*** (which we will review in Chapter 17). Remember that every organ system has a role to play in the maintenance of homeostasis.

What Can Happen if Homeostasis Is Disrupted?

If homeostasis is disrupted, a disease process can occur, and the organism can die as a result of this disruption.

What Can Cause a Disease Process?

Anything that disrupts homeostasis can cause a disease process.

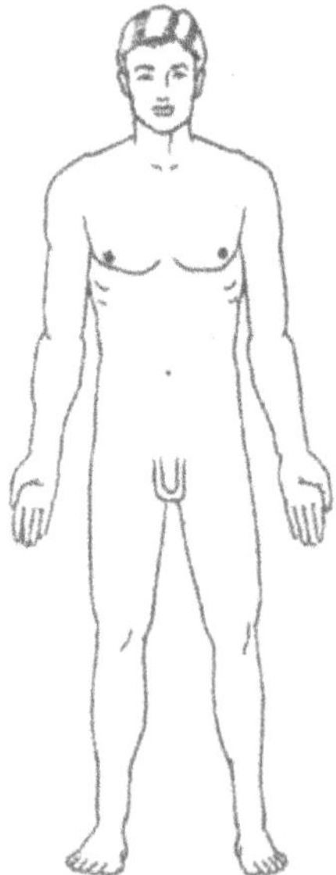

DEFINITION The integument (skin) and structures derived from it (hair, nails, and oil sweat glands).

FUNCTIONS Protects the body, regulates body temperature, eliminates wastes, and receives certain stimuli (tactile, temperature, and pain).

Figure 1.1 Integumentary system.

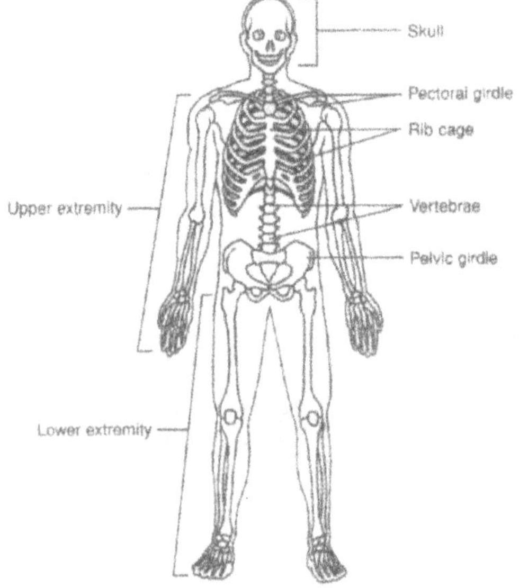

DEFINITION Bones, cartilage, and ligaments (which steady the bones at the joints).

FUNCTIONS Provides body support and protection, permits movement and leverage, produces blood cells (hematopoiesis), and stores minerals.

Figure 1.2 Skeletal system.

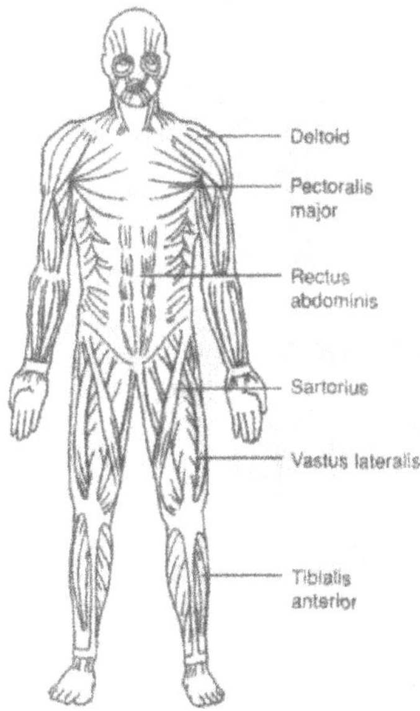

DEFINITION Skeletal muscles of the body and their tendinous attachments.

FUNCTIONS Effects body movements, maintains posture, and produces body heat.

Figure 1.3 Muscular system.

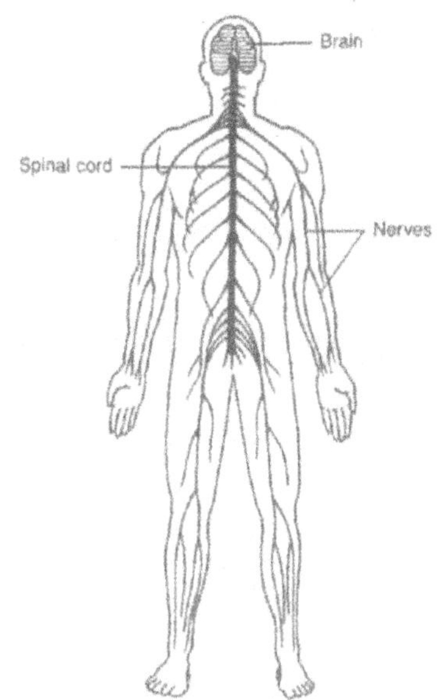

DEFINITION Brain, spinal cord, nerves, and sensory organs such as the eye and the ear.

FUNCTIONS Detects and responds to changes in internal and external environments, enables reasoning and memory, and regulates body activities.

Figure 1.4 Nervous system.

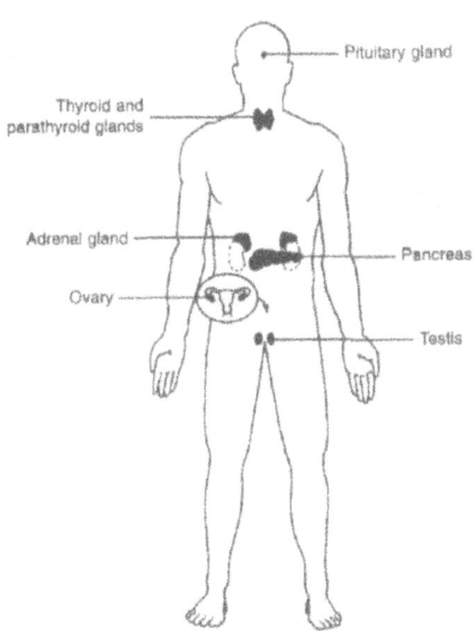

DEFINITION The hormone-producing glands.

FUNCTIONS Controls and integrates body functions via hormones secreted into the bloodstream.

Figure 1.5 Endocrine system.

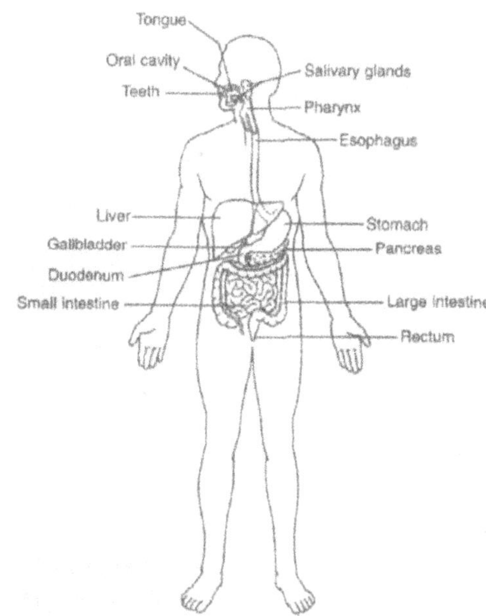

DEFINITION The body organs that render ingested foods absorbable.

FUNCTIONS Mechanically and chemically breaks down foods for cellular use and eliminates undigested wastes.

Figure 1.6 Digestive system.

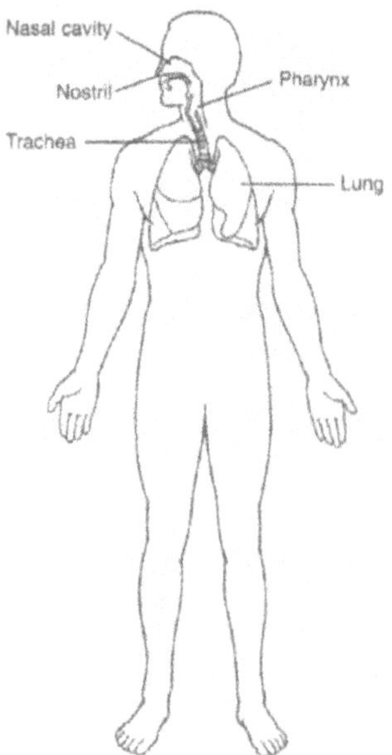

DEFINITION The body organs concerned with movement of respiratory gases (O_2 and CO_2) to and from the pulmonary blood (the blood within the lungs).

FUNCTIONS Supplies oxygen to the blood and eliminates carbon dioxide; also helps to regulate acid–base balance.

Figure 1.7 Respiratory system.

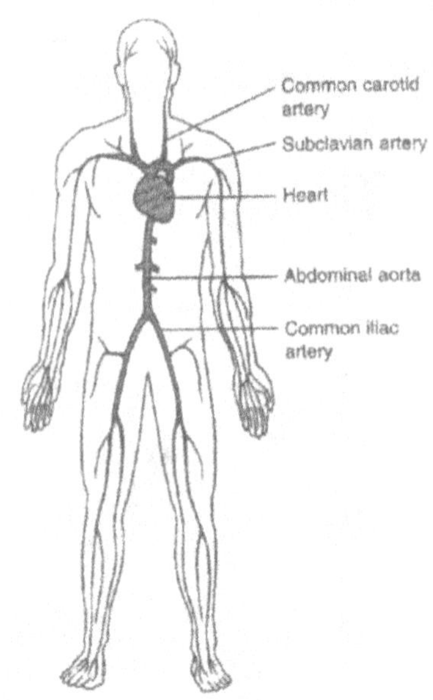

DEFINITION The heart and the vessels that carry blood or blood constituents (lymph) through the body.

FUNCTIONS Transports respiratory gases, nutrients, wastes, and hormones; protects against disease and fluid loss; helps regulate body temperature and acid–base balance.

Figure 1.8 Circulatory system.

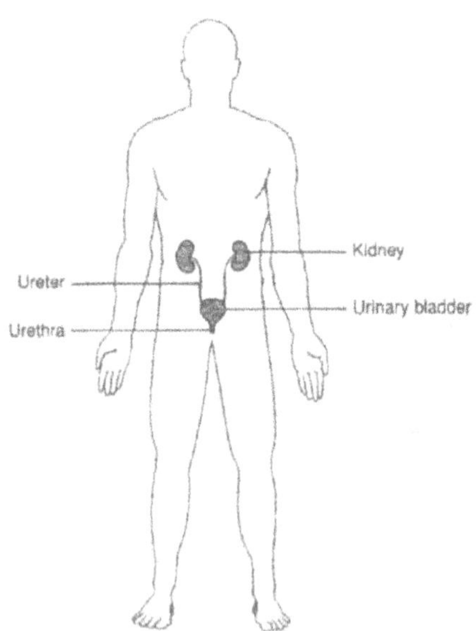

DEFINITION The organs that operate to remove wastes from the blood and to eliminate urine from the body.

FUNCTIONS Removes various wastes from the blood; regulates the chemical composition, volume, and electrolyte balance of the blood; helps maintain the acid–base balance of the body.

Figure 1.9 Urinary system.

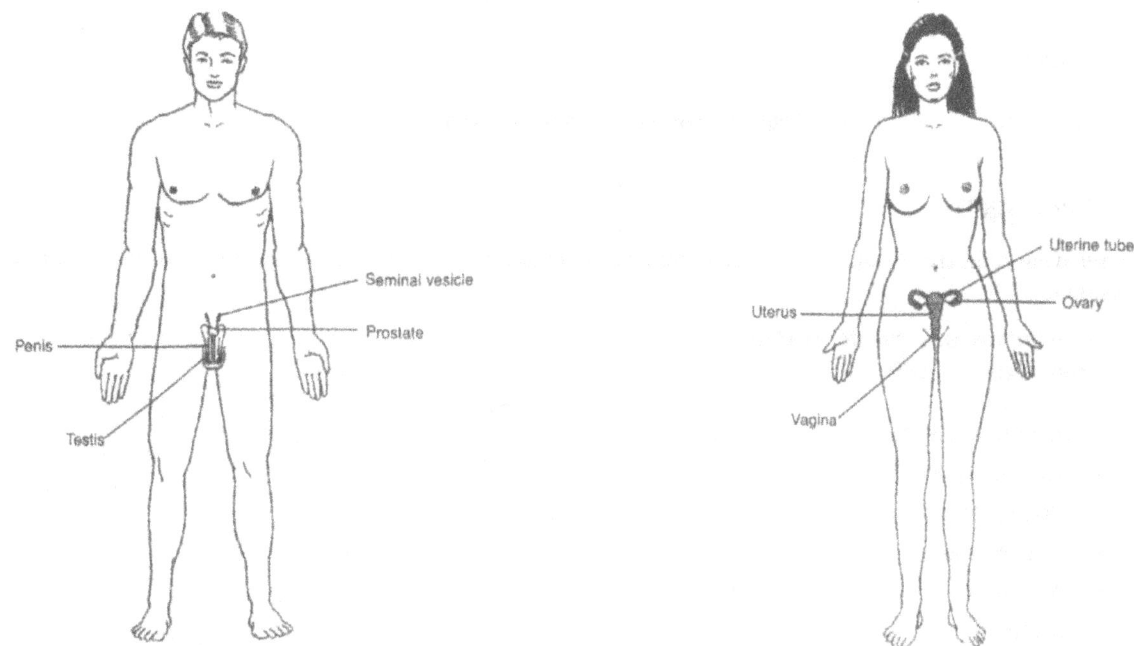

DEFINITION The body organs that produce, store, and transport reproductive cells (*gametes,* or sperm and ova).
FUNCTIONS Reproduce the organism, produce sex hormones.

Figure 1.10 Male and female reproductive systems.

What Can Disrupt Homeostasis?

Stress or stressors, such as an infection, can disrupt homeostasis.

What Is Stress?

Stress (which will be discussed in Chapter 4) can and will disrupt the homeostasis of the body and cause disease processes.

What Is a Disease?

A ***disease,*** or "dis-ease," is a disruption, disorder, stoppage, or interruption of the normal workings of the body. This means that the cells, tissues, organs, and organ systems are not working at their optimal level. A disease can present itself with symptoms and signs.

What Is a Symptom?

A ***symptom*** is a subjective finding, meaning that the patient will describe how he or she feels to the examiner.

What would be some examples of symptoms?
Examples of symptoms include

- Headaches (cephalgia)
- Joint pain (arthralgia)
- Stomachache
- Nervousness

- Anxiety
- Chills

Remember: These conditions cannot be read or measured by an examiner.

What Is a Sign?

A ***sign*** is an objective finding. This means that an examiner can observe, read, and measure the patient's condition.

What would be some examples of signs?
Examples of signs include

- Heart rate (pulse)
- Respiratory rate
- Blood pressure
- Temperature
- Skin color
- Swelling
- Edema

Remember: These conditions can be read and measured by the examiner.

1.2 Types of Diseases

Diseases can be named and broken down into different categories based on how, when, and where they affect the body.

What Is a Local Disease?

A ***local disease*** is a disease that affects one portion or a specific area of the body.

What would be an example of a local disease?
An example of a localized disease would be ***tinea pedis* or *athlete's foot***, a fungal infection that can be caused by *Epidermophyton floccosum*.

What Is a Systemic Disease?

A ***systemic disease*** is a type of disease that affects the entire body.

What would be an example of a systemic disease?
An example of a systemic disease would be ***multiple sclerosis***, an autoimmune disease in which the body's own defenses cannot distinguish between "self" and "nonself," or what are the person's own cells and what are foreign cells. In the case of multiple sclerosis, the body's own defensive cells attack the myelin sheath of the nerve cells (neurons).

What Is an Acute Disease?

An ***acute disease*** is a disease that begins quickly with signs and symptoms.

What would be an example of an acute disease?
An example of an acute disease would be the ***influenza virus***.

What Is a Subacute Disease?

A ***subacute disease*** is a disease that is in between an acute and a chronic disease. This form of disease is not as severe as an acute disease.

What would be an example of a subacute disease?
An example would be ***subacute thyroiditis***. Subacute thyroiditis is an inflammatory condition of the thyroid gland caused by a virus.

What Is a Chronic Disease?

A ***chronic disease*** is a disease that starts off slowly and lasts from months to years or even a lifetime.

What would be an example of a chronic disease?
An example of a chronic disease would be mononucleosis, caused by the ***Epstein-Barr virus***.

What Is an Autoimmune Disease?

An ***autoimmune disease*** occurs when the body's immune system attacks the body's own cells.

What would be an example of an autoimmune disease?
An example of an autoimmune disease would be ***rheumatoid arthritis***.

What Is a Cancerous Disease?

A ***cancerous disease*** occurs when there are mutations or abnormalities of cells and these cells grow uncontrollably. These cells can spread (metastasize) and affect other organs of the body.

What would be an example of a cancerous disease?
An example of a cancerous disease would be ***malignant melanoma***, a form of skin cancer.

What Is a Degenerative Disease?

A ***degenerative disease*** is a "wear and tear" type of disease. This can occur as a result of overuse syndrome, repetitive stress, or the aging process.

What would be an example of a degenerative disease?
An example of a degenerative disease would be ***osteoarthritis***.

What Is a Deficiency Disease?

Deficiency diseases occur when there is an insufficient dietary intake or malabsorption of nutrients, minerals, and/or vitamins.

What would be an example of a deficiency disease?
An example of a deficiency disease would be ***pernicious anemia*** due to a deficiency in vitamin B_{12}.

What Is a Genetic Disease?

Genetic diseases are diseases caused by abnormalities of the cell's genetic code. These diseases are also called ***hereditary diseases*** because they run in families and can be passed from one generation to another.

What would be an example of a hereditary disease?
An example of a hereditary disease would be ***sickle cell anemia.***

What Is an Infectious or Communicable Disease?

An ***infectious or communicable disease*** is a disease caused by bacteria, viruses, parasites, and/or fungi. Infectious diseases are contagious and can be transmitted from one person to another. These diseases can also be transmitted by animals or fomites (inanimate objects).

What would an example of an infectious or communicable disease?
An example of an infectious disease would be ***pharyngitis*** (strep throat), caused by the bacterium *Streptococcus pyogenes*.

What Is a Metabolic Disease?

Metabolic diseases disrupt normal chemical reactions that occur in the body.

What would be an example of a metabolic disease?
An example of a metabolic disease would be ***Graves' disease*** *or* ***hyperthyroidism,*** which is characterized by increased thyroid activity.

1.3 Disorders

What Is a Disorder?

A ***disorder*** is a dysfunction of a normal bodily function resulting in a disruption in homeostasis.

What Is a Traumatic Disorder?

A ***traumatic disorder*** is an injury that physically disrupts the normal working of the body.

What would be an example of a traumatic disorder?
Examples of traumatic disorders would include ***fractures*** and ***skin abrasions***.

What Is a Clinical Disease?

A ***clinical disease*** is a condition that presents with signs and symptoms.

What Is a Subclinical Disease?

A ***subclinical disease*** is a disease that does not present with signs and symptoms. Therefore, this type of disease is not clinically apparent.

What Is a Carrier?

A ***carrier*** is a person who is colonized by a disease-causing microorganism but does not exhibit signs or symptoms and may even have negative laboratory findings. This individual, however, can be contagious and can still infect others.

From a genetic point of view, a carrier is a person who possesses a genetic trait and can pass it on to his or her offspring, even though he or she may not exhibit the signs or symptoms associated with the trait.

What Is a Diagnosis?

A ***diagnosis*** is a decision as to the cause of a disease or health problem, based on patient history; physical examination; laboratory findings; or x-rays, MRIs, or CT scans.

What Is a Syndrome?

A number of signs and symptoms that together will present as a certain type of disease or abnormal condition are referred to as a ***syndrome***.

What Are Congenital Disorders?

Congenital disorders are abnormalities that present themselves at birth.

What would be an example of a congenital disorder?
An example of a congenital disorder would be ***trisomy 21*** or ***Down syndrome***.

TABLE **1.1 Review of Structures and Functions of the Human Body**

SYSTEM	STRUCTURES	FUNCTIONS
1. Integumentary system	Skin, hair, nails	Protection, maintains body temperature.
2. Skeletal system	Bones, cartilage, ligaments	Support, protection, movement, blood cell production.
3. Muscular system	Muscles, tendons	Movement, maintains organ volume, heat production.
4. Nervous system	Brain, spinal cord, nerves	Detects, interprets, and reacts to changes in the body's internal and external environments, reasoning, and memory.
5. Endocrine system	Hypothalamus, pituitary gland, thyroid gland, adrenal glands, thymus gland, pancreas	Secretes hormones which are chemical messengers which control and integrate organ activity.
6. Circulatory system	Heart, blood, blood vessels	Transports oxygen and nutrients to cells, transports carbon dioxide and wastes away from cells, regulates acid-base balance, protects against disease and fluid loss.
7. Lymphatic system	Lymphatic fluid, lymph vessels, tonsils, adenoids, thymus gland, red bone marrow, spleen, lymph nodes	Drains interstitial spaces, transports fat-soluble vitamins and dietary lipids, fights infection.
8. Respiratory system	Nose, mouth, pharynx, larynx, trachea, lungs	Oxygenates blood, eliminates CO_2, regulates acid-base balance.
9. Digestive system	Mouth, esophagus, pharynx, stomach, small intestine, large intestine, teeth, tongue, liver, gall bladder, pancreas	Ingests, breaks down, and absorbs food for cellular use, eliminates waste.
10. Urinary system	Kidneys, ureters, urinary bladder, urethra	Regulates fluid volume and electrolyte balance of blood, filters blood.
11. Reproductive system	Ovaries, testes	Produces male and female gametes and sex hormones, reproduces, and supports development of new individual.

1.4 Disease-Causing Agents

What Are Disease-Causing Agents?

A disease-causing agent is any pollutant or microorganism that can cause an infection.

What are some examples of disease-causing agents?
Examples of disease-causing agents are: bacteria, viruses, prions, fungi, parasites, and protozoa.

What Is a Pathogen?

A ***pathogen*** is a disease-causing agent.

What Is Pathology?

Pathology is the study of changes that cells and tissues undergo during a disease process or the disease state itself.

What Is a Pathologist?

A ***pathologist*** is a scientist who studies cells and tissue for changes that have occurred as a result of a disease process.

Bacteria

Most ***bacteria*** are harmless to humans. Some bacteria are helpful to humans. These bacteria are the "normal flora" that live in and on the surfaces of our bodies, such as in our intestines, on our skin, and in the female reproductive tract. Some bacteria can be used to produce foods, such as yogurt and cheese. Other bacteria can be harmful to humans. These bacteria can enter the body by various portals of entry, such as the following:

1. *Ingesting* improperly prepared foods [example: *Salmonella enterica*, the organism that causes food poisoning (gastroenteritis)].
2. *Inhaling* when an infected person coughs or sneezes (example: *Mycobacterium tuberculosis*, the organism that causes tuberculosis).
3. *Contact* with an infected person or object (example: *Staphylococcus aureus*, the organism that causes impetigo).

Viruses

Viruses are "nonliving" biological entities. They are considered nonliving because they need a host cell's biochemical "machinery" in order to replicate. Viruses contain either DNA or RNA, but not both. They can replicate by absorption, penetration, and uncoating. Some viruses attach themselves to the molecules located on the plasma membrane of the host cell. These molecules are important for normal cellular function. When they enter the cell by a process called *endocytosis*, the virus tags along and enters the cell. Other viruses attach themselves to the host cell's plasma membrane or cell wall, then inject their nucleic acid into the nucleus of that cell. In the host cell nucleus, the virus continues to replicate until the host cell bursts. All of the new viruses then in turn infect new host cells. Viruses can be transmitted from

- *Person to person.* An example would be the herpes virus type I or herpes simplex, which affects mucous membranes.
- *Animal or insect to person.* An example would be the rhabdovirus, which causes rabies. This virus is transmitted through the saliva of the infected animal and affects the brain of the new host.

Prions A prion is a very small substance that is made up of a protein that contains no nucleic acids. Prions can replicate and cause infection.

What are some examples of diseases caused by prions?
Prions can cause the neurological disorder ***Creutzfeldt-Jakob disease*** ("spongiform encephalopathy") in humans, ***scapies*** in goats and sheep, and ***mad cow disease*** ("bovine spongiform encephalopathy") in cattle.

Fungi (Yeast and Molds)
Many ***fungi*** enjoy a warm, moist environment. Relatively few of these organisms are harmful to humans. Those that are can be transmitted from

- *Person to person.* An example would be *Candida albicans*, which can cause thrush.
- *Object to person.* An example would be *Epidermophyton floccosum,* which causes *tinea pedis* or "athlete's foot." This organism is usually found in public showers and locker rooms.

Protists

Protists are parasites that can live in our bodies. Some of these disease-causing parasites can be transmitted to humans by

- *Contaminated food, water, and fecal matter.* An example would be *Entamoeba histolytica*, which causes dysentery.
- *Insect to human.* An example would be *Plasmodium falciparum*, which is transmitted by mosquitoes and causes malaria.
- *Human to human.* An example would be *Trichomonas vaginalis*, which affects the urinary tract and causes trichomoniasis, a sexually transmitted disease.

TABLE 1.2 Examples of Disease-Causing Organisms, Place of Infection, and Disease

ORGANISM	PLACE OF INFECTION	DISEASE
Bacteria		
Salmonella enterica	Intestines	Gastroenteritis
Myobacterium tuberculosis	Lung	Tuberculosis
Staphylococcus aureus	Skin	Impetigo
Viruses		
Herpes virus	Mucous membranes	Herpes simplex
Rhabdovirus	Brain	Rabies
Prions		
Infectious protein particle	Brain	Creutzfeldt-Jakob disease
Fungi		
Candida albicans	Mouth, skin	Thrush, dermatitis
Epidermophyton floccosum	Skin	Athlete's foot
Protists		
Entamoeba histolytica	Intestines	Ameboid dysentery
Plasmodium falciparum	Blood, circulatory system	Malaria
Trichomonas vaginalis	Genital tract	Trichomoniasis

Chapter 1 Review Questions

Fill In the Blank

1. The study of body structures is called ____________________.
2. The study of body function is called ____________________.
3. The steady state of the body is called ________________.
4. The two primary organ systems that maintain homeostasis are the ___________ system and the ___________ system.
5. ____________ disrupts homeostasis.
6. A disruption in the normal function of the body is called ____________________.
7. A disruption in the normal functions of the body presents as _________ and _________.
8. A sign is a(n) ______________finding.
9. A symptom is a(n) ________________finding.
10. A headache is an example of a(n) _____________ finding.
11. Blood pressure would be an example of a(n) ________________ finding.
12. This disease type affects a specific area of the body: _________________.
13. A(n) ______________disease affects the entire body.
14. This type of disease presents quickly with signs and symptoms: ______________.
15. A(n) ______________is a disease that starts slowly and lasts from months to years, or, in some cases, a lifetime.
16. This type of disease presents with signs and symptoms: ________________.
17. This type of disease would not present with signs and symptoms: ________________.
18. A person who possesses a disease-causing agent and is contagious but does not appear sick is called a(n) __________________.
19. A "wear and tear" type of disease is called a(n) _________________.
20. A decision based on patient history, physical exam, and laboratory findings is a(n) _______.
21. A(n) ______________is an abnormality of the normal function of an organ.
22. Signs and symptoms that present together are called _________________.
23. Genetic abnormalities present themselves at __________________.
24. Genetic abnormalities that present themselves at birth are called ________________.
25. A disease-causing agent is called a(n) ___________________.
26. The study of disease-causing agents is called ______________________.
27. A person who studies the changes that occur to cells and tissues as a result of disease is called a(n) ____________________.
28. Down syndrome would be an example of a(n) ________________disorder.
29. Multiple sclerosis would be an example of a(n) _______________disease.
30. Athlete's foot would be an example of a(n) ________________disease.

Matching

Which of the following are bacteria, viruses, fungi, or protists?

31. *Salmonella enterica* ______________________

32. Herpes ______________________

33. *Staphylococcus aureus* ______________________

34. *Candida albicans* ______________________

35. *Trichomonas vaginalis* ______________________

36. *Plasmodium falciparum* ______________________

37. *Epidermophyton floccosum* ______________________

38. *Mycobacterium tuberculosis* ______________________

39. Rhabdovirus ______________________

40. *Entamoeba histolytica* ______________________

Multiple Choice

41. Athlete's foot is caused by which type of organism?

A. Bacteria
B. Virus
C. Fungus
D. Parasite

42. A disease such as multiple sclerosis is a(n) ____________disease.

A. acute
B. subacute
C. local
D. systemic

43. An example of a genetic disorder would be __________.

A. food poisoning
B. rheumatoid arthritis
C. Down syndrome
D. osteoarthritis

44. A person who studies changes that cells undergo during a disease process is called a(n) ____________________.

A. endocrinologist
B. pathologist
C. epidemiologist
D. botanist

45. A "wear and tear" type of disease is called a ______________.

A. systemic disease
B. degenerative disease
C. congenital disease
D. pandemic disease

46. An example of a "wear and tear" type of disease would be ___________.

A. rheumatoid arthritis
B. osteoarthritis
C. systemic lupus erythematosus
D. amyotrophic lateral sclerosis

47. The two organ systems that maintain homeostasis are the ________ and the ___________ systems.

A. respiratory; circulatory
B. lymphatic; cardiac
C. endocrine; muscular
D. nervous; endocrine

48. The study of body structures is _____________.

A. physiology
B. anatomy
C. endocrinology
D. osteology

49. The study of body functions is __________.

A. physiology
B. anatomy
C. endocrinology
D. osteology

50. A decision based on patient history, physical exam, and laboratory findings would be a _____________.

A. diagnosis
B. syndrome
C. disease
D. symptom

Chapter 1: Review Questions and Answers

Fill In the Blank Answers

1. Anatomy
2. Physiology
3. Homeostasis
4. Nervous; endocrine
5. Stress
6. Disease
7. Signs; symptoms
8. Objective
9. Subjective
10. Subjective
11. Objective
12. Local disease
13. Systemic
14. Acute disease
15. Chronic disease
16. Clinical disease
17. Subclinical disease
18. Carrier
19. Degenerative disease
20. Diagnosis

21. Disorder

22. Syndromes

23. Birth

24. Congenital disorders

25. Pathogen

26. Pathology

27. Pathologist

28. Congenital

29. Systemic

30. Local

Matching Answers

31. Bacteria

32. Virus

33. Bacteria

34. Fungi

35. Protist

36. Protist

37. Fungi

38. Bacteria

39. Virus

40. Protist

Multiple Choice Answers

41. C

42. D

43. C

44. B

45. B

46. B

47. D

48. B

49. A

50. A

Epidemiology

Objectives

This chapter will introduce how diseases are spread from one person to another and how outbreaks of diseases are prevented and controlled.

Keywords:

Epidemiology
Epidemiologist
Etiology
Incidence rate
Prevalence rate
Infection
Morbidity rate
Mortality rate
Endemic disease
Sporadic disease
Epidemic disease
Pandemic disease
Common-source epidemic
Propagated epidemic
Pathognomonic
Immunity
Virulence
Sites of infection
Reservoirs of infection
Portal of entry
Portal of exit
Direct contact transmission
Indirect contact transmission
Droplet transmission
Waterborne pathogens
Airborne pathogens
Foodborne pathogens
Vector pathogens
Incubation period
Prodromal period
Period of illness
Period of decline
Period of convalescence
Communicable diseases
Vector control
Immunization
Quarantine
Isolation

2.1 Overview

What Is Epidemiology?

Epidemiology is the study of the causes, conditions, and distributions of diseases in a given population.

What Does an Epidemiologist Do?

An ***epidemiologist*** is a scientist who studies the causes and prevention of diseases.

What Is the Specific Cause of a Disease Called?

The specific cause of a disease is called its ***etiology***. The etiology of a disease-causing agent is the major concern of an epidemiologist. Epidemiologists are also concerned with the frequency of a disease in a given population.

What Does an Epidemiologist Have to Consider When Observing a Disease?

An epidemiologist must consider the:

- *Incidence rate.* The ***incidence rate*** of a disease is the number of *new* cases within a year.
- *Prevalence rate.* The ***prevalence rate*** of a disease is the total number of new and old cases of a disease in a given population reported in one year.

An epidemiologist must identify what causes and transmits diseases in order to control and prevent their spread.

What if There Is Infection?

If ***infection*** occurs, the frequency of illness and death must be studied.

What is the morbidity rate of a population?

- The ***morbidity rate*** is the number of people in a given population who have become ill per time period.

What is the mortality rate of a population?

- The ***mortality rate*** would be the number of people in a given population who have died per time period.

These rates are summarized in Table 2.1.

TABLE 2.1 Factors of Disease

Incidence rate	Number of new cases of a disease reported in one year
Prevalence rate	Number of new and old cases of a disease reported in one year
Morbidity rate	Number of people in a given population who have become ill per time period
Mortality rate	Number of people in a given population who have died per time period

2.2 Disease Classification

Epidemiologists measure the frequency of diseases in a given population with regard to distribution and the amount of damage the disease causes.

How Are Diseases Classified?

Diseases can be classified as *endemic, sporadic, epidemic,* and *pandemic.* These classifications are summarized in Table 2.2.

TABLE 2.2 Disease Classification

Endemic disease	A disease with a normal or average number of cases in a given population
Sporadic disease	A disease that infects in small numbers; sporadic diseases do not threaten a population
Epidemic disease	A disease where the normal or average number of cases is greater than that of an endemic disease
Pandemic disease	A disease that is distributed worldwide

What Is an Endemic Disease?

A disease that causes a normal or average number of cases in a given population is called an ***endemic disease.***

What would be an example of an endemic disease?
An example would be a seasonal-type disease, such as *chicken pox.*

What Is a Sporadic Disease?

A disease that occurs in small numbers of cases is called a ***sporadic disease.*** Sporadic diseases never threaten a population.

What would be an example of a sporadic disease?
An example of a sporadic disease would be improperly prepared food in a school or company cafeteria. Anyone eating the prepared food would become infected and feel sick. An organism that can cause food poisoning would be *Salmonella enterica.*

What Is an Epidemic Disease?

When the normal level of disease cases is greater than that of an endemic disease, the disease is called an ***epidemic disease.***

What would be an example of an epidemic disease?
An example of an epidemic disease would be a flu virus that infects an elementary school. Epidemic diseases are a significant health concern because of the high rate of infection. The school would most likely have to close to stop the spread of the disease.

What Is a Pandemic Disease?

When a disease is distributed worldwide, it is called a ***pandemic disease.***

What would be an example of a pandemic disease?
An example of a pandemic disease would be AIDS, which is caused by the HIV virus, or cholera, which is caused by the bacterium *Vibrio cholerae.*

2.3 Types of Epidemics

What Is a Common-Source Epidemic?

In a ***common-source epidemic***, large numbers of a population become infected by a common source.

What would be an example of a common-source epidemic?
An example of a common-source epidemic would be improperly handled food in a buffet. Everyone who eats this food on this particular day will become infected and feel sick.

What Is a Propagated Epidemic?

In a ***propagated epidemic***, person-to-person contact occurs. A person who is infected and feels sick infects a person who was not previously infected.

What would be an example of a propagated disease?
An example of a ***propagated epidemic*** would be an influenza outbreak.

What Does Pathognomonic Mean?

Pathognomonic refers to the specific characteristics of a disease.

What Is Immunity?

Immunity is specific resistance to a disease. It is the ability of a person to resist that disease.

What Is Virulence with Regard to a Disease-Causing Agent?

Virulence is the capacity of an organism to produce a disease.

2.4 Sites of Infection

What Are the Sites of Infection?

The ***sites of infection*** are the locations where organisms can infect a host organism. They are collectively called reservoirs of infections.

What are Reservoirs of Infection?

Reservoirs of infection can be human, animal, or nonliving.

What are human reservoirs?

- *Human reservoirs.* Humans can transmit disease-causing agents to other humans.

What is an example of a human reservoir?
An example of such a disease-causing agent would be *Neisseria meningitides.*

What are animal reservoirs?

- *Animal reservoirs.* Animals can transmit disease-causing agents to humans. Remember, many organisms infect both animals and humans.

What is an example of an animal reservoir?
An example of such a disease-causing agent would be the bacteria *Bacillus anthracis*, the organism that causes anthrax.

What are nonliving reservoirs?

- *Nonliving reservoirs.* Soil and water are examples of nonliving reservoirs. These areas make great places for microorganisms to multiply.

What would be an example of a soil and a water reservoir?
An example of a microorganism that is found in soil is *Clostridium tetani.* These bacteria cause tetanus. An example of a microorganism that is found in water is *Vibrio cholerae.* These bacteria cause cholera.

2.5 Types of Transmissions

What Is the Transmission of Diseases

A disease is transmitted when a disease-causing agent "gets out" (***portal of exit***) of the reservoir and "gets in" (***portal of entry***) to the host.

How Can Diseases Be Transmitted?

A disease-causing agent can be transmitted by direct or indirect contact.

What is a direct contact transmission?

- ***Direct contact transmission*** occurs when there is "skin-to-skin" contact.

What would be examples of direct contact transmission?

- Examples of such contact include shaking hands and kissing.

What are some diseases that can be transmitted this way?

- Diseases transmitted in this way include impetigo and herpes simplex virus infections.

What is indirect contact transmission?

- ***Indirect contact transmission*** occurs through inanimate objects.

What would be examples of indirect contact transmission?

- Examples of such contact include clothing, bedding, towels, and utensils.

What are some diseases that can be transmitted in this way?

- Diseases transmitted in this way include rhinovirus and tetanus.

What is droplet transmission?

- ***Droplet transmission*** occurs through the spread of fluid when an infected person coughs or sneezes on a noninfected person. Droplet transmission can also occur with "close contact speaking" with an infected individual.

What are examples of droplet transmission?

- Examples of transmission include coughing and close contact speaking.

What are some diseases that can be transmitted in this way?

- Diseases transmitted in this way include pneumonia and whooping cough.

How Do Disease-Causing Agents Get Spread to Infect Hosts?

Disease-causing agents or pathogens can spread through water, air, food, or vectors.

What Are Waterborne Pathogens?

Waterborne pathogens are those transmitted through contaminated water. The water can be contaminated by sewage (fecal material).

What is an example of a waterborne pathogen?
An example of a waterborne pathogen would be *Vibrio cholerae.*

What Are Airborne Pathogens?

Airborne pathogens are those transmitted through the air. They can cause infection in places where people are in close contact with one another or in buildings with central air conditioning and heating.

These buildings get little fresh air. Airborne pathogens can mix with dust. Walking, sweeping, and changing bed linens can agitate these dust particles and send them into the air, where they can be inhaled.

What is an example of an airborne pathogen?
An example of an airborne pathogen is *Mycobacterium tuberculosis.*

What Are Vector Pathogens?

Vector pathogens are those transmitted from living organisms, such as arthropods, to humans.

What are examples of vector pathogens?
Examples of arthropods are flies, mosquitoes, and ticks.

How do vectors transmit disease?
Vectors transmit disease in two ways:

- *Mechanical vector transmission.* With this method, the vector passively transmits disease with its body.

What is an example of a mechanical vector?

- An example of a mechanical vector would be a common housefly landing on your food after it landed on animal feces.

What is biological vector transmission?

- With this method, the vector actively transmits the pathogen. In biological vectors, the disease-causing agent will start its life cycle in the arthropod, then complete the life cycle once it has entered the body and has access to cells and tissues.

What is an example of biological vector transmission?

- An example of biological vector transmission would be a mosquito infecting a human with malaria.

The types of transmission are summarized in Table 2.3.

TABLE **2.3 Types of Transmission**

Direct contact transmission	Transmitted by skin-to-skin contact
Indirect contact transmission	Transmitted by inanimate objects
Droplet transmission	Transmitted through fluid droplets in air
Waterborne transmission	Transmitted through contaminated water
Airborne transmission	Transmitted through the air when mixed in dust particles
Foodborne transmission	Transmitted through improperly handled or cooked food
Vector transmission	Transmitted by living organisms, such as flies and mosquitoes

2.6 Development of Disease

How Do Diseases Develop?

If a person's resistance is low as a result of exhaustion, emotional stress, or trauma, he becomes more susceptible to becoming infected. Once the person is infected, the disease process begins.

First, there will be an ***incubation period***. *Remember*, this is the time between the initial exposure and the start of infection, which typically requires the multiplication of the organism, to the appearance of the signs and symptoms. The second stage will be the ***prodromal period***. The prodromal period will present with mild symptoms. The following stage is the ***period of illness***. This period represents the acute phase of the disease and will present with signs and symptoms. *Remember*, it is during the period of illness that the immune system responds to combat the disease-causing agent. The next stage is the ***period of decline***, when the signs and symptoms begin to subside and the person starts to feel better. *Remember*, the person can be susceptible to a secondary infection during this period.

The ***period of convalescence*** is the period of recovery. The person regains strength, and her body returns to a normal state. *Remember*, infection can, in some cases, be spread because the person who has recovered can still be harboring the disease-causing pathogen.

The periods of disease development are summarized in Table 2.4.

TABLE 2.4 Periods of Disease Development

Incubation period	The time between the initial exposure and the start of infection and the appearance of signs and symptoms
Prodromal period	Presents with mild signs and symptoms
Period of illness	Acute phase of the disease; will present with signs and symptoms
Period of decline	Signs and symptoms begin to decline
Period of convalescence	Recovery period

What Are Communicable Diseases and How Can We Control Them?

Communicable diseases are diseases that are spread or transmitted from one person to another. We can control the spread of these diseases by

- ***Vector control.*** Once the vector spreading the disease has been identified, methods to treat habitats and breeding grounds can be established.
- ***Immunization.*** The use of vaccines can be an effective way of controlling the spread of disease through artificially acquired active immunity. Vaccines are made up of killed, attenuated (less forceful or weakened), inactive, or fully virulent (strong or severe) organisms or toxoids (an exotoxin of a particular bacteria that has been altered so that it is not toxic, but will nonetheless stimulate the production of antitoxin in the person who received it through an injection).
- ***Quarantine.*** To quarantine humans and animals is to separate them from others. In case there is infection, this will prevent the spread of the disease to the general public.
- ***Isolation.*** Infected individuals can be prevented from making contact with the general public.

In quarantine there may or may not be an infected individual. In isolation there is definitely an infected individual whom is separated from noninfected individuals.

Chapter 2 Review Questions

Fill In the Blank

1. The study of the distribution and conditions of a disease in a given population is called _____.
2. A person who identifies, studies the causes of, and prevents diseases is called a(n) _____________.
3. A specific cause of disease is called ________________________.
4. The total number of new cases of a disease within a calendar year is called the _______________.
5. An epidemiologist is a person who identifies the causes and transmission of___________.
6. The total number of old and new cases of a disease is called the ____________________.
7. The number of people that have died as a result of a disease is called the __________________.
8. A disease with an average number of cases in a particular population is called a(n) ___________.
9. A(n) ___________ is a small number of isolated cases of a particular disease.
10. When the number of new cases of a disease in a particular population exceeds the average number of cases, it is a(n) _________________.
11. When a disease is distributed worldwide, it is called a(n) _______________disease.

12. When a given population suddenly becomes sick because of improperly handled food, it is called a(n) __________________epidemic.
13. A propagated epidemic occurs through what type of contact? __________________
14. This term refers to the specific characteristics of a diseases.
15. When a disease is considered contagious, it has the ability to __________________.
16. The time between initial exposure and infection is called ____________________.
17. When a person is symptomatic, she feels ______________________.
18. Diseases that are spread from one person to another are called________________.
19. The use of vaccines to control the spread of disease are called_____________.
20. When infected individuals are prevented from making contact with the general public:______________.

Matching

Match the following types of disease transmission.

21. Animal reservoir
22. Nonliving reservoir
23. Direct contact transmission
24. Indirect contact transmission
25. Droplet transmission
26. Vector transmission
27. Waterborne microorganisms
28. Portal of entry
29. Portal of exit
30. Airborne pathology

A. Skin-to-skin
B. *Vibrio cholerae*
C. Contaminated towels
D. Dog
E. Microorganism enters the body
F. Dust particles
G. Cough
H. Microorganism exits the body
I. Soil
J. Fly

Fill In the Blank

Types of diseases:

31. A disease that is worldwide: ____________________
32. Normal number of disease cases: ____________________

33. A disease that is widespread enough to cause a health concern: ___________________

34. A disease that occurs in small numbers: ___________________________

Matching

Match the reservoirs of infection:

35. Nonliving

36. Human

37. Animal

A. Rhinovirus

B. Tetanus

C. Anthrax

Multiple Choice

38. The number of people who have become ill in a given population is called the __________.

A. incidence rate

B. prevalence rate

C. morbidity rate

D. mortality rate

39. The total number of new and old cases of a disease in a given population is called the __________.

A. incidence rate

B. prevalence rate

C. morbidity rate

D. mortality rate

40. The total number of new cases of an infection is called the __________.

A. incidence rate

B. prevalence rate

C. morbidity rate

D. mortality rate

41. The number of people who have died because of a specific disease would be the __________.

A. incidence rate

B. prevalence rate

C. morbidity rate

D. mortality rate

42. When a pathogen is transmitted by skin-to-skin contact, it is called a(n) _______ transmission.

A. direct contact

B. indirect contact

C. droplet

D. airborne

43. When a pathogen gets transmitted by an inanimate object, it is called a(n) ______ transmission.

A. direct contact

B. indirect contact

C. droplet

D. airborne

44. An example of a pathogen that can become airborne would be __________.
   A. *Vibrio cholerae*
   B. *Escherichia coli*
   C. *Clostridium tetani*
   D. *Mycobacterium tuberculosis*

45. The period of a disease state in which the patient begins to feel better and regain strength is called the __________.
   A. incubation period
   B. prodromal period
   C. period of illness
   D. period of decline
   E. period of convalescence

46. The period of a disease state during which the patient's signs and symptoms begin to decline is called the __________.
   A. incubation period
   B. prodromal period
   C. period of illness
   D. period of decline
   E. period of convalescence

47. The period of a disease state during which the patient's immune system combats the disease-causing agent is called the __________.
   A. incubation period
   B. prodromal period
   C. period of illness
   D. period of decline
   E. period of convalescence

48. The period of a disease state during which the patient begins to present signs and symptoms is called the __________.
   A. incubation period
   B. prodromal period
   C. period of illness
   D. period of decline
   E. period of convalescence

49. The period from the time when the patient is initially exposed to the pathogen to the time signs and symptoms appear is called the __________.
   A. incubation period
   B. prodromal period
   C. period of illness
   D. period of decline
   E. period of convalescence

50. The spread of disease can be controlled and prevented by __________.
   A. vector control
   B. immunization
   C. quarantine
   D. isolation
   E. all of the above

Chapter 2: Review Questions and Answers

Fill In the Blank Answers

1. Epidemiology
2. Epidemiologist
3. Etiology
4. Incidence rate
5. Diseases
6. Prevalence rate
7. Mortality rate
8. Endemic disease
9. Sporadic disease
10. Epidemic disease
11. Pandemic disease
12. Common-source
13. Person-to-person
14. Pathognomonic
15. Spread
16. Incubation period
17. Sick
18. communicable diseases
19. Immunizations
20. Isolation

Matching Answers

21. D
22. I
23. A
24. C
25. G
26. J
27. B
28. E
29. H
30. F

Fill In the Blank Answers

31. Pandemic disease
32. Endemic disease
33. Epidemic disease
34. Sporadic disease

Match the Reservoirs of Infection Answers

35. B
36. A
37. C

Multiple Choice Answers

38. C
39. B
40. A
41. D
42. A
43. B
44. D
45. E
46. D
47. C
48. B
49. A
50. E

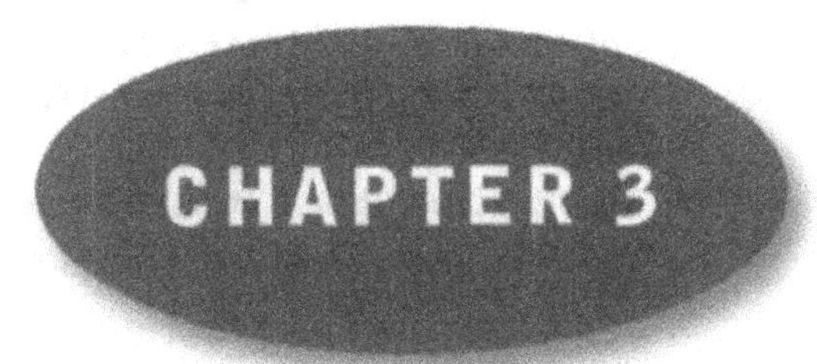

Cells and Tissues

Objectives

This chapter will review the structures that make up cells, cellular functions, cell division, and the phases of mitosis. Additional topics will include the four types of tissues that make up the human body, their structural makeup, their location, and their functions.

Keywords:

Cell
Plasma membrane
Cytosol
Centrosomes
Organelles
Cytoplasm
Nucleus
Endoplasmic reticulum
Ribosomes
Golgi complex
Lysosomes
Mitochondria
Peroxisome
Cytoskeleton
Connective tissue
Cilia
Flagellum
Cell division
Meiosis
Mitosis
Cytokinesis
Interphase
Prophase
Metaphase
Anaphase
Telophase
Tissues
Epithelial tissue
Muscle tissue
Nervous tissue
Loose connective tissue
Dense connective tissue
Dense regular connective tissue
Dense irregular connective tissue
Elastic connective tissue

3.1 Overview

What Is a Cell?

The ***cell*** is the smallest and most basic living, structural, and functional unit of the body.

What Are the Main Parts of the Cell?

The cell can be divided into three parts:

1. The ***plasma or cell membrane*** is the outer boundary of the cell. This structure separates the internal environment of a cell from its external environment. It also provides a gateway for materials to enter and exit the cell.
   - The fluid inside the cell is called *intracellular fluid.*
   - The fluid outside of the cell is called *extracellular fluid*. The two types of extracellular fluid are
     1. *Interstitial fluid* is the fluid in between cells within tissues.
     2. *Plasma* is the fluid portion of blood. Red blood cells, white blood cells, and platelets travel through the plasma.
2. ***Cytosol*** is the thick intracellular fluid that contains dissolved proteins and enzymes, nutrients, ions, and other small molecules that participate in metabolism (the chemical reactions that take place within the cell).
3. ***Organelles***, or "little organs," are highly organized membrane-bound structures that are specialized for specific cellular activities. Organelles are suspended in the cytosol. The term ***cytoplasm*** includes the cytosol and all the organelles except the ***nucleus***.

What Is the Plasma Membrane and What Does It Consist Of?

The ***plasma membrane*** is primarily composed of phospholipid molecules. These phospholipids provide the structural framework of the plasma membrane. They are arranged in two layers that are in a "back-to-back" formation, or a bilayer (see Fig. 3.1).

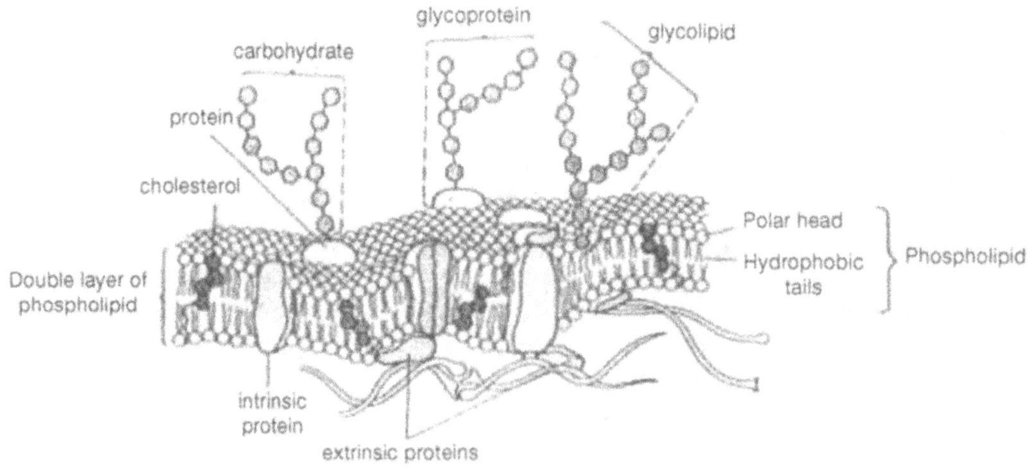

Figure 3.1 The structure of the cell membrane.

There are four types of lipid molecules that make up the plasma membrane bilayer. These are

- Phospholipids
- Cholesterol
- Glycolipids
- Glycoproteins

Some 75 percent of the membrane lipids are the phospholipids. Phospholipids contain both polar and nonpolar portions. The polar portions contain atoms that do not share their electrons equally. The atoms in the nonpolar portions share their electrons equally. The polar portions contain a phosphate-containing "head" that is said to be *hydrophilic*, or water-loving. The nonpolar portions contain two long fatty acid "tails" that are said to be *hydrophobic*, or water-fearing. Because "like seeks like" and because of the "back-to-back" orientation of these phospholipid molecules, their polar heads are positioned outward. The polar heads are always facing the watery fluid cytosol (intracellular fluid) on the inside or the extracellular fluid (interstitial fluid) on the outside. Molecules that have both polar and nonpolar portions are called *amphipathic*.

Cholesterol molecules are located within the plasma membrane and function in the stabilization of the phospholipid bilayer.

Glycolipids and glycoproteins are lipid and protein molecules that contain chains of carbohydrate molecules. These chemicals function as cell identity markers and are located within the plasma membrane.

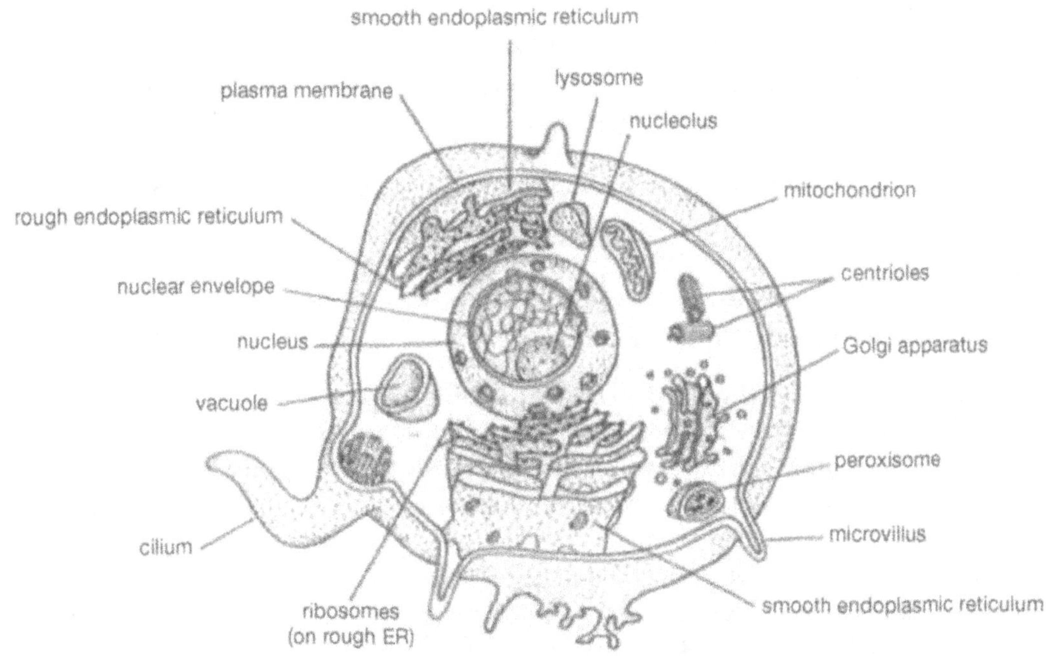

Figure 3.2 Cell organization.

3.2 Arrangement of Membrane Proteins

What Are Membrane Proteins, and How Are They Arranged?

The plasma membrane also contains membrane proteins that are divided into two categories:

1. *Integral proteins* that extend into or through the lipid bilayer
2. *Peripheral proteins* that associate with membrane lipids on the inner or outer surface of the membrane

Many integral proteins are glycoproteins, or proteins with sugary carbohydrate groups attached. The carbohydrate portions of glycolipids and glycoproteins form an extensive sugary coat called the *glycocalyx*.

Remember: This is important because the glycocalyx acts like a molecular "fingerprint" or "I.D. card" that enables cells to recognize each other and recognize foreign cells.

For example,

1. The ability of a white blood cell to detect a foreign glycocalyx is one way in which our immune system can respond to and destroy invading organisms.
2. The glycocalyx helps keep cells from being broken down and dissolved in the extracellular fluid.
3. The glycocalyx is involved in blood typing.

3.3 Functions of Membrane Proteins

What Are the Functions of Membrane Proteins?

1. Some of these proteins form *channels* through which specific substances, such as sodium and potassium, can pass.
2. Other membrane proteins act as *transporters*. Transporters bind to specific substances on one side of the plasma membrane and, by changing its shape, move the substance through to the other side.
3. Integral proteins called *receptors* serve as cellular recognition sites. These proteins recognize and bind a specific molecule.
4. Some integral and peripheral proteins are *enzymes* that speed up reactions inside or outside of the cell.
5. Membrane glycoproteins and glycolipids, which form the glycocalyx, are often *cell-identity markers*. They recognize cells of the same kind during tissue formation and respond to potentially dangerous foreign cells.
6. Some integral and peripheral proteins serve as *linkers*, linking cells together to form tissues.

3.4 Cell Structure

What Structures Make Up a Cell?

1. The ***plasma membrane*** encloses the cell's contents, creating a physical and chemical barrier that separates the cell's internal environment from the external environment.
2. ***Cytosol*** is the thick intracellular fluid of the cell, where many of the cell's chemical reactions occur.
3. ***Cytoplasm*** is the substance in which chemical reactions occur. It contains cytosol and all organelles except for the nucleus.
4. The ***nucleus*** contains hereditary material that controls cellular structure and cellular activities.
5. The ***endoplasmic reticulum*** (ER), or "highway of cells," forms a pathway for transporting molecules and provides a surface area for chemical reactions. The ER is also involved in synthesis, modification, sorting, packaging, and delivery of cellular products such as proteins and lipids. Also, the cytoskeleton may be considered a highway for vesicular transport within the cell.
6. ***Ribosomes*** are sites of protein synthesis. Some of them are located on the endoplasmic reticulum, giving it a "rough" appearance (rough endoplasmic reticulum). Smooth endoplasmic reticulum does not contain ribosomes. The smooth endoplasmic reticulum is the site for lipid synthesis and transportation, and also the place where many poisons are detoxified.
7. The ***Golgi complex***, the "UPS system" of cells, packages and delivers proteins and lipids.
8. ***Lysosomes***, the "digestive system" of cells, store digestive enzymes.
9. ***Mitochondria***, the "power house" of cells, produce ATP. ATP is the energy storage molecule of the cell.
10. ***Peroxisomes*** store enzymes that break down harmful by-products of cellular metabolism.
11. The ***cytoskeleton*** is the "skeleton" of the cell. It provides structural support and cell shape. Also, vesicles from the endoplasmic reticulum and the Golgi complex travel along the cytoskeleton.
12. ***Centrosomes*** serve as centers for the growth of microtubules involved in the movement of chromosomes during the mitosis phase of cell division.
13. ***Cilia*** are projections extending from the cell that move or sweep substances along the cell's surface.
14. The ***flagellum*** is a long projection that acts like a whip and moves the entire cell.

3.5 Cell Division

How Do Cells Divide?

Cells reproduce through ***cell division*** by two mechanisms:

1. *Reproductive cell division* is a mechanism through which the gametes (sperm and secondary oocytes) are produced by the gonads (testes and ovaries) in a two-step process called ***meiosis***.
2. *Somatic cell division* is a mechanism by which a single starting cell, called a *parent cell*, divides to produce two identical cells, called *daughter cells*. This process consists of a nuclear division called ***mitosis*** and a cytoplasmic division called ***cytokinesis***.

What Is the Cell Cycle?

The cell cycle is the life cycle of the cell and consists of the following phases:

- The G0–G1–S–G2 phase (which is collectively called the ***interphase***)
- The M phase or mitosis (which consists of four phases):
  1. Prophase
  2. Metaphase
  3. Anaphase
  4. Telophase
- The C phase or cytokinesis occurs when the plasma membrane and the cytosol divide, creating two daughter cells.

This process is shown in Figure 3.3.

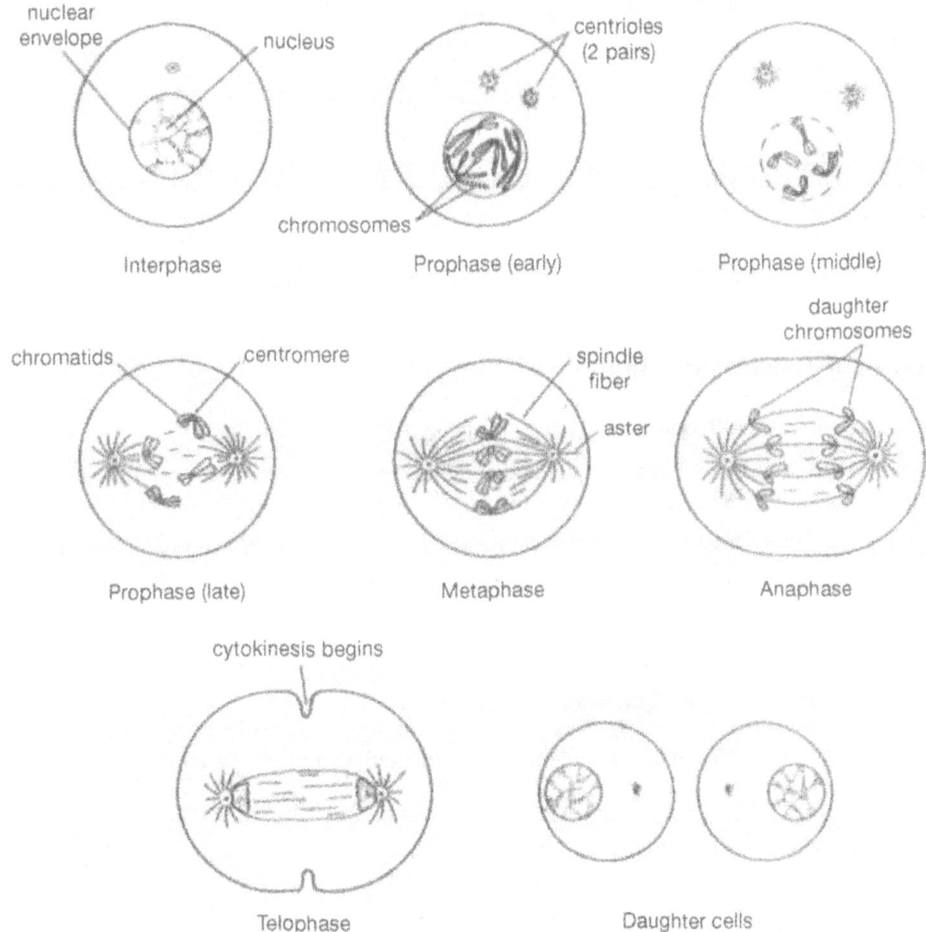

Figure 3.3 Cell mitosis.

Interphase

- *G0*. In this phase, the cell is metabolically active, although it is not concerned with division.
- *G1*. This is the primary growth phase of cells that have made the decision to divide; here the cytosol and organelles are replicated (copied).
- *S*. In this phase, the genetic information, or DNA, is replicated.
- *G2*. In this phase, chemicals, enzymes, and centrosomes are replicated.

Mitosis

- ***Prophase***. The nuclear envelope disappears, and the centrioles begin to migrate to opposite poles of the cell. Mitotic spindles begin to form, and chromatin fibers shorten, coil, and wrap around proteins called *histones* to form visible chromosomes (paired chromatids). *Kinetochores* (discs of protein) form and attach the chromosomes to the mitotic spindles.
- ***Metaphase***. Spindle fibers attach to the kinetochores to align the chromosomes along the equator of the cell.
- ***Anaphase***. The microtubules begin to shorten, resulting in the separation of the chromatids into chromosomes. These chromatids (now chromosomes) are pulled to opposite poles. As this happens, the cell plasma membrane begins to "pinch" inward, creating a "cleavage furrow."
- ***Telophase***. The chromosomes reach the opposite poles of the cell. The chromatids start to unwind into chromatin material (chromosomes disappear), and the nuclear envelope reappears. The cell plasma membrane continues to pinch inward.
- ***Cytokinesis***. The plasma membrane and cytosol separate, forming two identical daughter cells.

3.6 Tissues

What Are Tissues?

Tissues are groups of similar cells that work together to perform specific functions.

How Many Types of Tissues Are There?

1. ***Epithelial tissue*** covers body surfaces, lines hollow organs, and forms glands.
2. ***Connective tissue*** protects and supports the body and its organs. The many types of connective tissue bind some organs together, separate others, store energy, and help provide immunity.
3. ***Muscle tissue*** generates the physical force needed to make body structures move or contract.
4. ***Nervous tissue*** detects changes inside and outside of the body and responds to these changes by generating nerve impulses.

What Are the Characteristics of Epithelial Tissue?

Epithelial tissue can be divided into two types: covering or lining, and glandular. The characteristics of epithelial tissue are

1. Epithelial tissue has very little extracellular fluid between its cells because the cells are closely packed together.
2. The cells are arranged in continuous sheets in either single or multiple layers.
3. Epithelial tissue has nerve supply, but it is avascular (has no blood supply).

4. The cells of epithelial tissue have a high mitotic rate and can divide rapidly.
5. Epithelial tissue is the only tissue that makes direct contact with the external environment.

3.7 Epithelial Tissue

What Are the Functions of Epithelial Tissue?

The functions of the epithelial tissue are protection, filtration, lubrication, secretion, digestion, absorption, transportation, and excretion.

How Is Epithelial Tissue Classified?

Epithelial tissue is classified by the arrangement of its cell layers and the shapes of the cells (see Fig. 3.4).

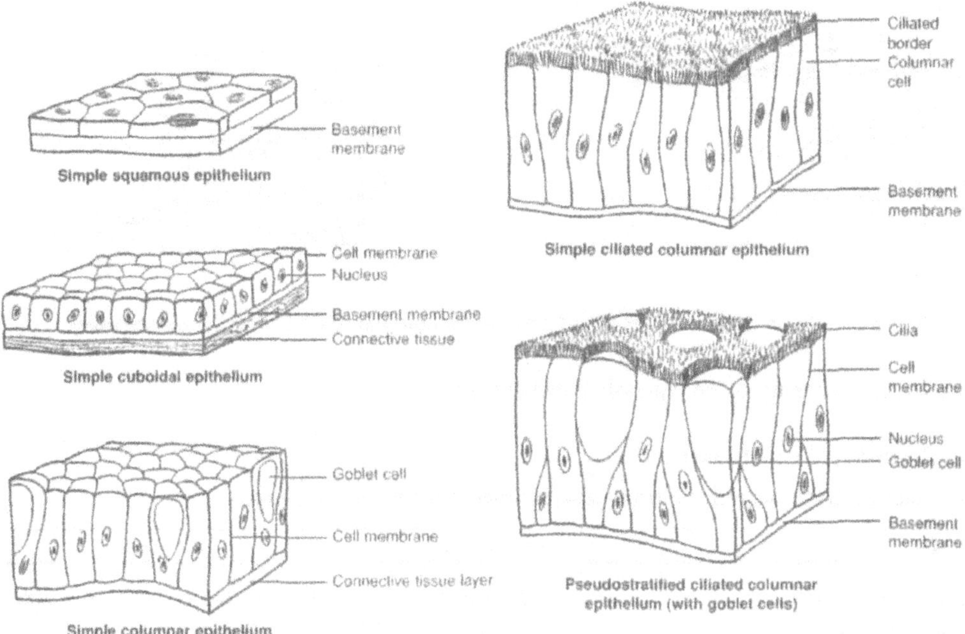

Figure 3.4 A comparison of simple epithelial tissues.

Arrangement of Layers

1. *Simple epithelium* is a single layer of cells. They function in diffusion, osmosis, filtration, and secretion.
2. *Stratified epithelium* consists of two or more layers of cells that protect underlying tissues where there is "wear and tear."
3. *Pseudostratified epithelium* contains only a single layer of cells but appears to have multiple layers because the nuclei exist at different levels.

Cell Shapes

1. *Squamous cells* are thin and flat and look like floor tiles or fried eggs. They allow for rapid transport of substances through them.
2. *Cuboidal cells* are shaped like cubes. They function in secretion or absorption.
3. *Columnar cells* are tall and cylindrical and protect underlying tissue. They function in secretion and absorption.
4. *Transitional cells* change shape and are used for stretching, expanding, and moving.

What are examples of epithelial tissues?
Examples include:

Simple Epithelium

1. Simple squamous epithelium
2. Simple cuboidal epithelium
3. Simple columnar epithelium

Stratified Epithelium

1. Stratified squamous epithelium
2. Stratified cuboidal epithelium
3. Transitional columnar epithelium (see Fig. 3.5)

Pseudostratified Columnar Epithelium

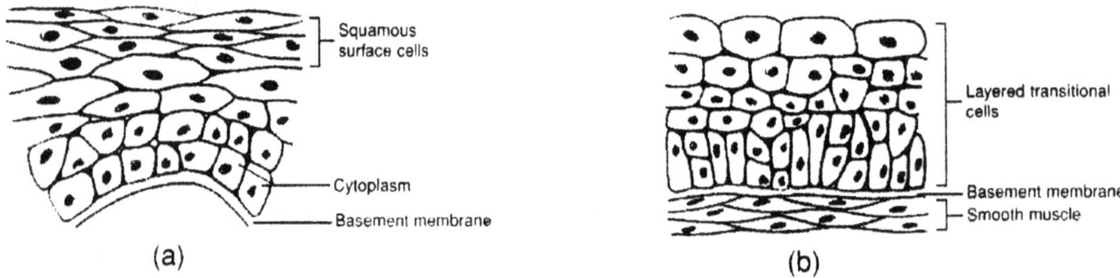

Figure 3.5 A comparison of stratified squamous epithelium and transitional epithelium.

Table 3.1 provides a summary of the types of epithelial tissue.

TABLE 3.1 Epithelial Tissue Review
Epithelial tissue functions: secretion, absorption, filtration, diffusion, and osmosis

TISSUE TYPE	LOCATION
Simple squamous epithelium	Glomerular capsule of kidney, blood vessels, lymph vessels
Simple cuboidal epithelium	Thyroid gland, kidneys, pancreas
Simple columnar epithelium	Intestines, gallbladder
Stratified squamous epithelium	External surface of skin, vagina, tongue
Stratified cuboidal epithelium	Sweat glands, male urethra
Transitional epithelium	Urinary bladder
Pseudostratified epithelium	Trachea

3.8 Connective Tissue

Connective tissue is the most abundant and widely distributed tissue in the body. It protects, supports, and separates structures and binds them together. It protects and insulates internal organs. Blood and lymphatic fluid are examples of fluid connective tissue and are the two major transport systems within the body. Adipose tissue (fat) is the major site of energy reserves.

1. Connective tissue contains cells, ground substance, and fibers. Fibers and ground substance form what is called the *matrix* and is located outside the cells.
2. Connective tissue does not occur on body surfaces or cavities.
3. Connective tissue has a nerve supply and is vascular, except for cartilage, which is avascular, and tendons and ligaments, which have little blood supply.

What Are the Cells That Make Up Connective Tissue?

The types of cells in connective tissue are as follows:

1. *Fibroblasts* secrete molecules that become the connective tissue's fibrous matrix.
2. *Macrophages* provide a vital defense for the body and are capable of engulfing bacteria and cellular debris by a process called phagocytosis (which means "the condition of a cell eating").
3. *Plasma cells* secrete antibodies and provide defense through immunity.
4. *Mast cells* are abundant alongside blood vessels. They produce histamine (a chemical that dilates blood vessels and increases their permeability during an inflammatory response) and heparin (a chemical that acts as an anticoagulant).
5. *Chondrocytes* form the cartilaginous matrix.
6. *Osteocytes* form the hard bony matrix.
7. *Adipocytes* store lipids (fats).
8. *Leukocytes* provide a defensive role during an immune response.

Macrophages, being differentiated monocytes, are leukocytes. Plasma cells, being lymphocytes, are also leukocytes.

What Is Ground Substance Made Of?

1. *Hyaluronic acid*, a viscous, slippery substance that lubricates joints
2. *Chondroitin sulfate*, a jellylike substance that provides support and adhesiveness
3. *Adhesion proteins* (such as fibronectin, laminin, collagen, and fibrinogen) that interact with plasma membrane receptors to anchor cells in position

What Fibers Are Located in Connective Tissue?

There are three types of fibers that are located in the matrix. These fibers give connective tissue structural support and strength.

1. *Collagen fibers* are very tough and have some flexibility. They consist of a protein called collagen. They are found in certain types of cartilage, tendons, and ligaments.
2. *Elastic fibers* provide strength and stretch. They consist of a protein called elastin. They are found in skin, blood vessels, and lungs.
3. *Reticular fibers* provide the framework of many soft tissue organs and provide strength and support. They consist of collagen with a coating of glycoprotein. They are found in the walls of blood vessels and around fat cells, nerve fibers, and skeletal and smooth muscle cells.

3.9 Types of Connective Tissue

What Are the Types of Connective Tissue?

The two major types of connective tissue are ***loose connective tissue*** and ***dense connective tissue.***

Loose Connective Tissue

1. *Areolar connective tissue* is one of the most widely distributed connective tissues of the body.

Where is areolar connective tissue located?

It is present in mucous membranes, in superficial regions of the dermis of the skin, and around blood vessels, nerves, and organs. With adipose tissue, it forms the subcutaneous layer between the skin and the underlying tissues.

2. *Adipose tissue* is fat tissue that stores triglycerides (fat). It provides insulation, energy reserve, support, and protection.

Where is adipose tissue located?
It is located around the kidneys and the heart, in yellow bone marrow, and behind the eyeball.

3. *Reticular connective tissue* provides framework and structure.

Where is reticular tissue located?
It is located in the liver, spleen, lymph nodes, and red bone marrow.

Dense Connective Tissue

1. ***Dense regular connective tissue*** is tough yet pliable. It is arranged in parallel patterns, and its strength withstands pulling along the axis of the fibers.

Where is dense regular connective tissue located?
It is found in tendons, aponeuroses, and ligaments.

2. ***Dense irregular connective tissue*** forms fasciae, the deeper region of the dermis, the pericardium, the periosteum of bone, and heart valves. It contains collagen fibers that are ***arranged in an irregular pattern.***

Where is dense irregular connective tissue located?
It is found where pulling forces are exerted in various directions.

3. *Elastic connective tissue* can be stretched and will snap back into shape.

Where is elastic tissue located?
It is found in the walls of elastic arteries and in the lungs and brachial tubes. It provides stretch.

The types of connective tissue are shown in Fig. 3.6. A review of the different types of connective tissue is given in Table 3.2.

Blood and lymph nodes are considered fluid-based connective tissue and will be discussed in Chapters 8 and 13. Bone is also considered connective tissue and will be discussed in Chapter 11.

TABLE 3.2 Connective Tissue Review

Connective tissue functions: protects, supports, insulates, separates, and binds structures together

TISSUE TYPE	FUNCTION/LOCATION
Loose Connective Tissue	
Areolar connective tissue	Mucous membranes around blood vessels, around nerves, subcutaneous region of the skin
Adipose connective tissue	Yellow bone marrow, around kidney, around heart
Reticular connective tissue	Liver, spleen, lymph nodes
Dense Connective Tissue	
Dense regular connective tissue	Tendons, ligaments, aponeuroses (broad, flat tendons)
Dense irregular connective tissue	Dermis of skin, fascia, pericardium, periosteum
Elastic connective tissue	"Elastic" arteries, lungs

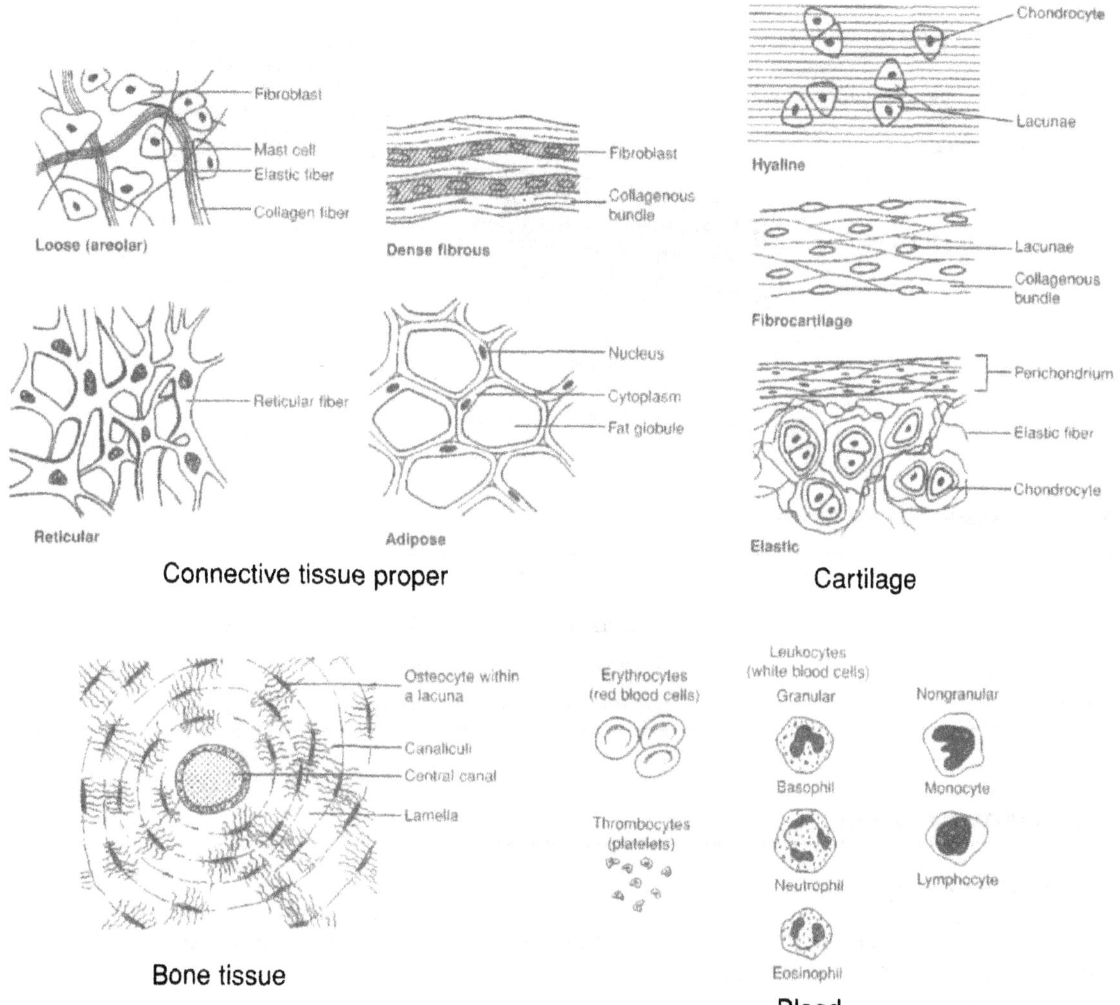

Figure 3.6 Types of connective tissue.

3.10 Muscle Tissue

What Is Muscle Tissue?

Muscle tissue consists of fibers (cells) that are modified for contraction. They provide motion, posture, and heat production.

How Is Muscle Tissue Classified?

There are three types of muscle tissue (see Fig. 3.7):

1. *Skeletal muscle* is voluntary (under conscious control) and is striated (consisting of contractile proteins). It is attached to bone and moves the joints of the skeleton.
2. *Cardiac muscle* is involuntary (under unconscious control) and is also striated. It is found in the walls of the heart.
3. *Smooth muscle* is involuntary and is nonstriated. Its movement is slow and "wavelike." It is located in the walls of hollow visceral organs.

The types of muscle tissue are summarized in Table 3.3.

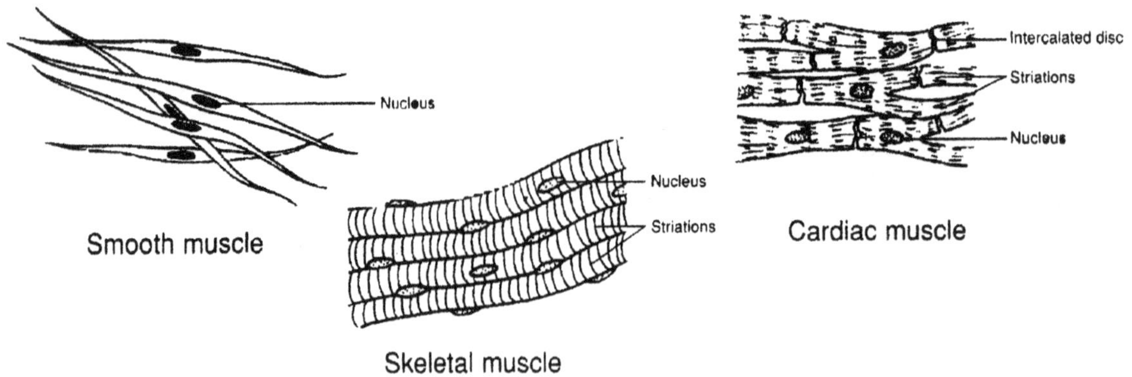

Figure 3.7 Types of muscle tissue.

TABLE 3.3 **Muscle Tissue Review**

TISSUE TYPE	FUNCTION/LOCATION
Skeletal muscle	Attached to bone and moves the joints of the skeleton
Cardiac muscle	Found in the walls of the heart
Smooth muscle	Located in the walls of hollow visceral organs

3.11 Nervous Tissue

What Is Nervous Tissue?

Nervous tissue detects changes inside and outside of the body, interprets those changes, and responds to these changes by generating nerve impulses.

There are two types of cells that make up nervous tissue.

1. *Neurons* are nerve cells. These cells elicit electrical impulses (action potentials). Their structure is shown in Fig. 3.8.
2. *Neuroglia* is the structure of supporting cells that protect the neurons.

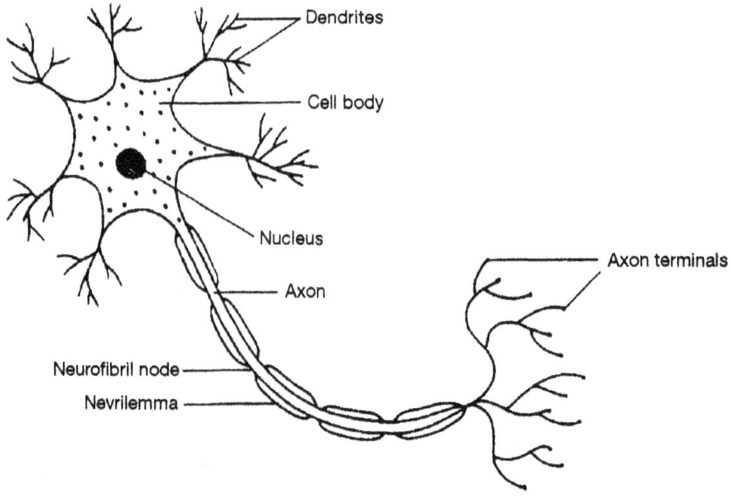

Figure 3.8 The structure of a neuron.

There are six types of neuroglia cells.

1. *Astrocytes* are involved with the blood-brain barrier, which prevents microorganisms and certain drugs from entering the brain from the blood.
2. *Oligodendrocytes* form the myelin sheath in the central nervous system.
3. *Microglia cells* are phagocytes that attack pathogens and other cellular debris.
4. *Ependymal cells* line the ventricles of the brain and are involved with the movement of cerebral spinal fluid.
5. *Neurolemmocytes* (Schwann cells) form the myelin sheath in the peripheral nervous system.
6. *Satellite cells* support cell bodies of neurons in the ganglions of the peripheral nervous system.

The types of neuroglia found in the central nervous system are shown in Fig. 3.9. The types of nervous tissue are summarized in Table 3.4.

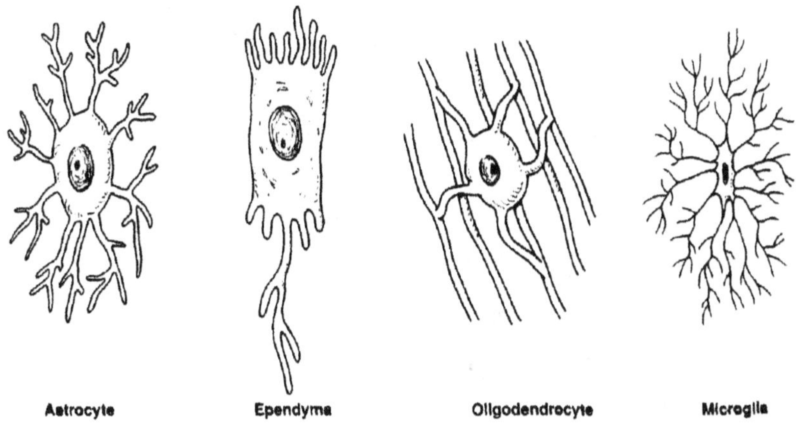

Figure 3.9 Types of neuroglia found in the central nervous system.

TABLE **3.4 Nervous Tissue Review**

TISSUE TYPE	FUNCTION/LOCATION
Neurons	Elicit electrical impulses (action potentials)
Neuroglia	Supporting cells that protect the neurons
Astrocytes	Form the blood-brain barrier
Oligodendrocytes	Form the myelin sheath in the central nervous system (CNS)
Microglia cells	Phagocytes that attack pathogens and cellular debris
Ependymal cells	Line the ventricles of the brain and circulate cerebral spinal fluid
Neurolemmocytes (Schwann cells)	Form the myelin sheath in the peripheral nervous system (PNS)
Satellite cells	Support cell ganglions of the peripheral nervous system

Chapter 3 Review Questions

Fill In the Blank

1. The basic structural and functional unit of life is called the ________________.
2. Structures within the cell that are specialized for specific cellular function are called __________.
3. The intracellular fluid of cells is called the ________________.
4. The fluid outside of cells is called ______________________.

5. The term used to describe the cytosol and all the organelles except for the nucleus is ____________.
6. This word means "water-loving": ______________________.
7. This word means "water-fearing": ______________________.
8. Membrane proteins that extend through the plasma membrane are ________________.
9. Molecular "fingerprints" or I.D. cards of the plasma membrane are called the ________.
10. The portion of a cell that separates the internal structure from the external environment is the ______________.
11. A pathway for transporting molecules within the cell is the ______________________.
12. These structures store digestive enzymes: ______________________.
13. These structures manufacture proteins: ______________________.
14. This structure packages and delivers large molecules: __________________.
15. These structures produce ATP: ______________________.
16. These structures contain enzymes that break down hydrogen peroxide: ______________.
17. This structure gives the cell support: ______________________.
18. This structure will move the entire cell: ______________________.
19. These structures can move substances along the surface of a cell: ________________.
20. This structure contains the hereditary material of the cell: ______________________.
21. The process by which cells reproduce is called ___________________________.
22. The type of cell division in which gametes are produced is called ___________________.
23. The type of cell division in which a single starting cell divides, producing two identical daughter cells, is called _________________.
24. Groups of similar cells form ____________________.
25. These tissues have a high mitotic rate: ______________________.
26. The most abundant type of tissue in the body is ____________________.
27. This type of tissue detects changes in the body's internal and external environment: _____________.
28. This type of tissue can generate force in order to move body structures: ____________________.
29. Tall cylinder-shaped cells that protect underlying tissue are called ______________________.
30. Tissues with two or more layers of flat epithelial cells are called ____________________.

Matching

31. The part of mitosis in which chromosomes become visible
32. The part of mitosis in which the chromosomes align along the equator of the cell
33. The part of mitosis in which the chromosomes separate and move to opposite poles of the cell
34. The part of mitosis in which the nuclear envelope reappears and the chromosomes disappear
35. The part of cell division in which the cytoplasm divides

A. Telophase
B. Metaphase
C. Cytokinesis
D. Prophase
E. Anaphase

Multiple Choice

36. A single layer of flat epithelial cells is called ___________.
    A. stratified squamous
    B. dense regular connective tissue
    C. simple squamous
    D. dense irregular connective tissue
    E. simple cuboidal
37. Epithelial cells that can change their shape are called ___________.
    A. cuboidal
    B. pseudostratified
    C. columnar
    D. transitional
    E. squamous
38. These cells store triglycerides and help insulate and protect body structures:
    A. adipose
    B. plasma cells
    C. fibroblasts
    D. macrophages
    E. mast cells
39. Which is *not* a component of connective tissue matrix?
    A. Hyaluronic acid
    B. Chrondroitin sulfate
    C. Collagen fiber
    D. Adhesive proteins
    E. Fibroblasts
40. Tendons would contain which type of connective tissue?
    A. Dense regular
    B. Dense irregular
    C. Areolar
    D. Elastic
    E. Reticular
41. Adipose would be considered ________________.
    A. dense regular connective tissue
    B. loose connective tissue
    C. dense irregular connective tissue
    D. reticular connective tissue
    E. muscle tissue
42. These are types of muscle tissue in the body: skeletal, cardiac, and ___________.
    A. elastic
    B. nervous
    C. adipose
    D. regular
    E. smooth

43. To which type of tissue would neuroglia cells belong?

A. Muscular
B. Epithelial
C. Nervous
D. None of these
E. All of these

44. Which type of connective tissue can stretch and "snap back" into shape?

A. Dense regular
B. Elastic
C. Dense irregular
D. Reticular
E. Areolar

45. Which type of connective tissue forms the periosteum of bone?

A. Dense regular
B. Elastic
C. Dense irregular
D. Reticular
E. Areolar

46. Which organelle is considered the "highway system" of the cell?

A. Nucleus
B. Golgi complex
C. Endoplasmic reticulum
D. Lysosome
E. Mitochondria

47. Which organelle is considered the "UPS system" of the cell?

A. Nucleus
B. Golgi complex
C. Endoplasmic reticulum
D. Lysosome
E. Mitochondria

48. Which organelles make protein?

A. Ribosomes
B. Peroxisomes
C. Lysosomes
D. Centrosomes
E. Nucleus

49. Which organelles contain digestive enzymes?

A. Ribosomes
B. Peroxisomes
C. Lysosomes
D. Centrosomes
E. Nucleus

50. Which organelles manufacture ATP?
   A. Nucleus
   B. Golgi complex
   C. Endoplasmic reticulum
   D. Lysosomes
   E. Mitochondria

Chapter 3: Review Questions and Answers

Fill In the Blank Answers

1. Cell
2. Organelles
3. Cytosol
4. Interstitial fluid
5. Cytoplasm
6. Hydrophilic
7. Hydrophobic
8. Integral proteins
9. Glycocalyx
10. Plasma membrane
11. Endoplasmic reticulum
12. Lysosomes
13. Ribosomes
14. Golgi complex
15. Mitochondria
16. Peroxisomes
17. Cytoskeleton
18. Flagellum
19. Cilia
20. Nucleus
21. Cell division
22. Reproductive cell division
23. Somatic cell division
24. Tissues
25. Epithelial tissue
26. Connective tissue
27. Nervous tissue
28. Muscle tissue
29. Columnar cells
30. Stratified squamous epithelium

Matching Answers

31. D
32. B
33. E
34. A
35. C

Multiple Choice Answers

36. C
37. D
38. A
39. E
40. A
41. B
42. E
43. C
44. B
45. C
46. C
47. B
48. A
49. C
50. E

Stress, Trauma, and Aging

Objectives

This chapter will discuss how cells and tissues react to stress, injury, and aging. It will also discuss the causes of cell and tissue injury and cell death.

Keywords:

Stress/stressor
Emotional stress
Physical stress
Chemical stress
Cellular adaptation
Hypertrophy
Atrophy
Hyperplasia
Hypoplasia
Metaplasia
Dysplasia
Aplasia
Agenesis

Local atrophy
Disuse atrophy
Pressure atrophy
Ischemic atrophy
Endocrine atrophy
Idiopathic atrophy
Cell injury
Physical injury
Toxic injury
Infectious injury

Ischemic injury
Hypoxia
Anoxia
Deficiency injury
Necrosis
Fat necrosis
Liquefaction necrosis
Gummatous necrosis
Caseous necrosis
Coagulation necrosis
Telomeres
Apoptosis

4.1 Overview

What Is a Stressor (or Stress)?

A ***stressor*** is anything that can disrupt homeostasis (the steady state of the body). ***Stress*** can cause a disease process.

How Many Types of Stress Are There?

There are three types of stress:

1. Emotional or psychological
2. Physical or physiological
3. Chemical

Some examples of ***emotional stress*** would be the loss of a loved one, "deadlines" at work, paying bills, and family illness. Some examples of ***physical stress*** would be poor ergonomics, trauma or injury, and repetitive motion. Some example of ***chemical stress*** would be smoking, drug abuse, alcohol abuse, industrial and environmental pollutants or toxins, and unhealthy foods.

How Can Organisms Combat Stress?

Organisms must be able to

1. Detect changes in their external environment, as well as changes that occur in their internal environment.
2. Interpret these changes.
3. React or respond and adapt to these changes. Cells that make up tissues can adapt to their environment by changing in size, number, and type.

What if the Stress Is Prolonged or Severe?

If the stress is prolonged or severe enough, the cells may be injured or destroyed.

4.2 Cellular Adaptation

What Is Cellular Adaptation, and What Are Some Examples?

Cellular adaptation is a process by which cells respond to stress.

What are examples of adaptation?
Examples of adaptation would include the following:

- ***Hypertrophy*** is the increase in the size of a cell and/or tissue mass. Hypertrophy can occur with a normal increase in workload.

  What would be an example of hypertrophy?

  An example of hypertrophy would be an increase in skeletal muscle mass with exercising. Or, it can occur as a result of an abnormal disease state.

  - ***What would be an example of an abnormal disease state?***

    An example of an abnormal disease state would be myocardial hypertrophy (enlarged heart muscle) caused by many years of high blood pressure.

- ***Atrophy*** is a decrease in the size of cells and tissues. This can result from nonuse, a decrease in blood flow, disruption of nerve innervation, and a reduction in endocrine secretions.

  - ***What would be an example of atrophy?***

    An example of atrophy would be the muscles of a paralyzed limb as a result of the loss of innervation.

- ***Hyperplasia*** is an increase in the number of cells in a given tissue as a result of overuse and hormone stimulation.

  - ***What would be an example of hyperplasia?***

    Examples of hyperplasia would include wound healing of the epidermis after repetitive stress and increases in the size of the breasts and the uterus during pregnancy.

- ***Hypoplasia*** is a decrease in the number of cells or cell production. Hypoplasia is not as severe as aplasia.
- ***Metaplasia*** is the replacement or conversion of cells. This happens when cells that are chronically irritated or inflamed are replaced by others that can handle the condition or are better suited for survival where other cells may die.
    - ***What would be an example of metaplasia?***

      An example of metaplasia would be the epithelial cells of the cervical mucosa changing to atypical cells in response to maturity changes and irritants to the vagina, such as changes in pH, hormone secretions, or trauma during sex and childbirth.
- ***Dysplasia*** is a change in the shape, site, and appearance of a cell as a result of abnormal or deranged growth.
    - ***What would be an example of dysplasia?***

      A dysplastic nevus, which is a mole or "birthmark" whose cells have changed to cancerous or precancerous cells.
- ***Aplasia*** is complete failure of cell production. With aplasia, the tissue or organ does not develop.
- ***Agenesis*** occurs when there is aplasia during fetal development. The complete absence of an organ will result from agenesis.
- ***Local atrophy*** can be caused by pressure, decreased blood flow (ischemia), or nonuse or disuse of the body part.
- ***Disuse atrophy*** occurs when there is a decrease in the size of a tissue or organ as a result of forced inactivity.
    - ***What would be an example of disuse atrophy?***

      The localized atrophy of a skeletal muscle as a result of a loss in motor nerve supply.
- ***Pressure atrophy*** occurs when there is a decrease in blood flow as a result of pressure. This pressure interferes with the normal circulation of blood to the cells and tissues, preventing these cells and tissues from receiving proper oxygen and nutrients.
- ***Ischemic atrophy*** can occur when pressure is placed upon blood vessels. This causes a decrease in blood supply to the tissue and organ. The result may be atrophy of the tissue and/or organ.
- ***Endocrine atrophy*** occurs when there is a decrease in hormone secretions.
    - ***What would be an example of endocrine atrophy?***

      Endocrine atrophy occurs if there is a decrease in pituitary gland (master gland) secretion. Other endocrine glands such as the thyroid gland may, over time, have atrophic changes.
- ***Ideopathic atrophy*** is a very rare form of atrophy of unknown cause.

Table 4.1 summarizes the types of changes in cell size discussed in this section.

TABLE 4.1 Examples of Change in Cell Size

Hypertrophy	Increase in cell and tissue size
Atrophy	Decrease in cell and tissue size
Local atrophy	Decrease in cell and tissue size resulting from localized pressure or localized ischemia
Disuse atrophy	Decrease in cell and tissue size resulting from forced nonuse
Pressure atrophy	Decrease in cell and tissue size resulting from a decrease in blood flow caused by pressure
Ischemic atrophy	Decrease in cell and tissue size resulting from insufficient blood flow
Endocrine atrophy	Decrease in cell and tissue size resulting from a decrease in endocrine gland secretion
Idiopathic atrophy	Atrophy of unknown cause

4.3 Cell Injury

What Is Cell Injury?

Cell injury occurs when the cells are damaged.
Cell injury will disrupt an individual's state of homeostasis because the injury can change the metabolic reactions that take place within the cell. The normal functions of these injured cells will be interfered with or interrupted, and this can lead to illness and a disruption in homeostasis.

What Can Cause an Injury to a Cell?

Cells can be impaired by physical agents, toxins, infection, ischemia, and deficiencies in nutrients and water. They can combat injury by using their cellular reserve chemicals to keep functioning properly or by adapting to the changes caused by the injury. If there is enough cellular reserve, the cell adapts; if there isn't, the cell dies. Cell death is called necrosis.

- *Physical agents.* ***Physical injury*** to cells can occur as a result of trauma, surgery, ultraviolet radiation, or therapeutic radiation.
- *Toxins.* ***Toxic injury*** can result from external or exogenous factors. These factors are environmental. Examples would include carbon monoxide poisoning, lead poisoning, alcohol, drugs, and silica dust. Internal or endogenous factors include genetic and metabolic disorders.
- ***Infectious injury.*** Organisms such as bacteria, protists, fungi, and viruses can cause cellular injury and cell necrosis. Viruses, for example, can cause mutations and interfere with normal cell synthesis.
- ***Ischemic injury.*** Ischemic injury results from a decrease in oxygen (***hypoxia***), absence of oxygen (***anoxia***), or carbon monoxide poisoning.
- ***Deficiency injury.*** Deficiency injury occurs when adequate amounts of nutrients, water, and even oxygen are not maintained.

Table 4.2 summarizes the various causes of cell injury.

TABLE 4.2 Causes of Cell Injury

INJURY	SOURCES OF INJURY
Physical injury	Trauma, surgery, radiation
Toxic injury	Alcohol, drugs, silica dust, carbon monoxide, lead poisoning
Infectious injury	Bacteria, protists, fungi, viruses
Ischemic injury	Hypoxia, anoxia
Deficiency injury	Decreased water, malnutrition

4.4 Necrosis

What Is Necrosis?

Necrosis is the death of a cell. This is the most serious effect of cell injury and is normally acute.

What are the types of necrosis?
The types of necrosis are

- **Fat necrosis.** Fat necrosis, or enzymatic necrosis, is most commonly a result of pancreatitis, a pancreatic disease. This disease causes a release of pancreatic enzymes that cause "self-digestion" of pancreatic cells.

- ***Liquefaction necrosis.*** In liquefaction necrosis, the dead tissue softens and liquefies. This type of necrosis can cause abscesses.
  - ***Where is liquefaction necrosis commonly seen?***

    This type of necrosis is most commonly seen in injuries to the central nervous system.
- ***Gummatous necrosis.*** This form of necrosis occurs as a result of syphilis, a sexually transmitted disease. Syphilis presents with both caseous and coagulation necrosis. A lesion that appears with syphilis is called a *gumma.*
- ***Caseous necrosis.*** The lesions of caseous necrosis have a "cheeselike" appearance. Caseous necrosis is seen in tuberculosis.
- ***Coagulation necrosis.*** Coagulation necrosis results from an *infarct*, or sudden "cutoff" in blood supply. This can occur in the heart and kidneys. Coagulation necrosis can also be caused by certain poisons, such as phenol and formaldehyde.

The different types of necrosis are summarized in Table 4.3.

TABLE 4.3 Types of Necrosis

Fat necrosis	Enzymatic necrosis; most commonly found in pancreatic disease
Liquefaction necrosis	Dead tissue liquefies; most commonly seen in injuries to the CNS
Gummatous necrosis	Can present with both caseous and coagulation necrosis. Mostly seen in syphilis.
Caseous necrosis	"Cheeselike" appearance; seen in tuberculosis
Coagulation necrosis	Results from the sudden cutoff of blood supply. Can be seen in the heart (myocardial infarct).

4.5 Aging and the Cell

All organisms age and eventually die. This is a natural process of life. As cells and tissues get older or age, they go through degenerative changes. These changes are believed to be predetermined genetically.

Damage to the plasma membrane, organelles, DNA, or RNA because of environmental factors can also shorten the life span of cells.

What Are Telomeres?

Telomeres are stretches of deoxyribonucleic acid that are arranged in a detailed sequence at the ends of chromosomes and protect the chromosomes from erosion during division. (They are part of the chromosome.)

What Happens When a Cell Ages?

As a cell ages, the telomeres start to shorten and eventually disappear completely. This, in turn, results in the erosion of chromosomal material.

What Is Apoptosis?

Apoptosis is a series of events that results in the death of cells when a specific signal is received or when a required signal is absent.

What would be examples of apoptosis?
Two examples are the apoptosis of cells between the digits in the developing fetal hand and the sudden dying off of lymphocytes when an immune response is finished.

Chapter 4 Review Questions

Fill In the Blank

1. Anything that can disrupt homeostasis is called ______________________.
2. Three types of stress are emotional, physical, and ________________.
3. The stress of losing a loved one would be an example of ___________ stress.
4. Trauma would be an example of _________________ stress.
5. Drug abuse and environmental pollutants are examples of ______________ stress.
6. A term used when there is an increase in cell size and tissue mass is ___________.
7. A term used to describe an increase in the number of cells in a given tissue as a result of overuse is _______________.
8. A term used to describe the replacement of cells as a result of chronic inflammation is ____________.
9. A decrease in the number of cells or cell production would be_____________.
10. A complete failure of cell production:_____________________.
11. The term used to describe a decrease in cell and tissue size is _________________.
12. The term used to describe a decrease in cell and tissue size resulting from localized pressure or ischemia is _______________.
13. A decrease in the size of a skeletal muscle as a result of a disruption of nervous innervation would be called _______________,
14. The atrophy of cells and tissues as a result of insufficient blood circulation is ____________.
15. The atrophy of cells and tissues as a result of a decrease in endocrine gland secretion is _______.
16. Atrophy of unknown cause would be termed _________________.
17. The replacement of cells is termed _________________.
18. The term used to describe aplasia during fetal life is __________________.
19. A change in the shape, size, and appearance of cells due to abnormal growth is called _________________.
20. The term used to describe the complete failure of cell production is ______________.

Matching

Match the types of cell injury.

21. Trauma
22. Malnutrition
23. Lead poisoning
24. Hypoxia
25. Bacteria
    - A. Physical injury
    - B. Toxic injury
    - C. Infectious injury
    - D. Ischemic injury
    - E. Deficiency injury

Match the types of cell necrosis.

26. Appearance of a gumma lesion
27. "Cheeselike" appearance
28. Enzymatic necrosis
29. Caused by a sudden infarct
30. Dead tissue softens and liquefies

A. Fat necrosis
B. Liquefaction necrosis
C. Gummatous necrosis
D. Caseous necrosis
E. Coagulation necrosis

Multiple Choice

31. An example of a physical agent that can cause a physical injury to a cell would be _________.

A. silica dust
B. a decrease in water
C. anoxia
D. a decrease in nutrients
E. radiation

32. An example of a toxic agent that can cause toxic injuries to a cell would be _________.

A. trauma
B. hypoxia
C. drugs
D. a decrease in nutrients
E. fungal infection

33. What would cause an infectious injury to a cell?

A. Anoxia
B. Radiation
C. Hypoxia
D. Bacteria
E. Lead

34. What would cause an ischemic injury to a cell?

A. Hypoxia
B. Anoxia
C. Carbon monoxide poisoning
D. None of the above
E. All of the above

35. Deficiency injury would be a result of _________.

A. malnutrition
B. lead poisoning
C. a virus
D. radiation poisoning
E. carbon monoxide poisoning

36. A form of necrosis that is associated with tuberculosis is __________.

A. coagulation necrosis
B. caseous necrosis
C. enzymatic necrosis
D. fat necrosis
E. gummatous necrosis

37. A form of necrosis commonly seen in injuries of the central nervous system is __________.

A. coagulation necrosis
B. caseous necrosis
C. liquefaction necrosis
D. fat necrosis
E. gummatous necrosis

38. A form of necrosis that occurs as a result of an infarct is __________.

A. coagulation necrosis
B. caseous necrosis
C. liquefaction necrosis
D. fat necrosis
E. gummatous necrosis

39. The form of necrosis associated with syphilis is __________.

A. coagulation necrosis
B. caseous necrosis
C. liquefaction necrosis
D. fat necrosis
E. gummatous necrosis

40. The form of necrosis associated with "self-digestion" is __________.

A. coagulation necrosis
B. caseous necrosis
C. liquefaction necrosis
D. fat necrosis
E. gummatous necrosis

41. All of the following are examples of chemical stress *except* __________.

A. trauma
B. toxins
C. smoking
D. alcohol
E. drug abuse

42. An example of emotional stress would be __________.

A. smoking
B. trauma
C. loss of a family member
D. pollutants
E. infection

43. Which of the following would *not* be an example of physical stress?
    - A. Poor ergonomics
    - B. Trauma
    - C. Pollutants
    - D. Injury
    - E. Repetitive motion

44. Alcohol abuse would cause which type of stress?
    - A. Emotional
    - B. Psychological
    - C. Physiological
    - D. Chemical
    - E. Physical

45. An industrial pollutant would cause which type of stress?
    - A. Emotional
    - B. Psychological
    - C. Physiological
    - D. Chemical
    - E. Physical

True/False

46. If stress is prolonged or severe enough, the cells can become injured or destroyed. ________
47. Stress cannot disrupt homeostasis. ___________
48. Cells can adapt to stress. ________________
49. Hypertrophy can occur with an increase in work or exercise. __________
50. Agenesis occurs when there is hyperplasia during fetal development. ________

Chapter 4: Review Questions and Answers

Fill In the Blank Answers

1. Stress
2. Chemical
3. Emotional
4. Physical
5. Chemical
6. Hypertrophy
7. Hyperplasia
8. Metaplasia
9. Hypoplasia
10. Aplasia
11. Atrophy
12. Local atrophy
13. Disuse atrophy
14. Ischemic atrophy
15. Endocrine atrophy
16. Idiopathic atrophy
17. Metaplasia
18. Agenesis
19. Dysplasia
20. Aplasia

Matching Answers

21. A
22. E
23. B
24. D
25. C
26. C
27. D
28. A
29. E
30. B

Multiple Choice Answers

31. E
32. C
33. D
34. E
35. A
36. B
37. C
38. A
39. E
40. D
41. A
42. C
43. C
44. D
45. D

True/False Answers

46. True
47. False
48. True
49. True
50. False

Hereditary and Genetic Control of Cellular Function

Objectives

This chapter will introduce the student to the study of heredity and explain how the inherited traits of parents are passed down to their children through the genes located in chromosomes.

Keywords:

Nucleic acids
Deoxyribonucleic acid (DNA)
Ribonucleic acid (RNA)
Gene
Chromosomes
Karyotype
Allele
Genotype
Phenotype

Autosomes

Sex chromosomes
Autosomal disorders
Trisomy 21 (Down syndrome)
Cri du chat (cry of the cat) syndrome
Autosomal dominant disorders
Huntington's chorea

Marfan's syndrome
Von Recklinghausen's disease
Osteogenesis imperfecta
Nonne-Milroy-Meige syndrome
Autosomal recessive disorders
Cystic fibrosis
Tay-Sachs disease
Gaucher's disease
Galactosemia
Alkaptonuria
Phenylketonuria
Sex chromosome disorders
Klinefelter's syndrome
Turner's syndrome
Hemophilia
Fabry's disease

5.1 Overview

What Are Nucleic Acids?

Nucleic acids are very large molecules made up of subunits called nucleiotides that consist of carbohydrates, a nitrogenous base, and a phosphate. There are different types of nucleic acids. Two of these are ***deoxyribonucleic acid*** and ***ribonucleic acid***.

What Is Deoxyribonucleic Acid?

Deoxyribonucleic acid, or ***DNA***, is our genetic material. This genetic material directs cellular function during the cell's life. DNA provides a blueprint for the production of protein.

What Is Ribonucleic Acid?

Ribonucleic acid, or ***RNA***, is responsible for the actual production of proteins from amino acids. Think of DNA as the "blueprints" or "plans" of the cell and RNA as the "foreman" or "boss" of the cell. RNA makes sure that the plans in the DNA are "constructed" properly. RNA uses the plans in the DNA to construct proteins from amino acids.

What Is a Gene?

A ***gene*** is a hereditary subunit or section of a DNA molecule. Genes produce products or perform functions. Genes pass on "formulations" called *traits* for the production of RNA, the synthesis of proteins, and the reproduction (copying) of DNA from one generation to the next.

What Is a Chromosome?

Chromosomes are DNA molecules that are tightly wound around proteins called *histones*. These chromosomes are organized in sections called *genes*. Different genes on a chromosome are responsible for different traits. These traits can be passed on from parent to offspring.

What would be examples of traits that are passed on from parent to offspring?
Examples of traits include eye color, hair color, height, and earlobe shape.

How Many Chromosomes Do Humans Have?

There are 46 chromosomes in a human cell. There are 22 pairs called homologous autosomes and a pair of sex chromosomes. The sex chromosomes are the X and Y chromosomes that distinguish males from females.

What Is a Karyotype?

A ***karyotype*** is a placement of a person's chromosomes that enables the viewing of them. It arranges a person's 22 paired chromosomes (autosomes) and sex chromosomes in order of size, shape, and banding patterns of each chromosome. Karyotyping is very useful because it can reveal a person's sex and whether he or she possesses too many, too few, or abnormally shaped chromosomes. Many hereditary disorders arise from abnormal numbers, shapes, and sizes of chromosomes.

How Can We Get Samples of Chromosomes?

Chromosome samples can be obtained from any cell that has a nucleus. Adult white blood cells are normally used, although chromosomes can also be obtained from the cells of embryos and fetuses.

What are the techniques used in obtaining fetal cells?
There are two techniques that are used in obtaining fetal cells:

1. ***Chorionic villi sampling***, or ***CVS***. Cells from the chorion are extracted and used. The chorion is the area where the placenta will form.
2. ***Amniocentesis***. Fetal cells are obtained from amniotic fluid.

What Is an Allele?
An ***allele*** is a version of a particular gene on a chromosome. Alleles represent certain traits. Humans have two alleles per trait, one inherited from each parent.

What Is a Genotype?
The ***genotype*** is the term used to describe the actual genes that a person's chromosomes contain.

What Is a Phenotype?
The ***phenotype*** is the expression or physical appearance of the individual.

What would be examples of phenotypes?
Examples of phenotypes would be blue eyes and blonde hair.

What Are Autosomes?
Autosomes are chromosomes that are not sex chromosomes.

What Are Sex Chromosomes?

Sex chromosomes are the X and Y chromosomes. These chromosomes decide whether a person is going to be male or female. They are also responsible for our sexual characteristics.

Sex Chromosome Inheritance
Women have two X sex chromosomes (XX), which means that the female gamete (ovum) always has an X chromosome. Males have one X and one Y sex chromosome (XY), which means that the male gamete (sperm) can have either an X or a Y chromosome. This means that the sex of the child is determined by the father.

5.2 Hereditary Abnormalities

What Are Autosomal Disorders?

Autosomal disorders appear when there are too many or too few chromosomes, a defect in the shape of the chromosome, or any number of other large or small mutations.

What are examples of autosomal dominant disorders?
Two examples of autosomal disorders are *trisomy 21 (Down syndrome)* and *cri du chat (cry of the cat) syndrome.*

Trisomy 21 (Down Syndrome)

What is Trisomy 21?
If there is an extra chromosome 21, the condition is called ***trisomy 21*** or ***Down syndrome***. Trisomy 21 means that there are three copies of chromosome 21. Down syndrome occurs when there is *nondisjunction*, that is, chromosomes or chromatids do not separate properly during meiosis.

What are the features of Down syndrome?
Children with Down syndrome have similar features, which include small mouth, protruding tongue, epicanthal folds (folds that occur in the inner eyelids), slanted eyes, short neck, short stature, short hands that contain a single crease in the palm (called a "simian crease"), mental retardation, and, in some cases, congenital heart disease.

Women over the age of 40 years have an increased chance of having a child with Down syndrome.

Cri du Chat Syndrome

What is cri du chat syndrome?
Cri du chat (cry of the cat) syndrome is so called because of the catlike cry of a child who has this condition. It is a disorder that occurs when there is a deletion of a short arm chromosome 5.

What are features of cri du chat syndrome?
Children with cri du chat syndrome have microcephaly (abnormally small brain) and mental retardation, "moon face," and wide eyes.

Table 5.1 summarizes these autosomal disorders.

TABLE 5.1 Autosomal Disorders

DISORDER	CHARACTERISTIC
Trisomy 21/Down syndrome	Small mouth, protruding tongue, short stature, simian crease, congenital heart disease, mental retardation
Cri du chat syndrome	Abnormally small brain, mental retardation

What Are Autosomal Dominant Disorders?

Autosomal dominant disorders will affect every generation. Only one copy of an abnormal gene is required. Parents with autosomal dominant disorders will pass along the disorder to at least half of their children.

What are examples of autosomal dominant disorders?
Examples of autosomal dominant disorders include *Huntington's chorea*, *Marfan's syndrome*, *Von Recklinghausen's disease*, *osteogenesis imperfecta*, and *Milroy's disease.*

Huntington's Chorea

What is Huntington's chorea?
Huntington's chorea is a progressive degeneration of the basal ganglia of the cerebrum.

What are the signs and symptoms of Huntington's chorea?
The signs and symptoms of Huntington's chorea include mental changes and involuntary shaking movements.

Marfan's Syndrome

What is Marfan's syndrome?
Marfan's syndrome is a hereditary connective tissue disorder. This disorder can present with ligament laxity and cardiovascular problems.

What are the features of Marfan's syndrome?
The features of Marfan's syndrome include long extremities and long phalanges.

Von Recklinghausen's Disease

What is Von Recklinghausen's disease?
Von Recklinghausen's disease is also called neurofibromatosis. It presents with benign nerve tumors (neurofibromas).

What are the signs and symptons of Von Recklinghausen's disease?
The signs and symptoms of Von Recklinghausen's disease include benign tumors on the trunk and extremities and "coffee-colored" skin spots called *café au lait spots.*

Osteogenesis Imperfecta

What is osteogenesis imperfect?
Osteogenesis imperfecta is a hereditary disorder that affects bone collagen and will cause the bone to be brittle. In severe cases, there may be spontaneous abortion, or the child may die at a very young age. If the child survives, he or she may be born with multiple skull, rib, and long bone fractures and brain damage as a result of trauma during labor. After birth, the child can have incomplete secondary ossification of the growth plates, stunted growth, and curvature of the vertebral column (scoliosis).

Nonne-Milroy-Meige Syndrome

What is Nonne-Milroy-Meige Syndrome?
Nonne-Milroy-Meige syndrome, also known as *Milroy's disease*, is a hereditary disorder that causes a congenital defect in lymphatic vessels. This defect will cause blockages in the lymphatic vessels, resulting in an increase of fluid in the extracellular spaces between cells (increase in interstitial fluid).

Table 5.2 gives a summary of these autosomal dominant disorders.

TABLE **5.2 Autosomal Dominant Disorders of Chromosomal Number or Structure**

DISORDER	CHARACTERISTIC
Huntington's chorea	Degenerative changes of the basal ganglion; involuntary shaky motions
Marfan's syndrome	Long extremities, long phalanges, ligament laxity, cardiovascular dysfunctions
Von Recklinghausen's disease	Benign tumors on trunk and extremities, café au lait spots
Osteogenesis imperfecta	Incomplete ossification of growth plates, brittle bones, fractures, scoliosis (curvature of the vertebral column)
Milroy's disease	Lymphatic vessel blockages, which cause an increase in interstitial fluid

5.3 Autosomal Recessive Disorders

What Are Autosomal Recessive Disorders?

Autosomal recessive disorders occur when there is a transfer of recessive alleles on an autosome.

Two copies must be present, meaning that they are inherited from both parents.

What are examples of autosomal recessive disorders?
Examples of autosomal recessive disorders include *cystic fibrosis*, *Tay-Sachs disease*, *Gaucher's disease*, *galactosemia*, *alkaptonuria*, and *phenylketonuria*.

Cystic Fibrosis

What is cystic fibrosis?
Cystic fibrosis is a hereditary systemic disease affecting many organ systems. The affected individual will have two abnormal genes, one defective gene from the mother and one from the father. The individual will experience excessive viscose endocrine secretions. These secretions will affect the lungs, pancreas, and digestive tract.

What are the signs and symptoms of cystic fibrosis?
The individual will present with thick respiratory mucus that is difficult to clear, making breathing difficult. He or she will have frequent respiratory infections, such as pneumonia and bronchitis. Decreased pancreatic exocrine secretions will cause malabsorption of the intestines, resulting in nutritional deficiencies. The individual may be thin, "fail to thrive," and have a delay in puberty. Individuals who suffer from cystic fibrosis are commonly of Caucasian decent and live to their mid-thirties.

Tay-Sachs Disease

What is Tay-Sachs disease?
Tay-Sachs disease is a hereditary disorder affecting chromosome 15. This disorder causes degeneration of the central nervous system. This occurs because there is an accumulation of *gangliosides* or *sphingolipids* in the neurons of the nervous system.

What are the signs and symptoms of Tay-Sachs disease?
Individuals will present with degenerative changes of the central nervous system, mental deterioration, and loss of eyesight. These individuals usually die before the age of four.

Gaucher's Disease

What is Gaucher's disease?
Gaucher's disease is an abnormal metabolic disorder affecting the breakdown of lipids. These lipids can build up in tissues and organs of the body and are called *cerebrosides* or *kersins*. The tissues affected are brain, bone, liver, and spleen.

What are the signs and symptoms of Gaucher's disease?
Signs and symptoms of Gaucher's disease include leukopenia, anemia, discoloration of the skin, an enlarged liver (hepatomegaly), an enlarged spleen (splenomegaly), and neurological problems with skeletal muscles.

Galactosemia

What is Galactosemia?
Galactosemia is an abnormal metabolic condition that occurs when the enzymes that convert the monosaccharide galactose to the monosaccharide glucose are missing.

What are the signs and symptoms of galactosemia?
The signs and symptoms of galactosemia include vomiting, diarrhea, anorexia, mental retardation, and failure to grow.

Alkaptonuria

What is alkaptonuria?
Alkaptonuria is an abnormal metabolic condition in which the amino acids phenylalanine and tyrosine are not totally broken down. The result is the buildup of homogentisic acid.

What are the signs and symptoms of alkaptonuria?
Signs and symptoms include increased levels of homogentisic acid, which will cause the urine to be dark and get darker and eventually turn black upon standing. Darkening of ligaments, tendons, fibrous connective tissue, and skin can also occur. This darkening in these areas of the body is called *ochronosis.*

Phenylketonuria

What is phenylketonuria?
Phenylketonuria, or ***PKU*** is an abnormal metabolic condition that occurs when phenylalanine (an amino acid) is not converted to tyrosine. This is the result of an enzyme deficiency.

What if phenylketonuria is not treated?
If it is not treated at an early age, phenylalanine can build up in the body. This can cause the demyelination of cerebral neurons, resulting in loss of coordination and balance, tremors, and mental retardation. The person can also present with eczema of the skin and an abnormal skin odor.

5.4 Sex Chromosome Disorders

What Are Sex Chromosome Disorders?

Sex chromosome disorders are disorders that affect the X and Y or sex chromosomes.

What are examples of sex chromosome disorders?
Examples would include *Klinefelter's syndrome*, *Turner's syndrome*, *hemophilia*, and *Fabry's disease*.

Klinefelter's Syndrome

What is Klinefelter's syndrome?
Klinefelter's syndrome occurs when there is an extra X chromosome present. Karyotyping will reveal a 47-chromosome XXY genotype.

What are the features of Kinefelter's syndrome?
Affected individuals will be tall, with abnormally long lower extremities, atrophic (small) testes, hypogonadism (decrease in the production of male sex hormones), infertility, and gynecomastia (enlargement of the breasts).

Turner's Syndrome

What is Turner's syndrome?
Turner's syndrome occurs when there is only the X chromosome present. Karyotyping will reveal a 45-chromosome X genotype.

What are the features of Turner's syndrome?
Affected individuals will present with small, nonworking sex organs (uterus, fallopian tubes, and ovaries). These individuals also will be short in stature; will have short, webbed necks; and will not go through puberty, grow breasts, or have a menstrual cycle.

Hemophilia

What is hemophilia?
Hemophilia is a set of hereditary disorders that affect the clotting of the blood. The individual can bleed excessively with even a minor wound.

What are the types of hemophilia?
There are two types of hemophilia:

1. ***Hemophilia A****, or* ***classic hemophilia***, is a genetic deficiency of clotting factor eight (factor VIII). The individual will bleed from minor wounds and have crippling joint problems as a result of bleeding into the joints. This is called *hemarthrosis.*
2. ***Hemophilia B****, or* ***Christmas disease***, is a genetic deficiency of clotting factor nine (factor IX). This form of hemophilia is clinically the same as hemophilia A.

Fabry's Disease

What is Fabry's disease?
Fabry's disease is a metabolic disorder that can cause an accumulation of glycolipids in the heart, kidneys, and brain.

What are the signs and symptoms of Fabry's disease?
The signs and symptoms of Fabry's disease include paresthesia (numbness) and causalgia (burning sensation) of the feet and hands, muscular abnormalities, abdominal pain, and death from organ dysfunction.

Table 5.3 summarizes the disorders linked to sex chromosomes.

TABLE 5.3 Sex-Linked Disorders

DISORDERS OF CHROMOSOME NUMBER	
Klinefelter's syndrome	Hypogonadism, gynecomastia, infertility, long lower limbs
Turner's syndrome	Small, nonfunctional female sex organs; short, webbed neck; short stature
DISORDERS THAT ARE SEX-LINKED RECESSIVE	
Hemophilia A	Classic hemophilia; there is a defect in clotting factor VIII
Hemophilia B	Christmas disease; there is a defect in clotting factor IX
Fabry's disease	A defect in the breakdown of glycolipids that causes a buildup in the heart, kidneys, and brain

Chapter 5 Review Questions

Fill In the Blank

1. Large molecules that contain carbohydrates, nitrogenous bases, and phosphates are called ____________________.
2. The nucleic acid that contains genetic material and directs cellular activity is _________.

3. The nucleic acid that is responsible for the formation of proteins is ________________.
4. These structures are composed of DNA molecules wound around histones: ___________.
5. Chromosomes are divided into sections called ____________________.
6. Human cells have ______________ chromosomes.
7. Eye color, hair color, and earlobe shape would be considered __________________.
8. We can view a person's chromosomes by viewing a(n) _______________________.
9. Which cells are normally used when sampling chromosomes? ________________.
10. Different versions of genes on a chromosome are called ____________________.
11. The term used to describe the actual genes that a person's chromosomes contain is ________.
12. The term used to describe the actual physical appearance of the individual is ________.
13. Women have a(n) ___________ genotype with regard to sex chromosomes.
14. Men have a(n) _____________ genotype with regard to sex chromosomes.
15. Trisomy 21 is an example of a(n) ______________________.
16. This autosomal dominant disorder is also called neurofibromatosis: ________________.
17. This autosomal dominant disorder will cause bones to be brittle: _________________.
18. This autosomal dominant disorder will cause blockages in lymphatic vessels: ________.
19. This autosomal recessive disorder affects chromosome 15 and causes degeneration of the central nervous system: _________________________.
20. This autosomal dominant disorder will present with elongated extremities and digits and can cause cardiovascular disorders: ______________________.

True / False

21. Autosomal chromosomes are the same as sex chromosomes.
22. An extra chromosome at chromosome 21 is called Down syndrome.
23. Children with Down syndrome have similar features.
24. Cri du chat syndrome is named for the catlike cry of these children.
25. Huntington's chorea is a disorder of the medulla oblongata.
26. Osteogenesis imperfecta causes coffee-colored spots.
27. Eye color would be an example of a phenotype.
28. Hair color would be an example of a genotype.
29. Males have XY chromosomes.
30. Females have XX chromosomes.
31. Amniocentesis is a technique used in obtaining fetal cells.
32. Blue eyes would be an example of a genotype.
33. Trisomy 21 is also known as Down syndrome.
34. Women over 40 years of age have an increased chance of having a child with Down syndrome.
35. Huntington's chorea is also called neurofibromatosis.

Matching

36. Huntington's chorea

37. Marfan's syndrome

38. Von Recklinghausen's disease

39. Osteogenesis imperfecta

40. Milroy's disease

41. Cystic fibrosis

42. Tay-Sachs disease

43. Galactosemia

44. Phenylketonuria

45. Klinefelter's syndrome

A. A condition in which phenylalanine is not converted to tyrosine
B. A disorder that makes bones brittle
C. A disorder in which galactose is not converted to glucose
D. A disorder that occurs when there is an extra X chromosome present in the male; XXY
E. A disease that affects the lymphatic vessels
F. An accumulation of gangliosides in the CNS
G. Neurofibromatosis
H. A disorder in which the individual will have thick respiratory mucus
I. A connective tissue disorder
J. Degeneration of the basal ganglia

Multiple Choice

46. A genetic disorder that affects the clotting of blood is __________.

A. Fabry's disease
B. Klinefelter's syndrome
C. hemophilia
D. alkaptonuria
E. galactosemia

47. A metabolic disorder affecting the breaking down of lipids is __________.

A. Klinefelter's syndrome
B. hemophilia
C. galactosemia
D. Fabry's disease
E. Gaucher's disease

48. This genetic disorder is characterized by hypogonadism, gynecomastia, small atrophic testes, and a tall build.

A. Klinefelter's syndrome
B. Turner's syndrome
C. Marfan's syndrome
D. Down syndrome
E. Huntington's disease

49. This genetic disorder causes a defect of the connective tissue.

A. Turner's syndrome
B. Cystic fibrosis
C. Marfan's syndrome
D. hemophilia
E. Huntington's disease

50. This genetic disorder can cause blockages in the lymphatic vessels.

A. Milroy's disease
B. Cystic fibrosis
C. Tay-Sachs disease
D. Fabry's disease
E. Marfan's syndrome

Chapter 5: Review Questions and Answers

Fill In the Blank Answers

1. Nucleic acid
2. Deoxyribonucleic acid
3. Ribonucleic acid
4. Chromosomes
5. Genes
6. 46
7. Traits
8. Karyotype
9. Adult white blood cells
10. Alleles
11. Genotype
12. Phenotype
13. XX
14. XY
15. Autosomal disorder
16. Von Recklinghausen's disease
17. Osteogenesis imperfecta
18. Milroy's disease
19. Tay-Sachs disease
20. Marfan's syndrome

True/False Answers

21. False
22. True
23. True
24. True
25. False
26. False
27. True
28. False
29. True
30. True
31. True
32. False
33. True
34. True
35. False

Matching

36. J
37. I
38. G

39. B

40. E

41. H

42. F

43. C

44. A

45. D

Multiple Choice Answers

46. C

47. E

48. A

49. C

50. A

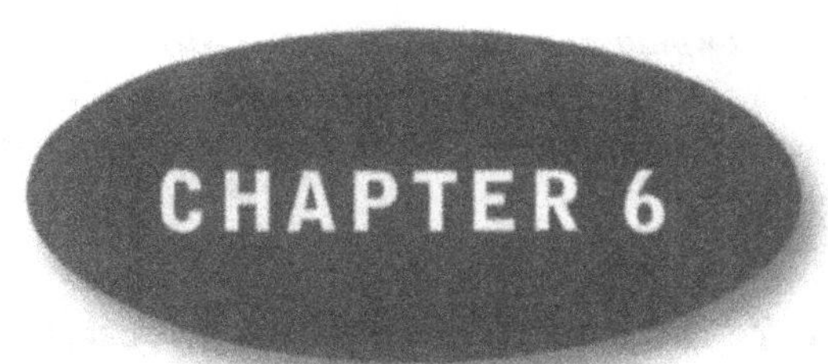

Congenital Disorders

Objectives

This chapter will discuss the causes of congenital disorders and give examples of congenital disorders.

Keywords:

Teratogen
Human immunodeficiency virus (HIV)
Acquired immunodeficiency syndrome (AIDS)
Syphilis
Chlamydia
Gonorrhea
Chickenpox
German measles
Fetal alcohol syndrome (FAS)
Arnold-Chiari deformity
Hydrocephalus
Spina bifida
Spina bifida occulta
Spina bifida cystica
Meningocele
Myelocele
Meningomyelocele
Cerebral palsy
Hirschsprung's disease
Klippel-Feil syndrome
Sprengel's deformity
Ventral septal defect

6.1 Overview

What Are Congenital Disorders?

Congenital disorders are disorders that are present at the time of birth. Some of these disorders, as seen in Chapter 5, are caused by genetic irregularities, while others are caused by chemicals, radiation, or microorganisms.

What Is a Teratogen?

A ***teratogen*** is anything that has the ability to cause a birth defect or congenital disorder.

Remember, anything that the mother is exposed to, eats, drinks, smokes, or injects into her body may, in fact, be a teratogen and affect the fetus.

Many things can be teratogens and cause harm to a fetus, leading to congenital disorders and birth defects.

What would be examples of teratogens?
Examples of things that can be teratogens include infectious diseases, nutritional deficiencies, chemicals, alcohol consumption, illegal drugs, and toxins found at home and at work.

6.2 Sexually Transmitted Infections That Can Cause Congenital Disorders

What Are Some Examples of Infectious Diseases That Can Cause Congenital Disorders?

Sexually transmitted infections (STIs) that can cause birth defects include human immunodeficiency virus (HIV), syphilis, gonorrhea, and chlamydia.

How Can These Diseases Affect a Fetus?

HIV

What is Human Immunodeficiency Virus?
Human immunodeficiency virus, the virus that causes ***acquired immunodeficiency syndrome (AIDS)***, can be passed from mother to fetus through the placenta. HIV is a RNA virus, which means that its genetic material consists of ribonucleic acid.

What are the signs and symptoms of HIV?
Signs and symptoms of HIV infection include night sweats, fever, and swollen cervical, axillary, and inguinal lymph nodes.

Syphilis

What is syphilis?
Syphilis is a bacterial infection caused by *Treponema pallidum.* Syphilis can be passed from an infected mother to the fetus through the placenta. Children born with syphilis can have multiple malformations and are usually born blind.

What are the stages of syphilis?
There are three stages of syphilis.

1. The first stage is *primary syphilis*. This stage presents with a hard ulcer called a *chancre* located at the site of the infection.
2. The second stage, called *secondary syphilis*, occurs around six weeks after infection and presents with a rash, especially on the palms of the hand or soles of the feet, hair loss, and gray patches on the mucous membranes.
3. The third stage is called *tertiary syphilis*. This is the most critical stage; it can develop after months or even years and will lead to death. Tertiary syphilis can affect the aorta, the main artery leaving the heart, and the nervous system. Tertiary syphilis will also present with large skin and organ lesions called *gummas*.

Chlamydia

What is Chlamydia?
Chlamydia is a bacterial infection caused by *Chlamydia trachomatis*. Chlamydia causes reproductive tract infections in both males and females and pelvic inflammatory disease in females. Babies born to mothers with chlamydia can have pneumonia and eye inflammation.

What are the signs and symptoms of chlamydia?
Although many people, especially women, are asymptomatic, the signs and symptoms of chlamydia include burning upon urinating and a mucoid discharge from the penis or vagina.

Gonorrhea

What is gonorrhea?
Gonorrhea is a bacterial infection caused by *Neisseria gonorrhoeae.*

What are the signs and symptoms associated with gonorrhea?
Gonorrhea causes a yellow-green urethral discharge and painful urination in males and pelvic inflammatory disease in males and females, although many women may be asymptomatic. Babies born to mothers with gonorrhea can get an infection of the eyes that can result in blindness. To prevent this, all babies' eyes are treated with antibiotic drops.

6.3 Other Infections That Can Cause Congenital Disorders

What Are Other Infections That Cause Congenital Disorders?

Chickenpox and German measles are infections that can cause congenital defects in a newborn.

Chickenpox

What is chickenpox?
Chickenpox is a viral infection caused by the varicella-zoster virus. The varicella-zoster virus is a DNA virus, meaning that its genetic material contains deoxyribonucleic acid.

What are the signs and symptoms associated with chickenpox?
Signs and symptoms include a pus-filled vesicular rash on the face and trunk of the body. This rash can cause intense itching.

Infection of a pregnant woman with chickenpox can cause encephalitis in the fetus.

German Measles

What is German measles?
German measles, also known as *rubella,* is caused by the rubella virus, an RNA virus.

What are the signs and symptoms associated with German measles?
German measles presents with a slight fever and a "red-spotted" rash that lasts for around three days.

German measles can be very dangerous to the fetus, especially if the mother is infected in her first trimester. This condition is called *congenital rubella syndrome* and can cause blindness, hearing loss, mental retardation, heart problems, premature delivery, and death of the fetus.

Table 6.1 summarizes the diseases discussed here that can cause birth defects.

TABLE 6.1 Diseases That Can Cause Congenital Disorders

DISEASE	SIGNS AND SYMPTOMS
Human immunodeficiency virus	Night sweats, fever, chills, swollen lymph nodes
Syphilis	Chancre, hair loss, rash on palms and soles, gray patches on mucous membranes, nervous system problems, lesions called gummas
Chlamydia	Burning sensation with urination and mucoid discharge
Gonorrhea	Painful urination and urethral discharge, blindness caused by infection during childbirth
Chickenpox	Vesicular rash on face and trunk
German measles (rubella)	Spotted rash with slight fever
Congenital rubella	Blindness, deafness, mental retardation, heart problems, premature delivery, and death of the fetus

6.4 Nutritional Deficiencies That Can Cause Congenital Defects

What Are Nutritional Deficiencies, and How Can They Cause Congenital Defects?

Deficiencies in nutrients, vitamins, and minerals can also cause congenital and birth defects. The following are some examples:

- *Vitamin B_6:* Vitamin B_6 is needed for normal cell metabolism. Without proper cell metabolism, cells will not divide or will not synthesize enzymes and hormones that are important for proper growth.
- *Folic acid:* Folic acid, also known as folate, is crucial for the production of DNA and cellular division.
- *Iron:* Iron is needed for red blood cell production, also known as erythropoiesis.
- *Calcium:* Calcium is needed for proper bone production and growth.

Table 6.2 summarizes the nutritional deficiencies that can lead to birth defects.

TABLE **6.2 Nutritional Deficiencies That Can Cause Congenital Defects**

NUTRIENT	FUNCTIONS
Vitamin B_6	Needed for proper cell metabolism
Folic acid	Needed for the production of DNA and cell division
Iron	Needed for red blood cell production
Calcium	Needed for proper bone production

6.5 Chemicals That Can Cause Congenital Disorders and Birth Defects

Can Smoking Cause Congenital Disorders and Birth Defects?

Chemicals taken into the body through cigarette smoking or inhaling second hand cigarette smoke can cause low birth weights, babies that are stillborn (born dead), and even sudden infant death syndrome (SIDS). Women who smoke cigarettes can also have babies born with physical malformations. Examples of these physical malformations would include cleft lips and cleft palates.

Can Drinking Alcohol Cause Birth Defects and Congenital Disorders?

Alcohol consumption can cause spontaneous abortions, low birth weights, and physical and mental abnormalities. Women who drink in excess or are alcoholics can deliver babies with ***fetal alcohol syndrome (FAS)***.

What are the signs and symptoms of fetal alcohol syndrome?

Babies with fetal alcohol syndrome will present with low birth weights; they will be small in stature and have malformations of the face and head; and they can be mentally retarded.

After babies are born with fetal alcohol syndrome, they will experience withdrawal symptoms. These symptoms include shaking, vomiting, and extreme irritability. These withdrawal symptoms are painful and are termed *delirium tremens*.

What Illegal Drugs Can Cause Congenital Disorders and Birth Defects?

Illegal drugs, like cocaine, can cause babies to be born with eye problems, coordination problems, and psychological problems. Cocaine can disrupt the mother's blood pressure, resulting in the disruption of the flow of oxygen to the fetus's brain.

Can Microorganisms Cause Congenital Disorders and Birth Defects?

Microorganisms can cause congenital disorders; for example, the parasite *Toxoplasma gondii* can cause toxoplasmosis. *Toxoplasma gondii* is a protozoan that can be transmitted by organ transplants, blood, or eating undercooked meat, and by a pregnant woman to her fetus. Pregnant women should avoid handling dirty kitty litter boxes. Exposure to cat fecal matter that contains *Toxoplasma gondii* can infect both mother and fetus, and can cause serious birth defects and possibly death to the fetus.

Can Chemicals Cause Congenital Defects?

Cleaning products found in the home and industrial toxins and chemicals found at work and colleges, such as benzene, asbestos, and formaldehyde, can all act as teratogens and should be avoided to prevent exposure.

6.6 Examples of Congenital Disorders

What Are Some Examples of Congenital Disorders?

Examples of congenital disorders are *Arnold-Chiari deformity, Spina bifida, Cerebral palsy, Hirschsprung's disease, Hydrocephalus, Klippel-Feil syndrome,* and *Sprengel's deformity.*

- ***Arnold-Chiari deformity.***

What is Arnold-Chiari deformity?
Arnold-Chiari deformity is a congenital malformation of both the medulla oblongata and the cerebellum of the brain. These structures of the brain will protrude inferiorly through the foramen magnum and into the spinal canal. This can be caused by ***hydrocephalus*** (an accumulation of cerebrospinal fluid in the ventricles of the brain). This accumulation of fluid is due to insufficient draining of cerebrospinal fluid from the ventricles. Hydrocephalus may be associated with or caused by spina bifida, lesions, or infections.

- ***Spina bifida.***

What is spina bifida?
Spina bifida is caused by agenesis (absence) of the posterior vertebral arches. There are two forms:

1. ***Spina bifida occulta.*** In this form, there is agenesis of the vertebral posterior arches, but there is no protrusion of the meninges or spinal cord.
2. ***Spina bifida cystica.*** This also involves agenesis of the vertebral posterior arches. The lumbar vertebrae are commonly affected. In spina bifida cystica, there can be protrusion of only the *meninges*, called ***meningocele.*** Protrusion of only the *spinal cord* is called ***myelocele.*** Protrusion of both the meninges and the spinal cord is called ***meningomyelocele.*** The term *cystica* means that these structures will be contained in a structure that looks like a cyst.

What are the signs and symptoms associated with spina bifida?
Signs and symptoms of spina bifida occulta include abnormal gait and loss of urinary control or incontinence.

- ***Cerebral palsy.***

What is cerebral palsy?
Cerebral palsy is a term that is used to describe a variety of conditions that cause brain damage. This damage occurs early in development and will affect motor function and coordination.

The cause is birth injury or oxygen deficiency during birth.

What are the signs and symptoms associated with cerebral palsy?
Cerebral palsy most commonly presents with a spastic "scissor like" gait; hemi- or paraplegia; or slow, snake-like, spastic, twisting movements of the upper extremities.

- ***Hirschsprung's disease.***

What is Hirschsprung's disease?
Hirschsprung's disease is congenital megacolon caused by the absence of normal bowel ganglion cells and nerve plexuses.

What are the signs and symptoms associated with Hirschsprung's disease?
Individuals will present with severely dilated colon, chronic constipation, impacted fecal matter, and diarrhea.

- ***Hydrocephalus.***

What is hydrocephalus?
Hydrocephalus is an accumulation of cerebrospinal fluid caused by a congenital drainage defect or obstruction of the third or fourth ventricle of the brain.

What are the signs and symptoms associated with hydrocephalus?
The most common sign is malformation of the skull.

- ***Klippel-Feil syndrome***

What is Klippel-Feil syndrome?

- Klippel-Feil syndrome is a congenital abnormality that presents with multiple blocks or fusions of the cervical region, causing a short, wide neck and central nervous system abnormalities. This may be accompanied by Sprengel's deformity.
- ***Sprengel's deformity.***

What is Sprengel's deformity?
Sprengel's deformity is a congenital elevation of the scapula.

- ***Ventral septal defect***

What is Ventral septal defect?
Ventral septal defect is the failure of the interventricular foramen to close, leaving a hole between the right and left ventricles.

Table 6.3 summarizes the congenital defects discussed here.

TABLE 6.3 Congenital Disorders

DISORDER	SIGNS AND SYMPTOMS
Arnold-Chiari deformity	Malformation of both the medulla oblongata and the cerebellum
Spina bifida	Agenesis of the posterior vertebral arches
1. Spina bifida occulta	Agenesis of the posterior vertebral arches with no protrusion of the meninges or spinal cord
2. Spina bifida cystica	Agenesis of the posterior vertebral arches; protruding structures are contained in a cyst like structure
3. Spina bifida cystica meningocele	Agenesis of the posterior vertebral arches with protrusion of the meninges
4. Spina bifida cystica myelocele	Agenesis of the posterior vertebral arches with protrusion of the spinal cord only
5. Spina bifida cystica meningomyelocele	Agenesis of the posterior arches with protrusion of both the meninges and the spinal cord
Cerebral palsy	Brain damage that occurs early in development and affects motor function and coordination
Hirschsprung's disease	Congenital megacolon
Hydrocephalus	Drainage defect in the third and fourth brain ventricles; causes malformation of the skull
Klippel-Feil syndrome	Multiple congenital blocks of the cervical region
Sprengel's deformity	Elevated scapula
Ventral septal defect	Failure of the interventricular foramen to close

Chapter 6 Review Questions

True/False

1. Any chemical or organism that has the ability to cause a birth defect or congenital disorder is called a teratogen.
2. An infectious disease can cause a birth defect.
3. Sexually transmitted diseases can cause congenital disorders.
4. Human immunodeficiency virus is a DNA virus.
5. Syphilis is a viral infection.
6. Syphilis can be passed from an infected mother to her fetus.
7. The second stage of syphilis is a chancre.
8. Chlamydia is caused by *Neisseria gonorrhoeae.*
9. Chickenpox is caused by the varicella-zoster virus.
10. Rubella is also called German measles.

Fill In the Blank

11. The organism that causes the disease syphilis is ______________________.
12. The virus that causes a deficiency in immunity is ____________________.
13. Tertiary syphilis presents with lesions called ____________________.
14. *Chlamydia trachomatis* causes the bacterial infection __________________.
15. *Neisseria gonorrhoeae* causes the bacterial infection ______________________.
16. The virus varicella-zoster causes ________________________.
17. The rubella virus causes ________________________.
18. An infection of German measles during fetal life is called ___________________.
19. The parasite that can be transmitted to pregnant women from a kitty litter box is _________.
20. Alcoholic women can deliver babies with ____________________.

Matching

21. Spina bifida occulta
22. Spina bifida cystica
23. Cerebral palsy
24. Hydrocephalus
25. Sprengel's deformity
26. Hirschsprung's disease
27. Klippel-Feil syndrome
28. Meningomyelocele
29. Ventral septal defect

30. Myelocele

A. Nonunion of the posterior vertebral arch with no protrusion of the meninges or spinal cord
B. Spinal cord structures contained in a structure that resembles a cyst
C. Congenital megacolon
D. Protrusion of the spinal cord
E. Condition caused by oxygen deficiency during birth
F. Congenital fusions of the cervical regions
G. An accumulation of cerebrospinal fluid caused by a drainage defect in the ventricles of the brain
H. A congenital failure of the interventricular foramen to close
I. A congenital defect causing the scapula to be elevated
J. Protrusion of both the meninges and the spinal cord

Multiple Choice

31. A congenital malformation of both the medulla oblongata and the cerebellum of the brain is called __________.

A. hydrocephalus
B. Klippel-Feil syndrome
C. Hirschsprung's disease
D. Sprengel's deformity
E. Arnold-Chiari deformity

32. An accumulation of cerebrospinal fluid in the ventricles of the brain can cause __________.

A. hydrocephalus
B. Klippel-Feil syndrome
C. Hirschsprung's disease
D. Sprengel's deformity
E. Arnold-Chiari deformity

33. Absence of the posterior vertebral arches is called __________.

A. cerebral palsy
B. spina bifida
C. hydrocephalus
D. Klippel-Feil syndrome
E. Sprengel's deformity

34. Protrusion of only the meninges is called __________.

A. myelocele
B. meningocele
C. meningomyelocele
D. spina bifida occulta
E. spina bifida cystica

35. Protrusion of only the spinal cord is called __________.

A. myelocele
B. meningocele
C. meningomyelocele
D. spina bifida occulta
E. spina bifida cystica

36. Protrusion of both the meninges and the spinal cord is called __________.
    A. myelocele
    B. meningocele
    C. meningomyelocele
    D. spina bifida occulta
    E. spina bifida cystica

37. If there is agenesis of the vertebral posterior arches and no protrusion, it is called _________.
    A. myelocele
    B. meningocele
    C. meningomyelocele
    D. spina bifida occulta
    E. spina bifida cystica

38. If there is agenesis of the vertebral posterior arches and protrusion of the meninges and/or the spinal cord in a cystlike sac, this is called __________.
    A. myelocele
    B. meningocele
    C. meningomyelocele
    D. spina bifida occulta
    E. spina bifida cystica

39. A term used to describe a variety of conditions that cause brain damage is __________.
    A. Hirschsprung's disease
    B. cerebral palsy
    C. hydrocephalus
    D. Sprengel's deformity
    E. Klippel-Feil syndrome

40. A congenital defect that causes the scapula to be elevated is __________.
    A. Hirschsprung's disease
    B. cerebral palsy
    C. hydrocephalus
    D. Sprengel's deformity
    E. Klippel-Feil syndrome

41. Congenital megacolon caused by the absence of normal bowel nerve plexuses is called __________.
    A. Hirschsprung's disease
    B. cerebral palsy
    C. hydrocephalus
    D. Sprengel's deformity
    E. Klippel-Feil syndrome

42. Congenital failure of the interventricular foramen to close is called __________.
    A. hydrocephalus
    B. cerebral palsy
    C. ventral septal defect
    D. Sprengel's deformity
    E. spina bifida

43. The human immunodeficiency virus is what kind of virus?

A. DNA
B. RNA
C. ATP
D. Bacterial
E. Fungal

44. Which type of organism is *syphilis*?

A. Virus
B. Fungus
C. Plant
D. Protist
E. Bacteria

45. Which type of organism is *Chlamydia*?

A. Virus
B. Fungus
C. Plant
D. Protist
E. Bacteria

46. How many stages of syphilis are there?

A. 1
B. 2
C. 3
D. 4
E. 5

47. Chickenpox and German measles are caused by __________.

A. viruses
B. fungi
C. bacteria
D. protists
E. parasites

48. Signs and symptoms of congenital rubella syndrome are __________.

A. loss of vision
B. hearing loss
C. heart problems
D. mental retardation
E. all of the above

49. Calcium is needed for proper bone production and growth.

A. True
B. False

50. Rubella is also known as __________.

A. syphilis
B. German measles
C. chickenpox
D. HIV
E. gonorrhea

Chapter 6: Review Questions and Answers

True/False Answers

1. True
2. True
3. True
4. False
5. False
6. True
7. False
8. False
9. True
10. True

Fill In the Blank Answers

11. *Treponema pallidum*
12. Human immunodeficiency virus
13. Gummas
14. Chlamydia
15. Gonorrhea
16. Chickenpox
17. German measles
18. Congenital rubella syndrome
19. *Toxoplasma gondii*
20. Fetal alcohol syndrome

Matching Answers

21. A
22. B
23. E
24. G
25. I
26. C
27. F
28. J
29. H
30. D

Multiple Choice Answers

31. E
32. A
33. B
34. B
35. A
36. C
37. D
38. E
39. B
40. D
41. A
42. C
43. B
44. E
45. E
46. C
47. A
48. E
49. A
50. B

New Growths: Cell Division and Differentiation

Objectives

This chapter will discuss "new growths": the abnormal growth of cells and how these new tumors affect the human body.

Keywords:

Neoplasia
Neoplasm
Tumor
Hyperplasia
Metaplasia
Dysplasia

Oncology
Benign tumors
Malignant tumors
Cancer

Embryonic tissue
Neoplastic tissue

Fibrous stroma

Vascular stroma

Angiogenesis
Metastasis
Primary site
Secondary site
Generation time
Doubling time
Pressure atrophy
Chemotaxis

7.1 Overview

What Is Neoplasia?

Neoplasia is the formation of new tissue. This process will involve an increase in the growth of tissues, creating a *"new mass" (neoplastic mass).*

What Is This Neoplastic Mass Called?

This neoplastic mass is called a ***neoplasm*** or new growth. New growths or masses are called ***tumors.***

What Happens When There Is an Increased Normal Workload and the Demand on Cells Increases?

When there is an increase in work, and thus demand, at the cellular level, ***hyperplasia*** occurs.

Remember from Chapter 4 that adaptive growth responses will cause hyperplasia, or an increase in the number of cells in a given tissue, as a result of overuse and hormone stimulation.

What Is an Example of Hyperplasia in the Body?

An example of hyperplasia in the body would be a thickening of the epidermis of the skin because of an irritation or friction from a high-heeled shoe, causing a callus.

What Happens When the Demand Is Prolonged or More Intense?

When demand at the cellular level is prolonged or more intense, *metaplasia* or *dysplasia* can occur.

What Is Metaplasia?

Metaplasia is the replacement or alteration of cells.

Remember, this happens when cells are chronically exposed to an unfavorable condition or are chronically irritated or inflamed.

Metaplasia occurs in the respiratory tract when substances, such as those produced by prolonged cigarette smoking, irritate the epithelial tissue that lines the respiratory tract. The normal tissue (ciliated pseudostratified columnar epithelium and goblet cells) is replaced with thicker, nonciliated epithelium. Ciliated epithelium and mucus from goblet cells clear microorganisms and debris particles that are inhaled into the respiratory tract. Metaplasia that occurs in epithelial tissue can usually be reversed.

What Is Dysplasia?

Dysplasia is a change in the size, shape, and appearance of cells.

Remember, this happens when cells are severely irritated for a long time.

Dysplasia results when there is a drastic increase in mitotic rates. Dysplasia is reversible, but this happens less than with metaplasia. When it is severe, dysplasia can look like tumors. Dysplasia can be seen in smokers who have chronic bronchitis. Sometimes these forms of tissue dysplasia are called *precancerous lesions*.

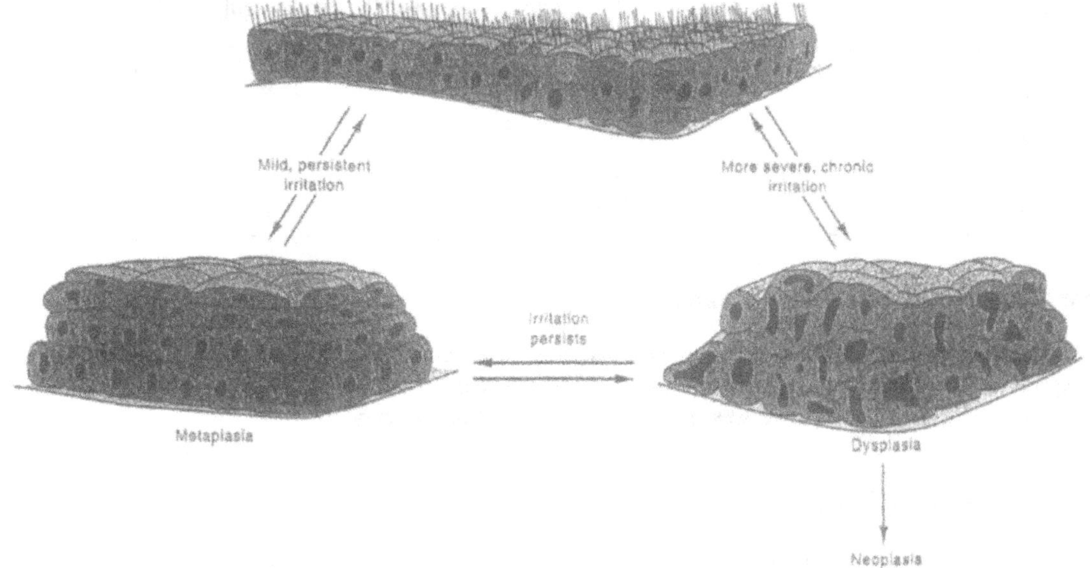

Figure 7.1 Metaplasia vs. dysplasia.

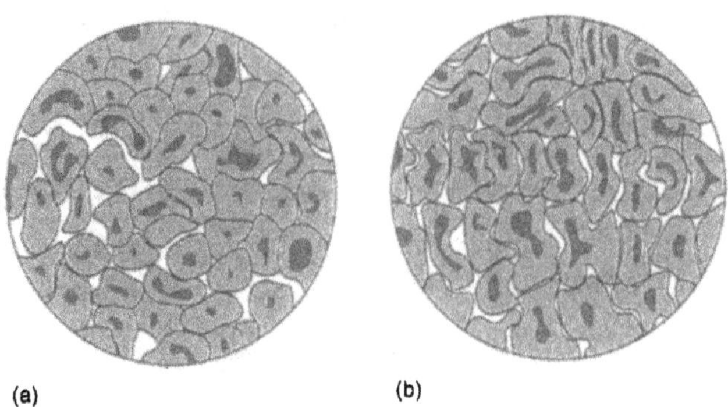

Figure 7.2 Dysplasia vs. neoplasia.

7.2 Tumors

What Is the Study of Tumors?

Oncology is the study of tumors. A person who studies tumors and treats people with tumors is called an *oncologist*.

What Are the Characteristics of Tumors?

Tumors can be either *benign* or *malignant.*

- ***Benign tumors*** grow very slowly, are localized, and do not spread to surrounding tissue.
- ***Malignant tumors*** grow fast and in a disorderly manner, are very aggressive, and spread to surrounding tissue.

The differences between benign and malignant tumors are summarized in Table 7.1.

TABLE 7.1 Differences between Benign and Malignant Tumors

	BENIGN TUMORS	MALIGNANT TUMORS
Structure of cells	Normal in shape	Larger and abnormal in shape
Structure of tissues	Regular and orderly	Irregular
Loss of function or differentiation	Minimal	Typical
Ability to metastasize	No	Yes
Rate of growth	Slow	Fast
Invasion of normal tissue	Slow	Fast
Prognosis	Good	Poor

What Does the Word Cancer Mean?

The word ***cancer*** means "crab" in Latin; it is used because of the crab claw–like extensions of malignant tumors. Malignant tumors can cause the death of the person if they are not treated in the early stages. They can not only spread to surrounding tissue, but also spread to different parts of the body.

How Do We Name Tumors?

The suffix "oma" at the end of a word denotes a tumor. If the tumor is benign, the root word will distinguish the neoplastic tissue.

What would be an example of a benign tumor?
An example of a benign tumor would be a *chondroma*, which is a benign cartilage tumor.
Malignant tumors are named according to their ***embryonic tissue*** of origin.

What Is Embryonic Tissue?

During development, an embryo has three primary tissue layers.

1. *Endoderm.* This provides the protective layer that lines internal surfaces.
2. *Mesoderm.* This provides cartilage and fibrous connective tissues.
3. *Ectoderm.* This provides the covering of outer body surfaces.

How Do We Name Cancerous or Malignant Tumors?

Tumors that are malignant and are found in tissue derived from the endoderm and the ectoderm are *carcinomas*. These carcinomas can be found in the epithelial layer of skin and the lining of the respiratory and digestive tracts. Malignant tumors of glandular tissues are called *adenocarcinomas*. Benign tumors of glandular tissues are called *adenomas*. Benign tumors that contain cysts are called *cystadenomas*. Malignant tumors of the mesoderm are called *sarcomas*.

What would be examples of sarcomas?
Examples of sarcomas would be

- *Chondrosarcomas:* malignant tumors of cartilage
- *Fibrosarcomas:* malignant tumors of fibrous connective tissue

Examples of tumor classification are given in Table 7.2.

TABLE 7.2 **Examples of Tumor Classification**

MALIGNANT TUMORS	BENIGN TUMORS	TISSUE TYPE
Carcinoma	Epithelioma	Epithelial tissue
Adenocarcinoma	Adenoma	Glandular tissue
Liposarcoma	Lipoma	Adipose (fat) tissue
Chondrosarcoma	Chondroma	Cartilage
Fibrosarcoma	Fibroma	Fibrous connective tissue

What Is the Structure of a Tumor?

Tumors have three principal structures: *neoplastic tissue, fibrous stroma,* and *vascular stroma.*

1. ***Neoplastic tissue.*** In *benign* tumors, the cells of the neoplastic tissue will look normal in size and shape and will also be arranged the same way as the cells of normal tissue. In *malignant* tumors, the cells will be very different in size, shape, and arrangement.
2. ***Fibrous stroma.*** Another part of a tumor is called the fibrous stroma. The fibrous stroma supports the tumor cells by forming a tissue "framework." As new tumor tissue is formed, the fibrous stroma will increase. Tumors that are malignant can release secretions that stimulate collagen production from fibroblasts and other components of the stroma.
3. ***Vascular stroma.*** The vascular stroma of the tumor provides the tumor's blood supply. The vascular stroma increases as the tumor's demand for blood flow increases. The process of forming new blood vessels in tumors is called ***angiogenesis***.

7.3 The Behavior of Tumors

How Do Tumors Behave?

Benign tumors grow faster than normal tissue but much more slowly than malignant tumors. The slow growth of benign tumors causes little damage to surrounding tissue. Benign tumors also have a fibrous capsule surrounding them, thus separating them from normal tissue. Malignant tumors, on the other hand, grow very fast and invade and disrupt normal structures and functions. Malignant tumors can also spread to other distant parts of the body. The spreading of malignant tumors to other distant parts of the body is called ***metastasis***. During metastasis, the tumor grows at its place of origin, which is called the ***primary site***. When tumor cells travel to other parts of the body, they make other tumors. These are called the ***secondary sites***.

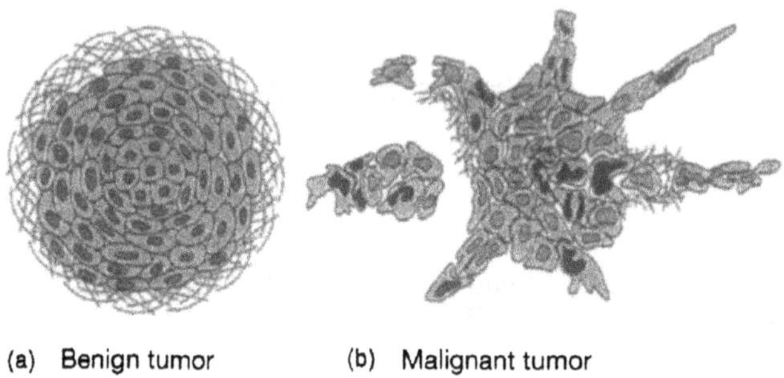

(a) Benign tumor (b) Malignant tumor

Figure 7.3 The Structure of a tumor.

What Is the Rate of Tumor Growth?

Tumor growth rates depend on two related things:

- ***Generation time*** is the amount of time between the division of cells.
- ***Doubling time*** is the amount of time it takes for the number of tumor cells to double in number or of the tumor itself to double in size. As new cells are produced, the doubling time can increase.

How Do Tumors Invade Normal Tissue?

There are a number of factors that can cause a tumor to invade normal tissue. One of these factors is ***pressure atrophy***. Pressure atrophy occurs when a tumor expands against normal tissue. This expansion can put pressure on normal tissue cells and the blood vessels that nourish them. This pressure ultimately causes apoptosis, the internal programmed death of cells. The death and eventual elimination of these cells permits their replacement by the growing tumor cells.

Another factor involved in the invasion of tumor cells, especially malignant tumor cells, is their ability to move and migrate into normal tissue cells. Normal tissue cells are bound tightly together. Malignant tumor cells, on the other hand, lose their adhesiveness, separate, and move into adjacent neighboring cells.

Tumor cells also invade adjacent normal tissue by the process of ***chemotaxis***. Chemotaxis is the chemical attraction that draws the tumor cells into the adjacent normal tissue.

How Do Tumor Cells Metastasize?

Tumor cells initially grow at the primary site and then, many times, penetrate through the blood vessels. The walls of capillaries and veins are very thin, allowing for penetration by aggressive tumor cells. Arteries, on the other hand, have thicker walls, making penetration less common.

When primary tumors penetrate blood and lymphatic vessels, the cells of the tumors break free, creating *emboli* that flow away from the primary site. These emboli become trapped at a distant site, and the cells begin to divide and grow, thus beginning the growth of a secondary tumor.

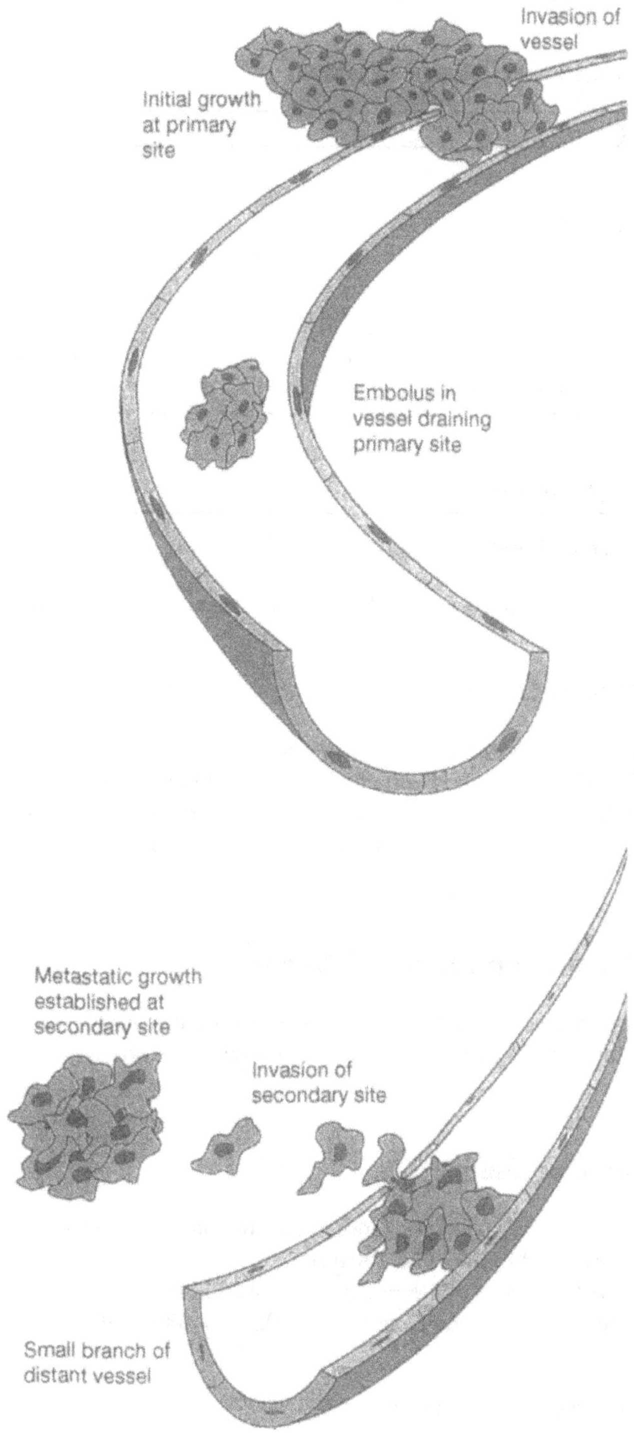

Figure 7.4 Metastasis by embolism.

Malignant tumors can also metastasize to other organs by penetrating through body cavities and the lumen of the gastrointestinal tract, ureters, bile ducts, oviducts, and other ducts. On rare occasions, tumors may metastasize as a result of surgery or biopsy. The procedures and instruments used may displace malignant cells to a secondary location. This type of metastasis is called *iatrogenic metastasis.*

Examples of metastases are given in Table 7.3.

TABLE 7.3 **Examples of Primary Tumor Metastasis**

SITES OF METASTASIS	PRIMARY TUMOR SITE
Bone, lymph nodes, brain	Breast cancer
Lymph nodes, spleen, liver, lung	Malignant melanoma
Bone, brain, liver, lung	Kidney cancer
Brain, lung	Osteosarcoma (bone cancer)
Bone	Prostate cancer
Lymph nodes, brain, liver, lung, ovaries	Colon cancer

7.4 The Effects of Tumors

What Are the Effects of Tumors?

Tumors can destroy tissue, compress organs, obstruct ducts, and cause infection, anemia, and pain.

How Do Tumors Destroy Tissue?

As tumors expand and invade normal tissue, they put pressure on cells. This pressure interferes with the normal daily activities of the cells. It also interferes with the blood supply to these cells, causing a reduction in the supply of nutrients and the removal of waste products. The steady expansion of the tumor and the deterioration of normal cell function will cause the death of normal cells. These dead cells will be replaced with tumor mass.

How Do Tumors Cause Compression of Organs?

The growth of the tumor will lead to the compression of neighboring tissue. A good example would be intracranial tumors. As these tumors grow and expand, they cause considerable distortion of the soft nervous tissue of the brain.

How Do Tumors Obstruct Ducts?

As tumors grow and spread to secondary locations, obstructions in the lumen of ducts can occur.

What would be examples of tumors that obstruct ducts?

Examples would include tumors of the respiratory bronchi that can stop air flow, tumors of the esophagus that can cause problems swallowing, and carcinomas arising in the epithelial mucosa.

How Do Tumors Cause Infections?

Malignant tumors can suppress the immune system by inhibiting the production of white blood cells (*neutrophils* and *monocytes*) in red bone marrow. When tumors grow near body surfaces, they interfere with the body's natural barrier that protects us from invading organisms. When this barrier is disrupted or damaged, microorganisms can gain access to the body and infect tissues.

Tumors can also affect normal mucus produced by goblet epithelial cells. This mucus prevents microorganisms from gaining access to the lungs. The flow of urine prevents microorganisms from the urethra and ureters from reaching the kidneys. Infections of the lungs and urinary system that can occur as a result of interferences of tumors are *pyelonephritis* and *bronchopneumonia.*

How Do Tumors Cause Anemia?

Anemia can be caused by a decrease in the number of red blood cells or a deficiency of hemoglobin. Anemia can also be caused by bleeding, which is the result of many malignant tumors. These tumors invade neighboring blood vessels and disrupt the walls, which will cause bleeding.

Tumors that affect bone marrow will cause a loss of platelet production. Loss or a decrease in platelets will cause bleeding because blood coagulation will be compromised. Tumors affecting the kidneys can disrupt the production of erythropoietin. Erythropoietin causes erythropoiesis, the stimulation of red bone cell production.

How Can Tumors Cause Pain?

Pain associated with tumors is severe and unrelenting. When tumors spread to bone, they can cause fractures. When tumors obstruct the walls of hollow organs, these walls can become stretched. Tumors in the vertebral column or in the skull can compress the spinal cord and brain.

What Effects Can Tumors Have on the Endocrine System and Hormone Secretion?

Tumors of endocrine tissue can cause uncontrolled hormone secretions. These uncontrolled secretions will result in the improper regulation of body systems. This will be very serious for the individual.

Chapter 7 Review Questions

Fill In the Blank

1. The formation of new tissue is called _______________.
2. What is a neoplastic mass? _______________.
3. An increase in the normal demand on cells will cause _____________.
4. Adaptive growth responses will cause ___________________________.
5. The replacement or conversion of cells is called _________________.
6. When cells are chronically exposed to an irritant or are chronically inflamed, __________ can occur.
7. Thickening of the epidermis of the skin would be an example of ___________.
8. Chronic cigarette smoking may cause a change from the normal ciliated pseudostratified epithelium to thicker, nonciliated epithelium, which would be an example of _____________.
9. A change in the site, shape, and appearance of cells is called ____________________.
10. Some forms of tissue dysplasia are called __________________.
11. Oncology is the study of ________________.
12. Tumors that do not spread to other tissues are called ______________ tumors.
13. Tumors that spread to other tissues are called __________________tumors.
14. What does the word *cancer* mean? ______________.
15. Which type of tumors can spread to different parts of the body?
16. Malignant tumors are named according to their _____________ tissue of origin.
17. The suffix "oma" denotes a(n) ________________tumor.

18. A benign tumor of cartilage would be called a(n) ____________________.

19. Embryonic tissue that provides a protective layer is called ____________________.

20. Embryonic tissue that provides fibrous connective tissue is called ______________.

21. Embryonic tissue that provides the covering of outer body surfaces is called _________.

22. Tumors that are malignant and are found in the endoderm and ectoderm are called _____.

23. Benign tumors of glandular tissues are called _________________.

24. Benign tumors of glandular tissues that contain cysts are called ___________________.

25. Malignant tumors of the mesoderm are called _________________.

26. Malignant tumors of fibrous connective tissue are called _________________.

27. Which structure supports tumor cells? _______________.

28. Which structure provides the tumor's blood supply? _______________.

29. The process of forming new blood vessels in tumors is called _________________.

30. The amount of time between the division of cells is called ____________________.

True/False

31. The term *neoplastic* means "new growth."

32. When there is an increase in the number of cells in a given tissue, this is called hypoplasia.

33. A callus would be an example of hyperplasia.

34. A decrease in the number of cells is called metaplasia.

35. Dysplasia is a change in the size, shape, and appearance of cells.

36. Tumors that grow very slowly and do not spread to the surrounding tissue are called benign tumors.

37. Malignant tumors grow very slowly and do not spread to the surrounding tissue.

38. In Latin, *cancer* means "crab."

39. Benign tumors of glandular tissues are called adenomas.

40. Malignant tumors that are found in the endoderm are called carcinomas.

Matching

41. Mesoderm

42. Fibrosarcoma

43. Adenocarcinoma

44. Epithelioma

45. Carcinoma

46. Replacement of cells

47. Lipoma

48. Liposarcoma

49. Adenoma

50. Fibroma

   A. Malignant tumor of fibrous connective tissue
   B. Malignant tumor of glandular tissue
   C. Embryonic cartilage
   D. Metaplasia
   E. Malignant tumor of epithelial tissue
   F. Benign tumor of fibrous connective tissue
   G. Benign tumor of adipose tissue
   H. Malignant tumor of adipose tissue
   I. Benign tumor of epithelial tissue
   J. Benign tumor of glandular tissue

Chapter 7: Review Questions and Answers

Fill In the Blank Answers

1. Neoplasia
2. A new growth
3. Hyperplasia
4. Hyperplasia
5. Metaplasia
6. Metaplasia
7. Hyperplasia
8. Metaplasia
9. Dysplasia
10. Precancerous lesions
11. Tumors
12. Benign
13. Malignant
14. Crab
15. Malignant tumors
16. Embryonic
17. Benign
18. Chondroma
19. Endoderm
20. Mesoderm
21. Ectoderm
22. Carcinomas
23. Adenomas
24. Cystadenomas
25. Sarcomas
26. Fibrosarcomas
27. Fibrous stroma
28. Vascular stroma
29. Angiogenesis
30. Generation time

True/False Answers

31. True

32. False

33. True

34. False

35. True

36. True

37. False

38. True

39. True

40. True

Matching Answers

41. C

42. A

43. B

44. I

45. E

46. D

47. G

48. H

49. J

50. F

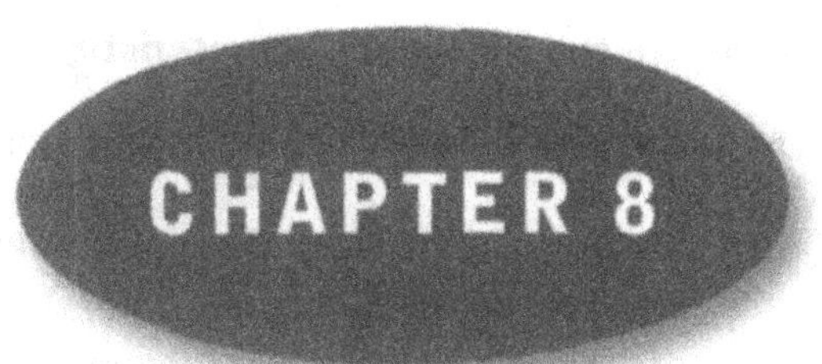

Blood and Blood Disorders

Objectives

The heart, blood, and blood vessels make up the cardiovascular system. This chapter will introduce the components of blood, the function of blood, and the blood vessels.

Keywords:

Hematology
Plasma
Formed elements
Erythrocytes
Leukocytes
Thrombocytes
Erythropoiesis
Polycythemia
Anemia
Neutrophils
Eosinophils
Basophils
B lymphocytes (B cells)
T lymphocytes (T cells)
Natural killer cells
Monocytes
Hemostasis
Hemophilia
Disseminated intravascular clotting
Thrombosis
Thrombus
Embolus
Embolism
Thrombocytopenia
Blood typing
Rh factor
Erythroblastosis fetalis
Sickle-cell anemia
Leukemia
Lymphocytic leukemia
Myeloid leukemia
Monocytic leukemia
Cyanosis
Septicemia
Thalassemia

8.1 Overview

What Is Hematology?

Hematology is the study, diagnosis, and treatment of blood disorders.

What Are the Functions of Blood?

The blood *transports* oxygen (from the lungs), nutrients (from the digestive tract), and hormones (from the endocrine system) to the cells of the body. The blood also removes carbon dioxide and wastes from the cells of the body.

The blood *regulates* pH through its buffer systems and temperature through its coolant and heat absorption properties.

The blood *protects* the body by preventing blood loss and fighting toxins and microorganisms through phagocytes and plasma proteins.

What Are the Physical Characteristics of Blood?

The characteristics of blood include the following:

- Blood viscosity is higher than that of water.
- Blood pH is 7.35–7.45.
- Blood temperature is 38°C or 100.4°F.
- Blood volume, in an average-sized adult, is 4 to 6 liters or 1.5 gallons.

How Can We Sample Blood?

Blood can be sampled by a finger stick, venipuncture from a vein, or arterial stick from an artery.

What Are the Components of Blood?

Blood is 55 percent ***plasma*** (the extracellular fluid in blood) and 45 percent ***formed elements***. Plasma is 92 percent water and 8 percent solutes.

What are the solutes in plasma?

The solutes in plasma include the following:

1. Proteins: albumins, globulins, and fibrinogen
2. Nutrients
3. Enzymes
4. Hormones
5. Respiratory gases
6. Electrolytes
7. Wastes

What are the formed elements in blood?

The formed elements include the following (each of these values is per microliter of blood):

1. 4.8–5.4 million ***erythrocytes*** or red blood cells
2. 5,000–10,000 ***leukocytes*** or white blood cells
3. 150,000–400,000 ***thrombocytes*** or platelets

Table 8.1 summarizes the components of blood. Figure 8.1 shows the appearance of the different types of blood cells.

TABLE 8.1 Components of Blood

Plasma 55%	• Water (92% of plasma)
	• Solutes (8% of plasma)
	• Proteins, nutrients, enzymes, hormones, respiratory gases, electrolytes, wastes
Formed elements (45%) (per microliter)	• Erythrocytes (red blood cells), 4.8–5.4 million
	• Leukocytes (white blood cells), 5,000–10,000
	• Thrombocytes (platelets), 150,000–400,000

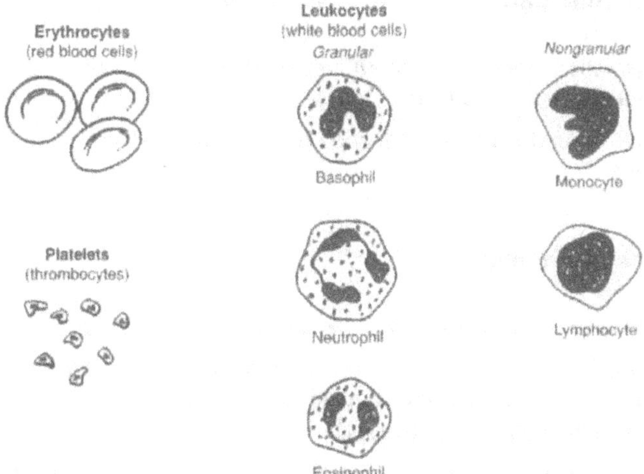

Figure 8.1 The appearance of blood cells.

8.2 Red Blood Cells

What Are Erythrocytes?

Erythrocytes are red blood cells. Red blood cells are biconcave cells that do not contain nuclei. They contain the red pigment hemoglobin, which transports oxygen (O_2) and carbon dioxide (CO_2). Red blood cells live 120 days. After 120 days, dead or worn-out red blood cells (RBCs) are trapped by phagocytes in the liver, spleen, or red bone marrow. The phagocytes "unzip" the RBC's plasma membrane and split apart the hemoglobin molecules.

The "*heme*" portion of the hemoglobin molecules contains iron (Fe^3+), which hooks up with a protein transporter called *transferrin.* Transferrin transports the Fe^3+ to the bone marrow to be reused. Fe^3+ is stored by an iron-storing protein called *ferritin*. Ferritin stores Fe^3+ in the liver, spleen, and muscle. The noniron portion of the heme molecule is converted to *bilirubin*, which travels to the liver and is one of the substances used in the synthesis of *bile*. Bile is secreted by the liver and stored in the gallbladder. When a human eats fats, the gallbladder contracts, releasing bile into the small intestine, where it emulsifies these fats. Some of the bilirubin gets converted into *urobilinogen* by bacteria in the large intestine. The urobilinogen gets absorbed into the blood, where it is converted to *urobilin*. This urobilin is filtered through the kidneys and excreted from the body in *urine*. Most of the urobilinogen stays in the large intestines, becomes *stercobilin*, and is excreted from the body in *feces*.

The "*globin*" of the hemoglobin molecules is made up of protein. This protein molecule is broken down into *amino acids* and is reused to make new protein.

In the red bone marrow of the long bones of the upper and lower extremities, ribs, sternum, and pelvis and the fetal liver and spleen, red blood cells are made. This process is called ***erythropoiesis***. In order to produce red blood cells, iron, globin, vitamin B_{12} (absorbed in the stomach), and erythropoietin (produced in the kidneys) are needed.

What Are Some Diagnostic Tests Used in the Measuring of RBCs?

- *Reticulocyte count.* A reticulocyte count measures the rate of erythropoiesis. A normal reticulocyte count is between 0.5 and 1.5 percent of all red blood cells. This means that the percentage of new reticulocytes that will become red blood cells and replace old red blood cells is between 0.5 and 1.5 percent of a blood sample. A person may show a high reticulocyte count if he or she is using iron supplements because of iron deficiency or show a low reticulocyte count if he or she is anemic because of malnutrition, leukemia, or the absence of intrinsic factor.
- *Hematocrit.* Hematocrit measures the percentage of red blood cells in whole blood. A normal or average hematocrit is 40 to 54 percent in males and 38 to 47 percent in females. A hematocrit is a useful test for diagnosing polycythemia and anemia.

What Are Some Conditions That Can Affect the RBC Count?

- ***Polycythemia.*** Polycythemia is an increased rate or large production of red blood cells in whole blood. This will cause an abnormally *high* hematocrit.
- ***Anemia.*** Anemia is a decrease in the rate of production or a loss of red blood cells. This will cause an abnormally *low* hematocrit.

What Are the Various Types of Anemia?

- *Hemorrhagic anemia* is caused by blood loss. This can be the result of trauma.
- *Pernicious anemia* is a form of nutritional anemia. It is a decrease in the production of red blood cells that occurs when there is a failure of parietal cells in the stomach to secrete intrinsic factor. Intrinsic factor is needed to absorb vitamin B_{12} in the stomach.
- *Nutritional anemia* is a decrease in the intake or absorption of vitamin B_{12}, iron, or folic acid that can result in a decrease in red blood cell production.
- *Aplastic anemia* is caused by the destruction of red bone marrow and its replacement by adipose tissue, fibrous connective tissue, or tumor cells. This destruction can be caused by radiation, chemicals, drugs, or chemotherapy. These toxins can also affect the production of red blood cells by hindering enzyme activity needed in hemopoiesis.

Table 8.2 summarizes the different types of anemia.

TABLE 8.2 Types of Anemia

TYPE	CHARACTERISTIC
Hemorrhagic	Caused by blood loss (trauma)
Pernicious	Caused by a decrease in vitamin B_{12} resulting from the failure of parietal cells to secrete intrinsic factor
Nutritional	Caused by a decrease in vitamin B_{12}, iron, or folic acid
Aplastic	Caused by the destruction of red bone marrow

8.3 White Blood Cells

What Are Leukocytes?

Leukocytes are white blood cells. The general functions of white blood cells are to fight infection, be involved in inflammation responses, attack foreign substances that enter the body, and attack abnormal self cells. Leukocytes live from seconds to years.

What Are the Types of White Blood Cells?

There are two main types of white blood cells (WBCs):

- *Granular leukocytes* have a grainy appearance. These include
  1. ***Neutrophils*** function in phagocytosis and destroy bacteria.
  2. ***Eosinophils*** function in allergic reactions, destroy parasites, and are involved in autoimmune diseases.
  3. ***Basophils*** function in allergic reactions and inflammation.

- *Agranular leukocytes* have a smooth-looking appearance. These include
  1. ***B lymphocytes (B cells)*** are involved in immune responses. These cells develop into *plasma cells* that secrete antibodies.
  2. ***T lymphocytes (T cells)*** are involved in immune responses. T cells mature in the thymus gland and attack invading viruses, spontaneously arising tumor cells, and transplanted tissue cells.
  3. ***Natural killer cells*** attack a variety of microorganisms that cause infection and certain types of spontaneously arising tumor cells.
  4. ***Monocytes*** are large phagocytes that function in phagocytosis of foreign cells, microorganisms, and dead or worn-out cells. Monocytes transform into macrophages. There are two types of macrophages:
     - *Wandering.* These macrophages circulate through the body, searching for foreign cells and dead or worn-out cells.
     - *Fixed.* These macrophages are secured in organs such as the spleen, liver, lymph nodes, and red bone marrow and "capture" or phagocytose foreign cells and dead or worn-out cells when they pass by.

Table 8.3 summarizes the different types of white blood cells.

TABLE 8.3 Types of White Blood Cells

TYPE	CHARACTERISTIC
Granular leukocytes	*Granular appearance*
Neutrophils	Phagocytosis of bacteria
Eosinophils	Destruction of parasites; involved in allergic reactions and autoimmune diseases
Basophils	Allergic reactions and inflammation
Agranular leukocytes	*Lack a granular appearance*
B lymphocytes	Involved in immune responses. Develop into plasma cells
T lymphocytes	Involved in immune responses. Mature in the thymus gland. Attack invading viruses, spontaneously arising tumor cells, and transplanted tissue cells
Natural killer cells	Attack microbes and certain tumor cells
Monocytes	Develop into macrophages, which are big phagocytes that attack worn-out, dead, or foreign cells

What Are Some Conditions That Can Affect White Blood Cell Counts?

- *Neutrophils* will increase in number with burns, stress, or bacterial infections and during an inflammatory response. They will decrease in number with exposure to drugs or radiation and with a decrease in vitamin B_{12}. Diseases that can increase the number of neutrophils are systemic lupus erythematosus, pneumonia, tonsillitis, and appendicitis.
- *Eosinophils* will increase in number with parasitic infections and allergies. They will decrease in number with stress and drugs. Diseases that will increase the number of eosinophils are autoimmune diseases, hay fever, and asthma.
- *Basophils* will increase in number with allergies, leukemia, and hypothyroidism (myxedema). They will decrease in number during ovulation and pregnancy and with stress and hyperthyroidism (Graves' disease). Diseases that will increase the number of basophils are kidney disease and hypothyroidism (myxedema).

- *Lymphocytes* will increase in number with certain forms of leukemia and viruses. They will decrease in number when there is immunosuppression and cortisol therapy. Diseases that will increase lymphocyte production are mononucleosis, mumps (myxovirus), and whooping cough (*Bordetella pertussis*).
- *Monocytes* will increase in number with certain viral, fungal, and bacterial infections and certain forms of leukemia. They will decrease in number with the suppression of red bone marrow and therapy with cortisol. Diseases that will increase the number of monocytes are tuberculosis (*Mycobacterium tuberculosis*) and typhus [some examples: *Rickettsia prowazekii, Rickettsia typhi,* and *Rickettsia rickettsii* (Rocky Mountain spotted fever)].

8.4 The Clotting of Blood

What Are Thrombocytes?

Thrombocytes or platelets develop under the influence of the hormone *thrombopoietin.* Thrombocytes form from megakaryocytes, which break into approximately 2,000 pieces. Each individual piece is surrounded by a cell plasma membrane and is called a platelet or thrombocyte. There are between 150,000 and 400,000 platelets per microliter in whole blood. Platelets are disc-shaped and exhibit many granules but do not contain nuclei. They live five to nine days. Dead, aged, or worn-out platelets are removed from the blood by fixed microphages in the spleen and liver. Platelets form a platelet plug to help stop the loss of blood when blood vessels are damaged, promote the contraction of the smooth muscle in blood vessels, and clot blood.

What Is Hemostasis?

Hemostasis refers to the stoppage of bleeding. If a blood vessel is damaged or broken, the loss of blood must be stopped quickly, and the clotting process must be very carefully controlled and localized.

What Are the Steps of Hemostasis?

Hemostasis involves the following processes:

- *Vascular spasm* is the contraction of the smooth muscle in blood vessels to stop the loss of blood.
- *Platelet plug formation* occurs when platelets adhere to the broken or damaged portion of a blood vessel to form a plug. This plug reduces the amount of blood loss at the area of damage.
- *Blood coagulation or clotting* involves a gel formation made up of fibrin (an insoluble protein) that traps the formed elements in the blood, forming a clot.

What Are Some Disorders That Affect the Clotting of Blood?

- ***Hemophilia*** is a hereditary defect in coagulation in which bleeding can occur spontaneously or after even minor trauma.
- ***Disseminated intravascular clotting***, or DIC, is a disorder affecting hemostasis. DIC is characterized by bleeding throughout the body and unregulated clotting of blood.
- ***Thrombosis*** is a condition in which there is clotting in an unbroken blood vessel.
- A ***thrombus*** is the actual clot. This can be a piece of debris, such as fat from a bone fracture, or even an air bubble.
- An ***embolus*** is a thrombus that has broken free and is traveling through the circulatory system.
- ***Embolism*** occurs when an embolus lodges or gets stuck in a blood vessel. This condition will impede or block the flow of blood. If this condition occurs in the lungs, it is called a *pulmonary embolism.* If it occurs in the brain, it is called a *cerebral vascular accident (CVA)* or *stroke.*
- ***Thrombocytopenia*** is a low platelet count, leading to bleeding from capillaries.

TABLE 8.4 **Functions of the Formed Elements Found in Blood**

ELEMENT	FUNCTION
Erythrocyte (RBC)	Carries oxygen and carbon dioxide
Leukocyte (WBC)	Fights infection; carries out an immune response
Thrombocyte	Clots blood and is important in the process of hemostasis (stopping bleeding)

8.5 Blood Types

What Is Blood Typing and How Does It Work?

Blood typing works on an antigen-antibody relationship. On the surface of red blood cells, there are genetically determined antigen groups called *agglutinogens* or *isoantigens.* The blood plasma contains genetically determined antibodies called *agglutinins* or *isoantibodies.* These agglutinins or isoantibodies will "attack" blood group antigens that the body does not normally have.

What Are the Blood Types and What Do They Mean?

The blood types are A, B, AB, and O. These groupings are based on antigen-antibody responses.

If an individual has *"type A" antigen* on his or her red blood cells, that person will have *"anti-B" antibodies* in the plasma. If an individual has *"type B" antigen* on his or her red blood cells, that person will have *"anti-A" antibodies* in the plasma. If an individual has *both* antigens, that person will have *"type AB" blood* and will have *no* antibodies. If an individual's red blood cells have *no* antigens, that person will have *"type O" blood.* Such a person will have *both* A and B antibodies in the plasma.

Remember:

- Individuals with type A blood can receive blood *only* from people with type A and type O blood.
- Individuals with type B blood can receive blood *only* from people with type B and type O blood.
- Individuals with type AB blood can receive blood from people with type A, type B, type AB, and type O blood because their plasma does not contain antibodies against these blood types.
- Individuals with type O blood can receive blood *only* from people with type O because type O has no antigens but has both antibodies in the plasma.

  Type O is the universal donor.

  Type AB is the universal receiver.

What Is Rh Factor?

Rh factor is another antigen that is either present or absent on a red blood cell. Unlike types A, B, and O, which are carbohydrates, Rh is a protein antigen. Rh was named after the Rhesus monkey, where this antigen was first discovered. If an individual has the antigen, that person is said to be Rh positive, and if an individual does not have the antigen, he or she is said to be Rh negative. This is where the positive and negative notation for blood type comes from.

Why Is Rh Important in Pregnancy?

If an Rh-negative female and an Rh-positive male conceive a child, there is a 50/50 chance that the child can have Rh-positive or Rh-negative blood. If the child is Rh-negative, it does not matter. If the child is Rh-positive, this can present a problem. The first Rh-positive baby's cells will enter the mother's circulatory system. The mother will, in turn, produce antibodies to fight the Rh-positive red blood cells. Every Rh-positive baby conceived after this will be attacked by the mother's antibodies. This condition is called ***erythroblastosis fetalis.***

8.6 Disorders That Can Affect Blood

What Are Other Disorders That Can Affect Blood?

Sickle-cell anemia is a hereditary disease in which there is a defect or abnormality of hemoglobin. The red blood cells become long, cigar-shaped structures that bend into "sickle-shaped" cells. These cells rupture or break apart very easily. People with this disease present with mild to severe anemia and jaundice (a yellow look to the skin and the sclera of the eyes), and can have fever and an increase in heart rate. Individuals with sickle-cell anemia experience joint pain, fatigue, and shortness of breath. These individuals can also have cell and tissue damage as a result of oxygen debt. Homozygous children (those inheriting two traits, one from each parent) will present with a more severe form of the disease. Heterozygous children (those inheriting one trait) will present with a less severe form of the disease.

Leukemia is the name given to a number of cancers affecting red bone marrow. The white blood cells divide rapidly and uncontrollably, thus interfering with the production of red blood cells, platelets, and normal white blood cells. As a result, blood oxygen levels decrease because the transport of oxygen is reduced. Blood clotting is disrupted and is abnormal, and these individuals do not fight infection properly and are more prone to infection and disease.

Leukemia is classified as being either acute or chronic.

- *Acute.* Symptoms come on rapidly. Children commonly have the acute form of leukemia.
- *Chronic.* Symptoms can take years to develop.

Risk factors for leukemia include chemotherapy and radiation therapy for treatment of other cancers, Down syndrome (genetic conditions), smoking, exposure to chemicals such as benzene, and infections such as the Epstein-Barr virus.

What Are the Different Types of Leukemia?

The different types of leukemia include lymphocytic leukemia, myeloid leukemia, and monocytic leukemia.

- ***Lymphocytic leukemia*** develops from lymphoid stem cells that normally develop into T lymphocytes and B lymphocytes.
- ***Myeloid leukemia*** develops from myeloid stem cells. These stem cells normally develop into granular leukocytes, neutrophils, eosinophils, and basophils.
- ***Monocytic leukemia*** also develops from myeloid stem cells. These stem cells normally develop into monocytes.

What Are Some Other Conditions Involving the Blood?

- ***Cyanosis*** is a bluish color in the skin and nail beds resulting from a decrease in oxygen in the blood.
- ***Septicemia***, or "blood poisoning," is caused by toxins or pathogenic bacteria located in the blood.
- ***Thalassemia*** is a genetic defect in the hemoglobin molecule that results from the faulty production of normal peptide chains. Usually patients are of Mediterranean descent. Individuals who are heterozygous will have one defective gene and are either asymptomatic or with minor symptoms. Homozygous individuals will have two defective genes and will present with symptoms. There are two types of thalassemia:
  - *Thalassemia major.* The individual has a more severe form of the disease and will present with symptoms. Thalassemia major is also called *Cooley's anemia.*
  - *Thalassemia minor.* With thalassemia minor, the individual presents with only minor symptoms or no symptoms.

The signs and symptoms include cephalgia (headache), nausea, anorexia, failure to thrive, fever, anemia, and an enlarged spleen (splenomegaly).

Chapter 8 Review Questions

Fill In the Blank

1. The study of blood is called ________________.
2. The pH of blood is ________________.
3. The temperature of blood is ________________.
4. The volume of blood is ________________.
5. The extracellular fluid of blood is called ________________.
6. The percentage of water in plasma is ______________.
7. Erythrocytes are ________________.
8. Leukocytes are ________________.
9. Thrombocytes are ________________.
10. Erythrocytes live ________________.
11. Thrombocytes live________________.
12. The primary function of red blood cells is to carry ___________ and ___________.
13. The primary function of platelets is to ________________.
14. The primary function of white blood cells is to ________________.
15. The process of making red blood cells is called ________________.
16. A test that indicates the rate of erythropoiesis, which is useful in the treatment of anemia, is ____________.
17. A test that measures the percentage of red blood cells in whole blood is ____________.
18. A neutrophil is an example of a(n) ____________________.
19. White blood cells that will increase in number with parasitic infections and allergies are ___________.
20. White blood cells that will increase in number with allergies, leukemia, and hypothyroidism are __________________.
21. Thrombocytes form from ________________.
22. The stoppage of blood loss is called ______________.
23. A hereditary defect in coagulation in which bleeding can occur spontaneously is called ______________.
24. The condition of a clot in an unbroken blood vessel is called a(n) ______________.
25. A clot that lodges or gets stuck in a blood vessel is called a(n) ______________.
26. Having a low platelet count is called ________________.
27. When an Rh-negative woman has an Rh-positive baby, the condition that can occur is _________.
28. A hereditary defect in the hemoglobin of red blood cells that changes their shape so that they look rod- or sickle-shaped is called ______________.
29. The name given to a number of cancers affecting red bone marrow is _________.
30. A bluish color in the skin and nail beds resulting from a decrease in oxygen in blood is called __________.

Matching

31. Polycythemia

32. Anemia

33. Hemorrhagic anemia

34. Pernicious anemia

35. Nutritional anemia

36. Aplastic anemia

37. Neutrophils

38. Eosinophils

39. Basophils

40. B cells

A. A decrease in RBCs
B. WBCs that function in the phagocytosis of bacteria
C. Caused by the destruction of red blood marrow
D. Caused by a lack of B_{12}
E. WBCs that function in destroying parasites
F. Caused by a decrease in iron or folic acid
G. WBCs that function in allergic reactions and inflammation
H. Caused by blood loss
I. Increased production of RBCs
J. Develop into plasma cells

True/False

41. Proteins are an example of solutes in plasma.

42. 40,000 is a normal leukocyte count in whole blood.

43. Red blood cells contain a nucleus.

44. Type O blood is the universal acceptor.

45. Type AB blood is the universal acceptor.

Multiple Choice

46. These blood cells live 120 days.

A. Thrombocytes
B. Leukocytes
C. Eosinophils
D. Erythrocytes
E. Platelets

47. Blood poisoning is called __________.

A. cyanosis
B. septicemia
C. leukemia

D. anemia
E. hemophilia

48. A problem with clotting would be __________.
A. cyanosis
B. septicemia
C. leukemia
D. anemia
E. hemophilia

49. Having a low red blood cell count would be __________.
A. cyanosis
B. septicemia
C. leukemia
D. anemia
E. hemophilia

50. A decrease in oxygen in blood would cause __________.
A. cyanosis
B. septicemia
C. leukemia
D. anemia
E. hemophilia

Chapter 8: Review Questions and Answers

Fill In the Blank Answers

1. Hematology
2. 7.35–7.45
3. 100.4°F or 38°C
4. 4–6 liters or 1.5 gallons
5. Plasma
6. 92 percent
7. Red blood cells
8. White blood cells
9. Platelets
10. 120 days
11. 5–9 days
12. O_2; CO_2
13. Clot blood
14. Fight infections
15. Erythropoiesis
16. Reticulocyte count
17. Hematocrit
18. White blood cell
19. Eosinophils
20. Basophils
21. Megakaryocytes
22. Hemostasis
23. Hemophilia
24. Thrombosis
25. Embolism
26. Thrombocytopenia
27. Erythroblastosis fetalis
28. Sickle-cell anemia
29. Leukemia
30. Cyanosis

Matching Answers

31. I

32. A

33. H

34. D

35. F

36. C

37. B

38. E

39. G

40. J

True/False Answers

41. True

42. False

43. False

44. False

45. True

Multiple Choice Answers

46. D

47. B

48. E

49. D

50. A

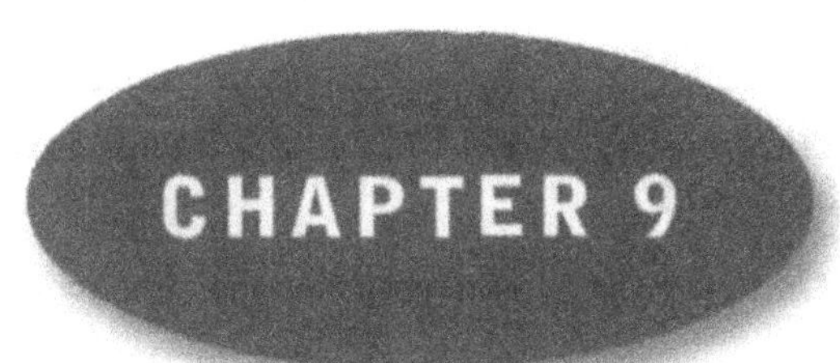

The Cardiovascular System

Objectives

This chapter will discuss the organization, structures, and functions of the heart and blood vessels. It will also examine the disorders and diseases associated with the heart, circulation, and blood pressure.

Keywords:

Cardiology
Mediastinum
Pericardium
Pericarditis
Cardiac tamponade
Epicardium
Myocardium
Endocardium
Endocarditis
Myocarditis
Atria

Auricles
Ventricles
Tricuspid valve
Bicuspid valve (mitral valve)
Pulmonary semilunar valve
Aortic semilunar valve
Rheumatic fever
Stenosis
Insufficiency
Myocardial infarction (MI)
Myocardial ischemia

Hypoxia
Angina pectoris
Ectopic pacemaker
Cardiac arrhythmias
Bradycardia
Tachycardia
Systole
Diastole
Stethoscope
Thrombophlebitis
Cerebral vascular accident (CVA)
Varicose veins
Transient ischemic attacks (TIAs)
Intracerebral hemorrhage
Subarachnoid hemorrhage
Berry aneurysm
Dissecting aneurysm
Arteriosclerosis
Atherosclerosis
Hypertension (high blood pressure)

9.1 Overview

What Is the Study, Diagnosis, and Treatment of Diseases That Affect the Cardiovascular System?

The study of the cardiovascular system and the treatment of diseases of that system is called ***cardiology.***

Where Is the Heart Located?

The heart is located in the ***mediastinum.*** The mediastinum is located between the lungs, anterior to the vertebral column and posterior to the sternum. About two-thirds of the heart's entire mass is located to the left of the midline of the trunk.

The heart is the "hub" or center of the cardiovascular system.

What Is the Pericardium?

The ***pericardium*** is a saclike structure that surrounds or encloses the heart.

What Is the Pericardium Composed Of?

The pericardium is composed of a fibrous outer layer called the *fibrous pericardium* and an inner *serous pericardium.* The inner serous pericardium is composed of a *parietal layer* and a *visceral layer.* The visceral layer is also called the *epicardium.* In between the parietal and visceral layers of the serous pericardium is a space called the *pericardial space.* This space contains *pericardial fluid.* The pericardial fluid reduces friction when the heart beats.

What Is a Condition That Affects the Pericardium of the Heart?

Inflammation of the pericardium is called ***pericarditis.*** Pericarditis can occur with trauma, infection, and heart attacks.

What are the signs and symptoms of pericarditis?
Signs and symptoms include sharp chest pain described as a "stabbing" sensation, difficulty breathing while lying down, fever, and fatigue.

Pericarditis can result in ***cardiac tamponade***, which is pressure around the heart caused by bleeding in the pericardial cavity.

What Are the Walls of the Heart Called, and Where Are They Located?

The heart wall contains three layers.

What are the three layers of the heart?
These layers are

- ***Epicardium.*** The epicardium makes up the external wall and is also called the visceral portion of the serous pericardium. This layer gives the heart its slick, smooth appearance.
- ***Myocardium.*** The myocardium is the middle layer that makes up the bulk of the heart. This layer is made up of cardiac muscle and provides the contractions that pump the blood.
- ***Endocardium.*** The endocardium forms the inner smooth lining of the heart.

What Types of Tissue Make Up These Layers?

The epicardium is composed of connective tissue. The myocardium is composed of muscle tissue. The endocardium is composed of endothelial tissue.

Figure 9.1 shows the structures of the heart.

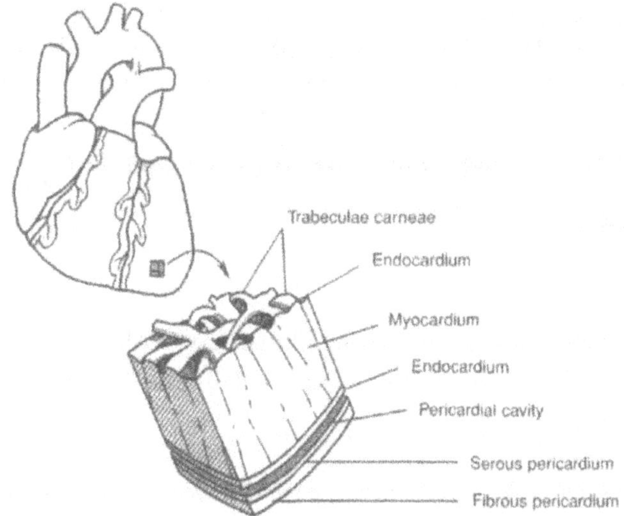

Figure 9.1 The heart wall, the pericardial cavity, and the pericardium.

What Are Some Examples of Disorders That Can Affect Heart Tissue?

Disorders that can affect heart tissue include endocarditis and myocarditis.

- ***Endocarditis***

What is endocarditis?
Endocarditis involves the inflammation of the endocardium and valves of the heart. Endocarditis is typically caused by a bacterial infection.

What are the signs and symptoms associated with endocarditis?
The signs and symptoms include rapid and irregular heartbeats, tiredness and fatigue, fever, chills, and sweating at night.

- ***Myocarditis***

What is myocarditis?

Myocarditis involves the inflammation of the myocardium of the heart.

This condition can occur as a result of a virus infection, a bacterial infection (such as *Streptococcus pyogenes*), which causes *rheumatic fever*, or chemical and radiation exposure.

What are the signs and symptoms associated with myocarditis?
The signs and symptoms of myocarditis include rapid and irregular heartbeat, tiredness and fatigue, slight chest pain, pain in the joints, and loss of breath.

What Are the Chambers of the Heart?

The heart is a hollow organ and contains four chambers. There are two upper chambers called ***atria***; there is a left and a right atrium. Each of these atria has an appendage or "overflow sac" called an ***auricle***; there is a right and a left auricle. The heart contains two lower chambers called the ***ventricles***; there is a right and a left ventricle.

What Is the Function of Heart Valves?

Heart valves prevent the backflow of blood when it flows out of a chamber.

What Are Heart Valves Made Up Of?

The heart valves are made up of dense irregular connective tissue, *chordae tendineae*, and papillary muscles. When the papillary muscles relax, the chordae tendineae loosen, causing the valves to open. When the papillary muscles contract, the chordae tendineae tighten, causing the valves to close. Heart valves open and close in response to pressure changes that occur as a result of cardiac muscle contractions and relaxations.

What Are the Heart Valves Called, and Where Are They Located?

There are two types of heart valves.

- *Atrioventricular valves.* These include the
  1. ***Tricuspid valve***, located between the right atrium and the right ventricle.
  2. ***Bicuspid valve** or **mitral valve***, located between the left atrium and the left ventricle.
- *Semilunar valves.* These include the
  1. ***Pulmonary semilunar valve***, located between the right ventricle and the pulmonary trunk.
  2. ***Aortic semilunar valve***, located between the left ventricle and the aorta.

Figure 9.2 shows the internal anatomy of the heart.

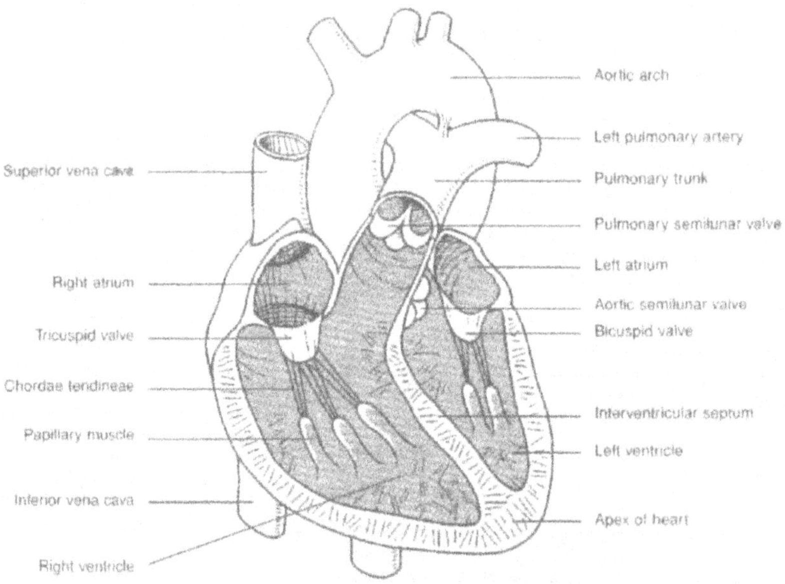

Figure 9.2 Internal anatomy of the heart.

What Are Some Conditions That Can Affect the Heart Valves?

Conditions that can affect the heart valves include infections, stenosis, and insufficiency.

- ***Infections.***

What would infect heart valves?
Infections such as ***rheumatic fever***, a bacterial infection caused by *Streptococcus pyogenes*, can damage and destroy the heart valves, especially the bicuspid valve and the aortic semilunar valve.

- ***Stenosis.***

What is stenosis and what complication would it cause?
Stenosis is a narrowing of a heart valve. This decreases the flow of blood through the valve. An example would be mitral stenosis, where the opening of the mitral valve narrows, obstructing the flow of blood.

- ***Insufficiency.***

What is insufficiency and what complication would it cause?
Insufficiency is a condition in which the valves do not or cannot completely close. Insufficiency would occur with a mitral valve prolapse. This condition occurs when one or both cusps prolapse or protrude into the left atrium every time the heart contracts. It will cause the blood to backflow into the left atrium.

How Does Blood Travel through the Heart?

Deoxygenated blood [blood carrying carbon dioxide (CO_2)] from the systemic circulation enters the superior and inferior vena cava. Blood from the superior and inferior vena cava and the coronary sinus (carrying deoxygenated blood from heart tissue) travels

1. Into the right atrium
2. Through the tricuspid valve
3. Into the right ventricle
4. Through the pulmonary semilunar valve
5. Into the pulmonary trunk
6. Which splits into the right and left pulmonary artery into the lungs

In the lungs, the blood enters the pulmonary capillaries. Here CO_2 diffuses out of the blood and O_2 diffuses into the blood.

Oxygenated blood from the lungs travels back to the heart by the right and left pulmonary veins

1. Into the left atrium
2. Through the bicuspid (mitral) valve
3. Into the left ventricle
4. Through the aortic semilunar valve
5. Into the aorta, which distributes it throughout the body

The aorta has four divisions:

1. *Ascending.* The ascending aorta travels superiorly from the left ventricle to the arch.
2. *Arch.* From the arch, the aorta travels inferiorly.
3. *Thoracic.* The thoracic portion travels inferiorly through the thoracic cavity.
4. *Abdominal.* The abdominal portion travels inferiorly through the abdominal cavity.

How Does Heart Tissue Get Oxygenated Blood and Nutrients Delivered and Deoxygenated Blood and Wastes Removed?

The *right and left coronary arteries* branching from the ascending aorta deliver oxygenated blood and nutrients to heart tissue. The coronary sinus (which is a large vein) removes deoxygenated blood and wastes from the heart tissue. The coronary sinus delivers blood rich in CO_2 back to the right atrium, and the whole process begins again.

9.2 Cardiac Diseases and Disorders

What Are Some Examples of Cardiac Diseases or Disorders?

Examples of cardiac diseases and disorders would include *myocardial infarctions*, *myocardial ischemia*, *hypoxia*, and *angina pectoris*.

- ***Myocardial infarction***, or ***MI***.

What is a myocardial infarction?
Also known as a heart attack, myocardial infarction is the death of heart tissue. This is mostly due to clogging or obstruction in the coronary artery that stops the normal flow of oxygenated blood to the heart. The tissue that dies is replaced with scar tissue. This scar tissue cannot contract, causing a decrease in heart muscle strength. If the area of the myocardial infarction is large enough, it can disrupt the normal conduction system of the heart and result in the sudden death of the individual.

- ***Myocardial ischemia.***

What is myocardial ischemia?
Myocardial ischemia is the result of a partially obstructed coronary artery that causes a reduction of blood flow to the myocardium.

- ***Hypoxia.***

What is hypoxia?
Hypoxia is a reduction in oxygen supply. This is caused by ischemia. Hypoxia will weaken the cells and tissues.

- ***Angina pectoris.***

What is angina pectoris?
Angina pectoris is chest pain resulting from an inadequate flow of oxygen to the heart; it is associated with myocardial ischemia. The signs and symptoms of angina pectoris present as a tightness in the chest (the individual feels as if the chest is being crushed). Symptoms occur during activity or exertion and stop with rest. Pain can also be referred to the lateral aspect of the left arm to the elbow and the neck up to the chin. Sometimes there are no signs or symptoms of this condition. This is referred to as *silent myocardial ischemia*. This is extremely dangerous because the individual will have no warning signs of an impending heart attack.

What Are the Pacemaker and Conduction System of the Heart?

The heart contains specialized tissues that cause spontaneous electrical impulses called *action potentials*. These action potentials stimulate cardiac muscle fibers to contract. The cardiac muscle fibers (or cells) are called *autorhythmic cells* because they contract repeatedly and rhythmically. These cells act like a "pacemaker" and conduction system, sending an electric current through a series of nodes in the heart.

What Are the Nodes That Make Up the Conduction System of the Heart?

The nodes that make up the conduction system of the heart are as follows:

- The *sinoatrial node* or *SA node* is located in the wall of the right atrium and initiates the cardiac action potential (electrical impulse). The SA node will initiate action potentials 90 to 100 times per minute. When we are at rest, the neurotransmitter acetylcholine is released by the *parasympathetic division of the autonomic nervous system*, which lowers the rate of impulses to 75 times per minute. (The average heart rate is around 75 beats per minute.) The SA node is called the *pacemaker* of the heart.
- The *atrioventricular node* or *AV node* receives the electrical impulse (action potential) from the SA node and passes it on to the *atrioventricular bundle*.
- The *atrioventricular bundle* or *AV bundle* is also referred to as the *Bundle of His*. The AV bundle is the electrical connection between the atria and the ventricles and is located in the upper portion (superior portion) of the interventricular septum.

- *Right and left bundle branches.* The electrical impulses from the AV bundle travel to the right and left bundle branches and through the interventricular septum toward the apex (inferior portion) of the heart.
- *Conduction myofibers or Purkinje fibers.* The Purkinje fibers receive the impulses from the right and left bundle branches and send the impulses through the ventricular heart muscles.

Figure 9.3 shows the conduction system of the heart.

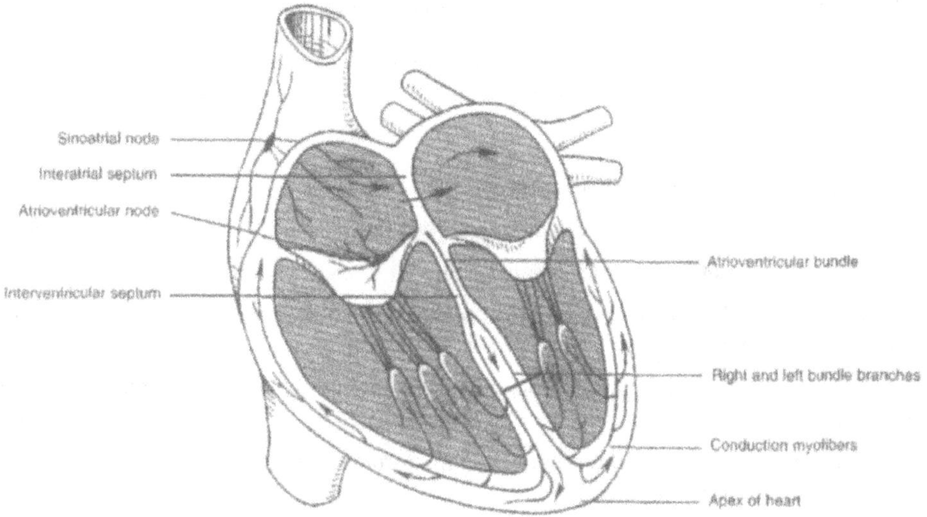

Figure 9.3 The conduction system of the heart.

How Long Does It Take for an Electrical Impulse to Travel through the Heart?

About 200 milliseconds after the atria contract, the ventricles contract.

What Is a Condition That Can Affect the "Pacemaker" of the Heart?

A condition that may develop is an ***ectopic pacemaker.*** This is a place other than the SA node that abnormally becomes self-excitable. Ectopic pacemakers can cause extra heartbeats and even "pace" the heart muscle. Causes of an ectopic pacemaker include electrolyte imbalance, hypoxia, drugs, alcohol, caffeine, nicotine, and digitalis.

9.3 Heart Muscle Physiology

How Does Heart Muscle Contract?

The electrical impulses started at the SA node travel down the conduction system of the heart and excite the contractile fibers (cells) of the heart. The contractile fibers of the heart have a resting membrane potential of around −90 mV. When these fibers are stimulated, their fast "voltage-gated" Na^+ (sodium) ion channels open. Na^+ ions rush in, since sodium is a cation (a positively charged ion). This *depolarizes* the contractile fiber. The cytosol (the intracellular fluid of the cell) is more electronegative than the extracellular fluid (interstitial fluid). Sodium is more abundant outside of the cell. When the gates open, sodium travels down the gradient from a region of higher sodium concentration (interstitial fluid) to a region of lower concentration (intracellular fluid). This is called *facilitated diffusion*. After a couple of milliseconds, the sodium channels inactivate, drastically slowing and thus decreasing the flow of sodium into the fibers.

The next phase is the *plateau phase*. Here the cell plasma membrane becomes permeable to calcium ions (Ca^{2+}). The calcium ion channels open, allowing calcium ions to enter the cell. This process maintains depolarization. At the same time, potassium (K^+) channels open.

This causes the next phase, the recovery of the resting potential, called *repolarization*. Here the sodium channels remain closed, the calcium channels close, and more potassium channels open, causing more outflow of potassium.

This whole process of the contractile fibers depolarizing to repolarizing takes 0.3 second.

How Can We Measure Electrical Impulses in the Heart?

Electrical changes in the heart can be recorded by an *electrocardiogram*, also known as an ECG or EKG. An ECG/EKG is a very good diagnostic tool in revealing acute MI, myocardial ischemia, and ventricular aneurysms.

A normal ECG or EKG consists of a

- *P wave*, which represents atrial depolarization
- *QRS complex*, which represents ventricular depolarization
- *T wave*, which represents ventricular repolarization
- The *P-Q interval* or *P-Q segment* is the time period between the excitement of the atria and the excitement of the ventricles.
- The *S-T interval* or *S-T segment* represents the time when the ventricular contractile fibers are fully depolarized.
- The *Q-T interval* or *Q-T segment* represents the time from the beginning of ventricular depolarization to the end of ventricular repolarization.

What Are Some Disorders That Can Cause an Irregular ECG/EKG?

- *Enlarged P waves* may indicate an enlarged atrium.
- *No P waves* or small, irregular P waves that appear "sawtooth" can indicate atrial fibrillation.
- *Enlarged Q waves* can indicate an acute myocardial infarction.
- *Enlarged R waves* can indicate enlarged ventricles.
- *Flattened T waves* could indicate insufficient oxygen as a result of coronary artery disease.
- *Elevated T waves* may indicate high levels of potassium in the blood.
- *A long P-Q interval* could indicate rheumatic fever or coronary artery disease.
- *An elevated S-T segment* indicates an acute myocardial infarction.
- *A depressed S-T segment* indicates an insufficient supply of oxygen to heart muscle.
- *A lengthened Q-T interval* can be the result of damage to the heart muscle, conduction problems, or a decrease in normal blood flow to heart muscle.

What Is Arrhythmia?

Any deviations from the normal rate of the heart or the normal electrical impulses of the conduction system are called ***cardiac arrhythmias.***

What are the signs and symptoms associated with cardiac arrhythmias?
The signs and symptoms of cardiac arrhythmias include rapid or slow heart rate, heart flutters, chest pain, shortness of breath, fainting, and dizziness.

What would be the causes of cardiac arrhythmias?
The causes of cardiac arrhythmias include an improper flow of electrical impulses through the heart as a result

of high blood pressure, heart attack, heart ischemia, coronary artery disease, cardiomyopathy, heart valve dysfunction, smoking, drugs, alcohol, caffeine, and genetic disorders.

What are the types of arrhythmias?
There are two types of arrhythmias: Rate arrhythmias and conduction arrhythmias.

- *Rate arrhythmias.* Rate arrhythmias include bradycardia and tachycardia.

What is bradycardia?

1. ***Bradycardia*** is a slow resting heart rate or pulse that is less than 50 beats per minute. The cause of bradycardia is increased or excessive vagus nerve (cranial nerve X) stimulation. Cranial nerve X is part of the parasympathetic subdivision of the autonomic nervous system. Drugs and a decrease in body temperature can also cause bradycardia.

What is tachycardia?

2. ***Tachycardia*** is a fast or rapid heart rate or pulse greater than 100 beats per minute. The cause of tachycardia is increased or excessive sympathetic stimulation (subdivision of the autonomic nervous system). The ingestion of drugs or caffeine and an increase in body temperature can also cause tachycardia.

- *Conduction arrhythmias.* Conduction arrhythmias include:

1. *Abnormal sinoatrial node* rhythms.
2. *Ectopic pacemakers* caused by heart damage, ischemia, nicotine, coffee, alcohol, anxiety, and abnormal pH.
3. *Blockages* of normal impulses traveling through the conduction systems. Causes are destruction resulting from an infarct, increased vagal stimulation, and infection.

What Are Premature Heartbeats and How Do They Appear on an ECG/EKG?

Premature heartbeats are caused by ectopic pacemakers. Ectopic pacemakers cause early waves in the cycle.

- *Atrial premature complex* or atrial premature depolarization is caused by the premature depolarization of an atrial ectopic pacemaker. This may cause an interval of atrial fibrillation or flutter. Atrial fibrillation will interfere with normal heart function.
- *Atrioventricular node premature depolarization* is caused by the premature depolarization of an ectopic pacemaker in the atrioventricular node. This causes a normal QRS complex on an ECG/EKG with no P wave.
- *Premature ventricular depolarization (PVD)* or premature ventricular complexes (PVCs) begin from a ventricular ectopic pacemaker. The ECG/EKG shows no P waves, a wide QRS complex, and commonly an inverted T wave (an alteration of ventricular repolarization).

What Are Fibrillations or Flutters and What Do They Show on an ECG/EKG?

- *Atrial fibrillation* is a common atrial arrhythmia caused by the disorganization of electrical impulses in the atria. The ECG/EKG shows no P wave and a normal appearance of the QRS complexes and T waves, although they have irregular rhythms.
- *Ventricular fibrillation* is caused by uncoordinated and disorganized electrical impulses in the ventricles. This is a very serious condition. The blood pressure will rapidly drop, and death will occur without defibrillation.
- *Ventricular tachycardia* occurs when there is one ectopic pacemaker in the ventricles. This condition is serious because it can cause cardiac output to decrease. Ventricular tachycardia can develop into ventricular fibrillation (the QRS complex can be lengthened more than 0.12 second).

What Is a Cardiac Cycle and What Does It Consist Of?

A cardiac cycle consists of a contraction, called ***systole***, and relaxation, called ***diastole***. The phases of the cardiac cycle include relaxation, ventricular filling, and ventricular systole or contraction. A complete cardiac cycle takes 0.8 second. The beats occur approximately 75 times per minute.

How Can We Listen to the Heart?

In order to listen to these heart sounds, an instrument called a ***stethoscope*** is used.

What Are the Sounds That Are Heard through a Stethoscope Called and What Do They Mean?

The sounds heard through a stethoscope are the closing of the heart valves.

The *S1 sound* is the first heart sound that is heard. It represents the closing of the atrioventricular valves. These valves close after ventricular systole begins. The *S2 sound* is the second heart sound that is heard. It represents the closing of the semilunar valves. These valves close at the end of ventricular systole. When blood flows through smoothly, the only sounds heard will be the S1 and S2 sounds. If the valves are damaged as a result of a disease process or if they fail to open or close completely, turbulence in the flow of blood occurs. This turbulence can be heard, and this sound is called a *heart murmur*.

What Is Cardiac Output, and How Is It Calculated?

Cardiac output is the amount of blood pumped or ejected from the left ventricle in a minute. Cardiac output (CO) = stroke volume (SV) × heart rate (HR).

What is stroke volume?

Stroke volume is the amount of blood pumped or ejected by the left ventricle during each systole or contraction.

Heart rate is how many times the heart beats in a minute.

If the HR = 75 beats per minute and SV = 80 mL per beat, CO = (75 beats/min) × (80 mL/beat) = 6,000 mL/min = 6.0 L/min.

What Are Blood Vessels and Their Function?

Blood vessels transport oxygen, nutrients, and hormones to the cells of the body and carry carbon dioxide and wastes away from the cells of the body.

Types of blood vessels include:

1. Arteries
2. Arterioles
3. Capillaries
4. Venules
5. Veins

What Are Blood Vessels Composed Of?

The walls of arteries and veins contain the same layers, or *tunicae*.

What layers do tunicae have?

These layers include

- The *tunica externa* or tunica adventitia is the outermost connective tissue layer, which contains collagen and elastic fibers.
- The *tunica media* is the middle layer and is the thickest layer, containing elastic fibers and smooth muscle.

- The *tunica interna* or tunica intima is the innermost layer. This layer makes contact with the blood. The tunica interna is composed of endothelium, which is made up of squamous epithelial cells.

The walls of arteries are thicker and more elastic than those of veins. Arterial blood is under pressure as a result of the pumping power of the heart. Also, the smooth muscle of the arteries will contract and relax as a result of sympathetic and parasympathetic innervation. These contractions and relaxations will cause the *lumen* of the arteries to vasodilate and vasoconstrict.

What Is the Lumen?

The lumen of blood vessels is the "hole" through which the blood flows.

What Are the Functions of the Blood Vessels?

The functions of the blood vessels are as follows:

- *Arteries* carry blood away from the heart.
- *Arterioles* are very small, almost microscopic blood vessels. They regulate the flow of blood from arteries to capillaries.
- *Capillaries* are made of only tunica interna (intima) and *do not* contain a tunica externa or tunica media. These microscopic blood vessels exchange blood gases and materials between the blood and the tissues of the body. Capillaries branch in between the cells that make up tissues, forming a capillary network. This network increases the surface area, allowing the rapid exchange of large amounts of material between the blood and the tissues. Capillaries connect arterioles to venules.
- *Venules* are small, almost microscopic veins and are formed by a group of capillaries. Venules merge together to form veins.
- *Veins* carry blood toward the heart. They consist of the same tunicae as arteries, although they have a thinner tunica media and tunica externa. The blood in veins is not under as much pressure as it is in arteries. Veins have valves along their lumen that prevent the backflow of blood.

The principal arteries and veins of the body are shown in Figures 9.4 and 9.5.

Remember: Blood is *pumped* through arteries, *flows* through veins, and *oozes* through capillaries.

What Is Edema?

Edema is a swelling caused by an increase in extracellular fluid. Edema can be due to a buildup of capillary pressure because of an obstruction in a vein, heart failure, or an increase in the permeability of the capillary walls.

How does edema occur?
When the balance between interstitial fluid and plasma is disrupted, edema occurs.

How Can Circulation Be Checked?

Circulation is checked by taking a pulse. A pulse is the expansion and elastic recoil of the arterial walls every time the heart pumps. This alternating expansion and recoil within the walls of an artery represents the heartbeat because the arterial walls "pulse" every time the left ventricle of the heart pumps.

The normal or average pulse rate (heart rate) is between 60 and 80 beats per minute.

What Is Blood Pressure?

Blood pressure is the mounting pressure placed by blood on the arterial walls every time the left ventricle contracts. Blood pressure is measured using a device called a *sphygmomanometer* or *blood pressure cuff* and a stethoscope.

Blood pressure is measured using the brachial artery in adults and the femoral artery in infants and small children.

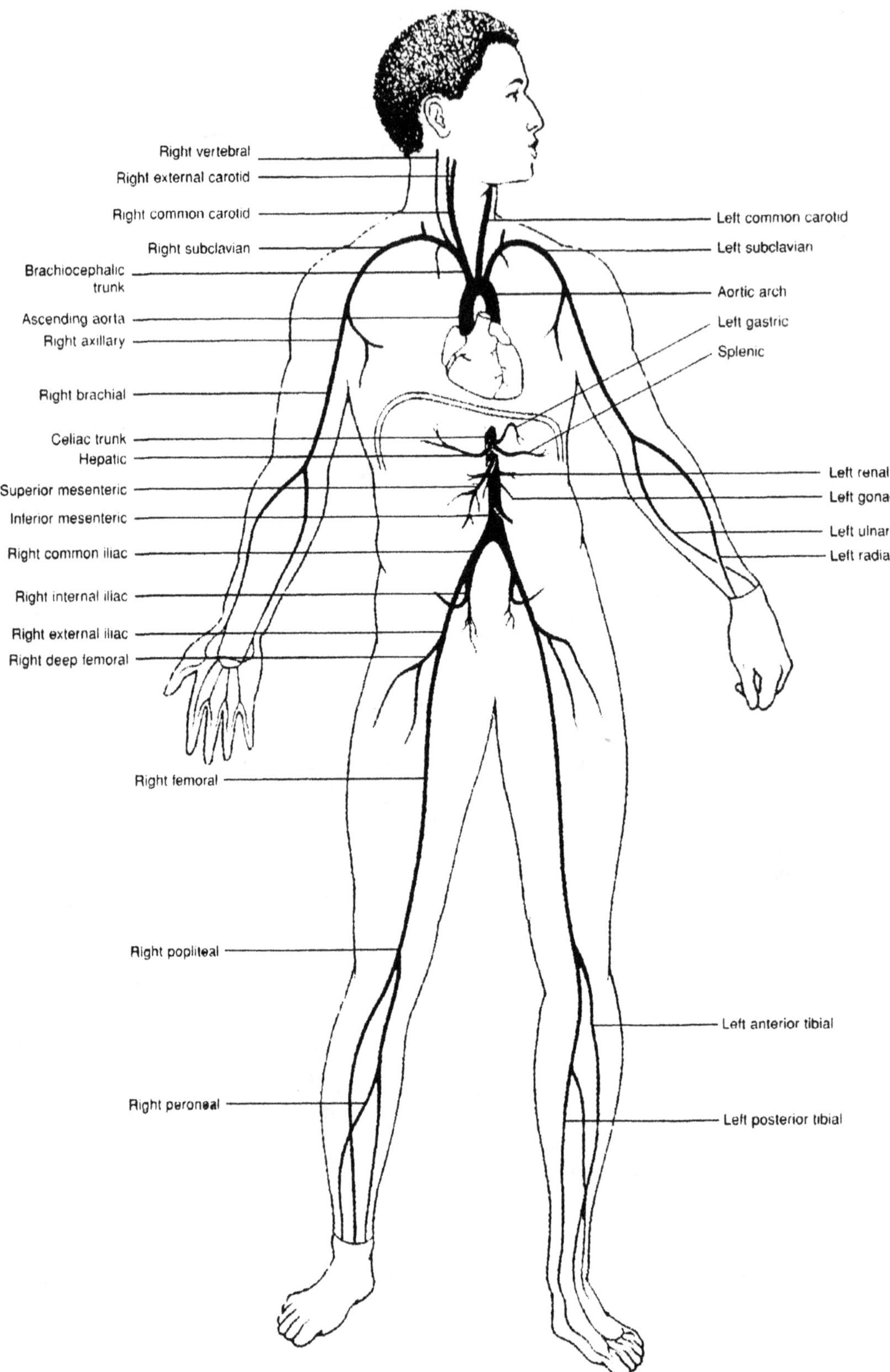

Figure 9.4 Principal arteries of the body.

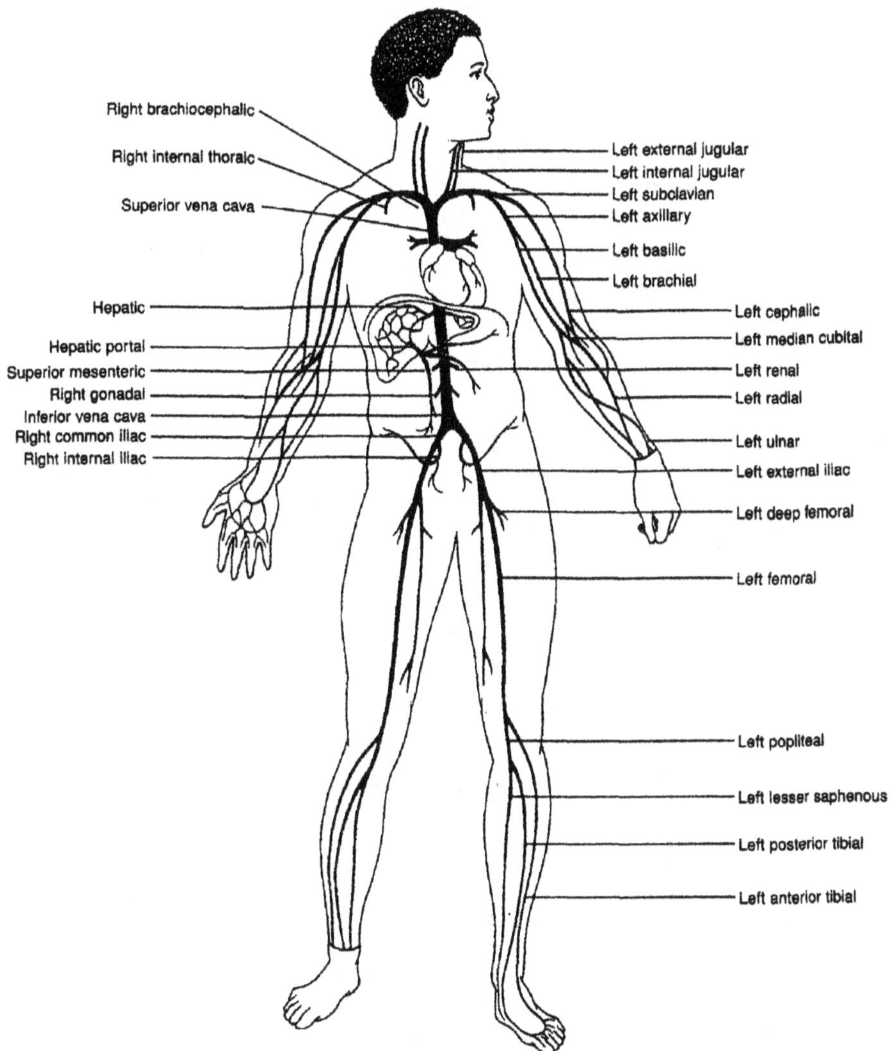

Figure 9.5 Principal veins of the body.

When a person is listening for the blood pressure, the sounds that are heard are called *Korotkoff sounds*. The first sound that is heard with cuff pressure is called the *systolic pressure*. Systolic blood pressure represents the force of the blood during ventricular contraction. As the pressure in the cuff decreases, the sound that is heard will decrease in loudness. When the cuff pressure stops constricting, the artery sounds will stop. The last sound that is heard is called the *diastolic pressure* and represents the force of the blood during ventricular relaxation.

What Is a Normal or Average Blood Pressure?

Normal or average blood pressure is

- For males, 120/80 mmHg
- For females, 110/70 mmHg

What do the top and bottom numbers in a blood pressure represent?
The top number represents systolic blood pressure; the bottom number represents diastolic blood pressure.

9.4 Pathologies Associated with Circulation

What Are Examples of Pathologies That Can Occur in the Cardiovascular System?

Examples of pathologies that can occur in the cardiovascular system would include ***thrombophlebitis, varicose veins, transient ischemic attacks, intracerebral hemorrhages, subarachnoid hemorrhages, dissecting aneurysms, arteriosclerosis, atherosclerosis,*** and ***hypertension.***

What is thrombophlebitis?
Thrombophlebitis occurs as a result of inflammation and blood clotting in a vein. This condition is common in the veins of the lower extremities (legs). If these clots break free, an embolism can occur if the broken piece obstructs a blood vessel. If the obstruction occurs in the lungs, it is called a *pulmonary embolism*. If the obstruction occurs in the coronary arteries, it can cause a *myocardial infarction* or *heart attack*. If the obstruction occurs in the cerebral artery of the brain, it will cause a ***cerebral vascular accident (CVA)*** or *stroke*.

What causes thrombophlebitis?
The causes of thrombophlebitis include family history, trauma, varicose veins, cancer, paralysis of the upper or lower extremities, oral contraceptives, and postmenopausal estrogen replacement drugs.

What are the signs and symptoms associated with thrombophlebitis?
The sign and symptoms of thrombophlebitis commonly include pain, tenderness, swelling, and redness at the affected area.

What are varicose veins?
Varicose veins are more commonly seen in women. These dilated and twisted veins occur in the lower extremities. The causes of varicose veins include venous valve damage, sitting and/or standing for long periods of time, family history, obesity, pregnancy, hormonal replacement drugs, and the loss of vein elasticity.

What are the signs and symptoms associated with varicose veins?
The signs and symptoms of varicose veins include leg pain and discomfort and enlarged, dark-looking veins.

What is a transient ischemic attack?
Transient ischemic attacks (TIAs) are caused by brief, temporary disturbances of cerebral circulation. TIAs present as brief episodes of impaired neurological function.

What are the signs and symptoms associated with transient ischemic attacks?
The signs and symptoms of TIAs include unilateral blindness on the same side as the TIA, contralateral body paralysis, and slurred speech.

What is a intracerebral hemorrhage?
Intracerebral hemorrhage is bleeding into the brain, commonly caused by high blood pressure.

What is a subarachnoid hemorrhage ?
Subarachnoid hemorrhage is bleeding into the arachnoid space of the meninges, commonly caused by a ***berry aneurysm***. Berry aneurysms are small lesions in the *circle of Willis* of the brain. These aneurysms can burst and leak into the subarachnoid space of the meninges.

What is a dissecting aneurysm?
A ***dissecting aneurysm*** is a longitudinal tear of the ascending portion of the aorta. Dissecting aneurysms present as severe chest pain and pressure. When the aorta ruptures, blood fills the pericardium, causing pressure on the heart. Cardiac tamponade and death occur.

What is arteriosclerosis?
Arteriosclerosis is hardening and thickening of the arteries.

What is atherosclerosis?
Atherosclerosis is clogging of the arteries caused by atheromas or fibrous plaques in the tunica intima. These plaques consist of cholesterol, fats, lipids, and debris resulting from necrosis. Atherosclerosis is commonly seen in the large arteries of the lower extremities, the coronary arteries, and the circle of Willis in the brain. Atherosclerosis is serious because it can lead to ischemia of the heart, heart attacks, and stroke.

What are the risk factors of atherosclerosis?
Risk factors include high blood pressure, high cholesterol, smoking, obesity, and diabetes mellitus.

What is hypertension?

Hypertension or ***high blood pressure*** is a consistent resting blood pressure of 140/90 mmHg or higher. High blood pressure is called the "silent killer" and can lead to kidney failure, CVAs, heart attack, and heart failure. In some individuals, the cause may be unknown. Known factors include narrowing of arteries, oral contraceptives, medicines for colds, drugs, sleep apnea, smoking, obesity, high salt (sodium) intake, excessive alcohol consumption, stress, diabetes, endocrine disorders, kidney disease, and pregnancy.

What are the signs and symptoms associated with hypertension?

The signs and symptoms of hypertension include headaches (cephalgia), dizziness, fatigue, muscle cramping, excessive sweating, and irregular heartbeats.

Chapter 9 Review Questions

Fill In the Blank

1. The __________ is the center of the cardiovascular system.
2. The study, diagnosis, and treatment of diseases that affect the cardiovascular system is called ______________.
3. The heart is located in the ______________.
4. A "saclike" structure that surrounds the heart is the ______________.
5. Inflammation of the pericardium caused by infection, trauma, or a heart attack is called __________.
6. Pressure on the heart valve causes ______________.
7. The layer of the heart that is made up of cardiac muscle is the ______________.
8. Rheumatic fever can cause inflammation of the myocardium. This is called __________.
9. Narrowing of heart valves, possibly as a result of scar tissue, is called ______________.
10. A myocardial infarction is also called a(n) ______________.
11. A partially obstructed coronary artery that causes a decrease or reduction in the flow of blood to the myocardium is called ______________.
12. The two upper chambers of the heart are called ______________.
13. The two lower chambers of the heart are called ______________.
14. The valve between the right atrium and the right ventricle is called the ______________.
15. The bicuspid valve is also called the ______________.
16. The valve between the right ventricle and the pulmonary trunk is called the __________.
17. Chest pain resulting from inadequate oxidation to the heart is called ______________.
18. The structure referred to as the pacemaker of the heart is the ______________.
19. The AV bundle is also known as the ______________.
20. How long does it take for an electrical impulse to travel through the heart?

Matching

21. Ectopic pacemaker
22. Enlarged P waves
23. "Sawtooth" P wave

24. Flattened T wave
25. ECG
26. Arrhythmias
27. Tachycardia
28. Bradycardia
29. PVD
30. Ventricular fibrillation
    A. Electrocardiogram
    B. Any deviation from a normal electrical impulse
    C. May indicate an enlarged atrium
    D. Slow resting heart rate
    E. Can indicate atrial fibrillation
    F. Premature ventricular depolarization
    G. Disorganized electrical impulses in the ventricles
    H. A place that becomes self-excitable
    I. Rapid resting heart rate
    J. Can indicate insufficient O_2

True/False

31. Listening to the heart sounds is called Korotkoff.
32. Normal blood pressure in a male is 120/80 mmHg.
33. Normal blood pressure in a female is 110/70 mmHg.
34. The top number in blood pressure is the diastolic pressure.
35. The systolic blood pressure represents the force of blood during ventricular contraction.
36. Inflammation and blood clotting in a vein is called a myocardial infarction.
37. An embolism in the brain is called a stroke.
38. A stroke is called a cerebral vascular accident.
39. Varicose veins are more commonly seen in women.
40. A berry aneurysm will not cause a subarachnoid hemorrhage.
41. Angina pectoris is chest pain resulting from inadequate oxygen to the heart.
42. Cardiac muscle fibers are called autorhythmic cells because they contract repeatedly and rhythmically.
43. Blood in veins is under pressure.
44. Edema is swelling resulting from an increase in blood in the extracellular spaces.
45. Pulse rate is measured by a sphygmomanometer.

Multiple Choice

46. This condition is commonly seen in women and is the result of venous valve damage.
    A. Varicose veins
    B. CVA
    C. TIA

D. MI
E. Aneurysm

47. A small lesion in the circle of Willis is called a(n) __________.
A. subarachnoid hemorrhage
B. intracerebral hemorrhage
C. dissecting aneurysm
D. berry aneurysm
E. CVA

48. Bleeding into the brain, commonly caused by high blood pressure, is called a(n) __________.
A. berry aneurysm
B. dissecting aneurysm
C. subarachnoid hemorrhage
D. transient ischemic attack
E. intracerebral hemorrhage

49. Hardening and thickening of arteries is called __________.
A. atherosclerosis
B. TIA
C. CVA
D. arteriosclerosis
E. aneurysm

50. High blood pressure is called __________.
A. tachycardia
B. bradycardia
C. hypertension
D. CVA
E. TIA

Chapter 9: Review Questions and Answers

Fill In the Blank Answers

1. Heart
2. Cardiology
3. Mediastinum
4. Pericardium
5. Pericarditis
6. Cardiac tamponade
7. Myocardium
8. Myocarditis
9. Stenosis
10. Heart attack
11. Myocardial ischemia
12. Atria
13. Ventricles
14. Tricuspid valve
15. Mitral valve
16. Pulmonary semilunar valve
17. Angina pectoris
18. Sinoatrial node
19. Bundle of His
20. 200 milliseconds

Matching Answers

21. H
22. C
23. E
24. J
25. A
26. B
27. I
28. D
29. F
30. G

True/False Answers

31. False
32. True
33. True
34. False
35. True
36. False
37. True
38. True
39. True
40. False
41. True
42. True
43. False
44. False
45. False

Multiple Choice Answers

46. A
47. D
48. E
49. D
50. C

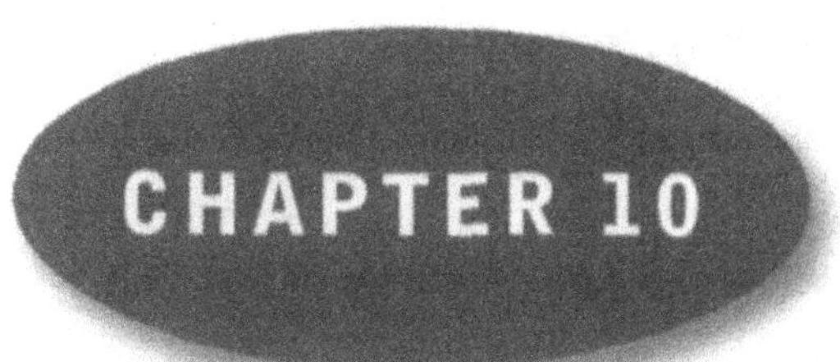

The Integumentary System

Objectives

This chapter will discuss the structures of our largest organ, the skin. We will also discuss the functions of these structures and the diseases associated with the integumentary system.

Keywords:

Dermatology
Epidermis
Dermis
Hypodermis
Keratinocytes
Melanocytes
Langerhans' cells
Merkel cells
Cyanosis
Jaundice
Erythema
Albinism
Ecchymosis
Petechiae
Purpura
Cellulitis
Impetigo
Folliculitis
Scarlet fever
Erysipelas
Herpes simplex
Varicella-zoster
Warts
Dermatophytes
Fungal infections (dermatomycoses)
Parasitic infestations
Dermatitis
Skin cancer

10.1 Overview

What Are the Structures That Make Up the Integumentary System?

The structures that make up the *integumentary system* are the skin, hair, nails, and glands.

Why Is Skin Considered an Organ?

Skin is considered an organ because it consists of different tissues that are joined together to perform specific activities.

What Is Dermatology?

Dermatology is the study, diagnosis, and treatment of skin disorders.

What Are the Functions of the Skin?

The functions of the skin are as follows:

- Skin functions in the *regulation of temperature*. When you get hot, the blood vessels of the skin dilate. When the blood gets close to the surface of the skin, heat leaves the body. When you are cold, the blood vessels of the skin constrict, holding the heat in.
- Skin provides a *protective barrier* and is our first line of defense against invading microorganisms. The top layer of skin also protects against ultraviolet radiation.
- Skin *detects changes* through sensory receptors for heat, cold, touch, pressure, and pain.
- The skin's dermis layer is a *reservoir for blood.*
- When it is exposed to sunlight, the skin *produces vitamin D*, which is needed in the absorption of calcium.
- The skin also *excretes waste products* through the process of sweating.

What Are the Layers of the Skin?

The skin has three main layers:

- The ***epidermis***, which is the top layer and is above the dermis. *Epi* means "above."
- The ***dermis***, which means "skin" and is the middle layer.
- The ***hypodermis*** or *subcutaneous region*, which is the bottom layer.

10.2 The Epidermis

What Types of Tissue Make Up the Epidermis?

The epidermis contains epithelial tissue. It is *avascular* (having no blood supply) and has a nerve supply.

What Kinds of Cells Make Up the Epidermis?

The types of cells that make up the epidermis are keratinocytes, melanocytes, Langerhans' cells, and Merkel cells.

What are keratinocytes?

- ***Keratinocytes.*** These cells produce a "waterproof" protective protein called *keratin*. This keratin helps to protect the skin from wear and tear and waterproofs it.

What are melanocytes?

- ***Melanocytes.*** These cells that produce a black or brown pigment called *melanin*. This pigment absorbs ultraviolet light radiation produced by the sun. This radiation can be very damaging to the cells of underlying tissue.

What are Langerhans' cells?

- ***Langerhans' cells.*** These cells are produced in red bone marrow and migrate to the epidermis, where they fight infection during an immune response.

What are Merkel cells?

- ***Merkel cells.*** These cells are located in the deepest portion of the epidermis and supply sensory reception.

The types of cells that make up the epidermis are summarized in Table 10.1.

TABLE 10.1 Cells That Make Up the Epidermis

CELLS	FUNCTION
Keratinocytes	Waterproof and protect
Melanocytes	Protect against ultraviolet radiation
Langerhans' cells	Fight infection during an immune response
Merkel cells	Sensory reception

What Are the Layers of the Epidermis?

The epidermis contains five layers or *strata*. From the deepest layer to the most superficial, they are as follows:

1. *Stratum basale.* This layer consists of cuboidal or columnar cells called keratinocytes. These cells undergo mitosis and divide. This layer contains melanocytes, Langerhans' cells, and Merkel discs for touch sensation.
2. *Stratum spinosum.* This layer consists of 8 to 10 rows or layers of cells that are polyhedral, or have "many sides." These keratinocytes are tightly packed together.
3. *Stratum granulosum.* This layer consists of 3 to 5 rows of cells that release a water repellant.
4. *Stratum lucidum.* This layer contains 3 to 5 rows of dead flat keratinocytes. It is found in areas of "hairless" skin, such as the palms of the hands and the soles of the feet.
5. *Stratum corneum.* This layer contains 25 to 30 layers of flat dead cells that are filled with keratin. The cells of this layer are shed and replaced by the cells from deeper layers.

The layers of the epidermis are summarized in Table 10.2 and shown in Figure 10.1.

TABLE 10.2 Layers of the Epidermis

LAYER	CHARACTERISTIC
Stratum basale	Deepest layer, keratinocytes that undergo mitosis
Stratum spinosum	8 to 10 layers of tightly packed polyhedral cells
Stratum granulosum	3 to 5 layers of cells that release a water repellant
Stratum lucidum	3 to 5 layers of dead flat keratinocytes; found on the palms of the hands and the soles of the feet
Stratum corneum	25 to 30 layers of flat dead cells that are filled with keratin

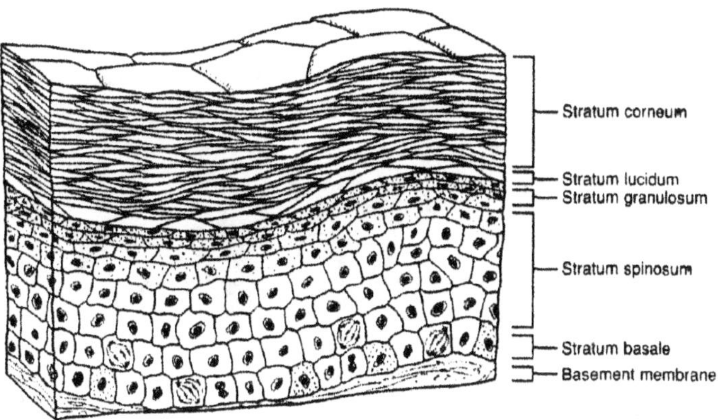

Figure 10.1 Layers of the epidermis.

How Do We Replace These Cells?

A hormone called *epidermal growth factor* stimulates the growth and cell division of epithelial and epidermal cells during tissue development, tissue repair, and tissue replacement.

10.3 The Dermis and Subcutaneous Region

What Kind of Tissues Make Up the Dermis Layer of Skin?

The dermis is composed of connective tissue containing collagen and elastic fibers. The dermis has two regions.

What two regions form the dermis?

1. *Papillary region.* This is the superficial region of the dermis and contains elastic fibers. The papillary region contains dermal papillae. These dermal papillae create indentations of the epidermis, causing an increase in surface area. These indentations contain *Meissner's corpuscles*, which are sensory receptors for touch.
2. *Reticular region.* This is the deep region of the dermis and consists of dense, irregular connective tissue. This region also contains nerves, hair follicles, oil glands, sweat gland ducts, and small amounts of adipose (fat) tissue.

What Types of Tissue Make Up the Subcutaneous Region of Skin?

The subcutaneous layer of skin consists of areolar connective tissue and adipose tissue. This layer also contains *Pacinian corpuscles*, which are sensory receptors for pressure.

The structure of the skin is shown in Figure 10.2.

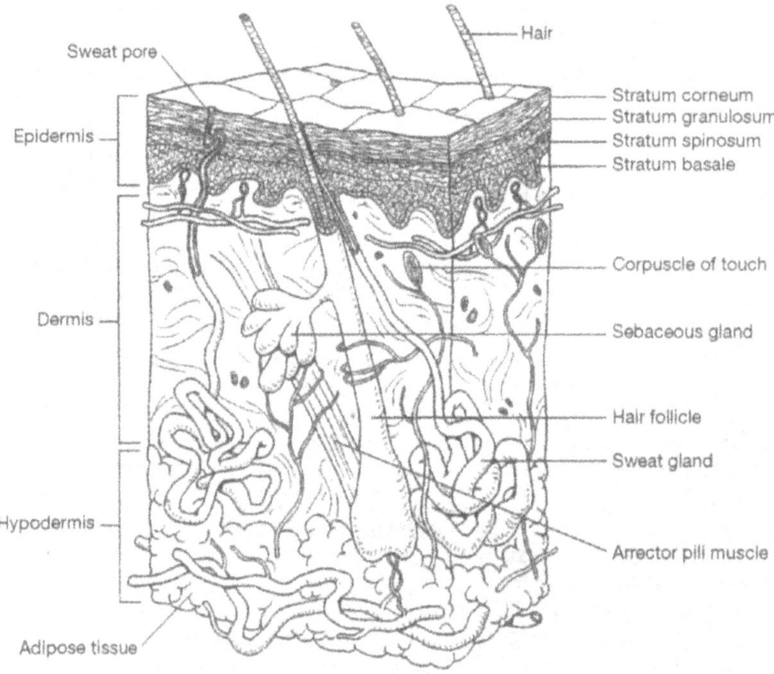

Figure 10.2 The skin.

10.4 Skin Color

The color of skin can be an important indicator of homeostatic imbalances.

What Are the Pigments That Make Up Skin Color?

There are three pigments that make up skin color:

- *Melanin* is a yellow to black pigment. The more melanin a person has, the darker that person's skin will be. An accumulation of melanin in patches causes *freckles.* Melanin can be found in mucous membranes.
- *Carotene* is a yellow-orange pigment that is located in the dermis and subcutaneous regions of the skin that contain adipose tissue and the stratum corneum layer of the epidermis.
- *Hemoglobin* is the pigment that carries oxygen on red blood cells. This pigment gives skin its "pinkish" color.

What Are Some Abnormalities Associated with Skin Color?

When there is a decrease in the amount of oxygen in the blood, the skin can have a pale or bluish appearance. This blue color of skin is called ***cyanosis.*** Cyanosis can occur with the presence of lung and heart disease.

When there are imbalances or malfunctions of the liver as a result of a pathology, the skin and the whites of the eyes (sclera) can turn yellow in color. This is called ***jaundice.***

The skin may be red and sweating during ***heat exhaustion*** and pale and dry with ***heat stroke***. When a person gets "sunburn," there is trauma to the blood vessels, which creates redness. This redness is called ***erythema.***

The enzyme tyrosinase converts tyrosine to the pigment melanin. When there is a genetic defect in this enzyme, the condition ***albinism*** will occur. Without melanin, there will be no skin or hair pigmentation.

10.5 Skin Lesions

What Are Other Variants of the Skin?

Any variant of the skin is called a *lesion*. Lesions can be listed as primary, secondary, and tertiary.

What Are Examples of Primary Lesions?

Some examples of primary lesions are

- *Bulla.* A bulla is an elevated, fluid-filled blister.
- *Macule.* A macule is a flat discoloration in skin color, like a mole or a freckle.
- *Nodule.* A nodule is a solid mass that can be palpated. It is a small, round elevation, usually larger than 6 cm.
- *Papule.* A papule is a solid elevated mass that is smaller than a nodule.
- *Plaque.* A plaque tends to be small and scaly, with some elevation.
- *Pustule.* A pustule is an elevated pus-filled lesion, usually the result of an infection.
- *Tumor.* A tumor is an elevated palpable mass caused by abnormal tissue growth.
- *Vesicle.* A vesicle is a fluid-filled blister.
- *Wheal.* A wheal is a palpable elevated lesion, also called a hive; it is normally the result of stress or an allergic reaction.

Types of primary skin lesions are summarized in Table 10.3.

TABLE 10.3 Primary Skin Lesions

LESION	CHARACTERISTICS
Bulla	Fluid-filled blister
Macule	Flat mole or freckle
Nodule	Large elevated mass larger than 6 cm
Papule	Solid elevated mass that is smaller than a nodule
Plaque	Small, scaly mass with some elevation
Pustule	Elevated pus-filled lesion
Tumor	Elevated mass caused by abnormal tissue growth
Vesicle	Fluid-filled blister
Wheal	Hive

What Are Examples of Secondary Lesions?

Some examples of secondary lesions are

- *Crust.* Crust is the result of either dried pus or dried blood on the surface of the skin.
- *Erosion.* Erosion is the result of friction on the surface of the skin. This friction wears away the top layer of skin.
- *Excoriation.* An excoriation is a shallow cut or scratch.
- *Keloid.* A keloid is a larger growth of scar tissue.
- *Scale.* Scales are dry patches of surface epithelial cells.
- *Ulcer.* Ulcers are the result of tissue loss caused by a type of pressure injury.

Types of secondary skin lesions are summarized in Table 10.4.

TABLE 10.4 Secondary Skin Lesions

LESION	CHARACTERISTICS
Crust	Dried pus or blood
Erosion	Result of friction on the skin
Excoriation	Shallow cut or scratch
Keloid	Large growth of scar tissue
Scale	Dry patches of epithelial cells
Ulcer	Tissue loss because of pressure or injury

What Are Examples of Tertiary Lesions?

Some examples of tertiary lesions are

- ***Ecchymosis.*** An ecchymosis is a bruise.

What causes an ecchymosis?
Trauma can cause an ecchymosis.

- ***Petechiae.*** Petechiae are vascular lesions that present as small "pinpoint" hemorrhages on the surface of the skin.

What can cause petechiae?
Petechiae could be the result of a blood or vascular disorder.

- ***Purpura.*** A purpura is a small bruise on the surface of the skin. It is usually red or purple in color.

What can cause a purpura?
Purpura can be the result of a blood clotting problem.
Types of tertiary skin lesions are summarized in Table 10.5.

TABLE 10.5 Tertiary Lesions

LESION	CHARACTERISTICS
Ecchymosis	Bruise
Petechiae	Small pinpoint vascular lesions
Purpura	Small bruise that can be the result of clotting problems

10.6 Hair

What Are the Components of Hair?

A hair or pili consists of the following parts:

- *Shaft.* The shaft is superficial to the surface of the skin.
- *Root.* The root penetrates the dermis and hypodermis layers of skin.
- *Hair follicle.* The hair follicle is made up of epithelial cells. As these cells divide, they push the old cells to the surface, causing hair to get longer. This is called the *growth stage*. The hair follicle surrounds the hair root. During the *resting stage* of hair growth, the cells do not divide and the follicles atrophy. *Arrector pili muscles* in the dermis layer are connected to hair follicles. When these muscles contract, they pull on the hair follicle, making the hairs stand up. When hair follicles die, *alopecia* or baldness occurs.

10.7 Glands

What Are the Glands Associated with Skin?

The glands associated with the skin are as follows:

- *Sebaceous glands.* Sebaceous glands are oil glands. These glands secrete sebum and open up into hair follicles and on the skin.
- *Sudoriferous glands.* Sudoriferous glands are sweat glands. Sweat glands empty onto the skin's surface. There are two types of sweat glands:
  1. *Eccrine glands* are located all over the skin. They are especially numerous on the palms of the hand and the soles of the feet.
  2. *Apocrine glands* are located in the skin of the armpit (axilla) and the pubic (groin) region.
- *Ceruminous glands.* Ceruminous glands are located in the skin of the ear and produce cerumen or earwax.

What Is Acne?

On occasion, excess sebum from sebaceous glands and dead cells from skin clog pores. This creates a good environment for bacteria growth. The bacteria can cause irritation, resulting in the inflammation of the follicles and sebaceous glands. This condition is called *acne vulgaris* or acne.

10.8 Nails

What Are Nails Made From?

Nails are made of hardened epithelial tissue. They protect the distal ends of fingers and toes. Nails consist of a *nail root*, which is embedded in the cuticle and contains keratinocytes. These keratinocytes divide, making the nails grow. The white region of the nail that looks like a half moon is called a *lunula*, which means "little moon." The *nail body* is the portion of the nail that can be seen.

The *free nail border* is the portion that extends distally past the fingers and toes and can be cut or trimmed. The structure of a nail is shown in Figure 10.3.

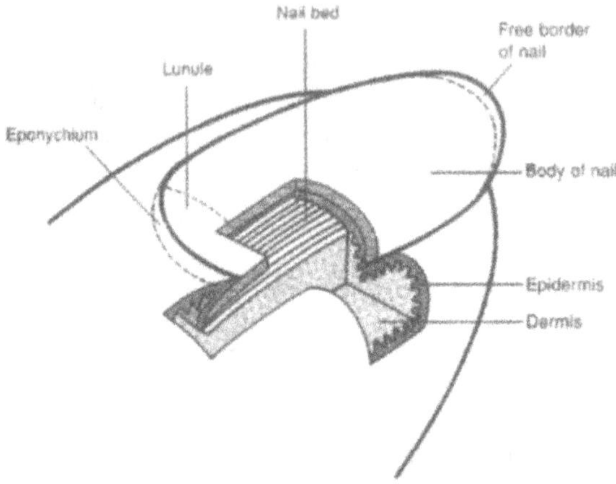

Figure 10.3 The structure of a nail.

What Are Some Conditions That Can Cause Irregularities of Nails?

Examples of conditions that can affect the nails are

- *Club nails.* Club nails occur when the base of the nail is greater than 180 degrees. This condition can be caused by lung cancer, heart disease, hypoxia, and liver cirrhosis.
- *Spoon nails.* Spoon nails are indentations of the nail bodies. This can be caused by anemia.
- *Bean's lines.* Bean's lines are transverse depressions in the nail bed. They are the result of an acute illness.
- *Paronychia.* Paronychia is inflammation of the skin around the nails. This can be caused by an abscess.
- *Leukonychia.* Leukonychia or white spots or lines on the nail is caused by trauma or by aggressive nail filing.

10.9 Pathophysiology

What Conditions or Pathogens Can Affect the Skin?

No other organ can be visually inspected, is exposed to infection or disease, or can be injured like skin. Skin can be damaged by trauma, sunlight, microorganisms, and environmental and industrial pollutants.

What Would Be an Example of a Condition That Can Damage Skin?

Burns can damage skin and can be caused by exposure to sun, steam, heat or flame, chemicals, and electricity. Burns are classified by the depth of the tissue damage they cause.

- *First-degree burn.* A first-degree burn will cause damage to the top layer of the epidermis. This type of burn will present as a redness or hyperemia.
- *Second-degree burn.* A second-degree burn will cause damage to both the epidermis and the dermis. Blistering of the skin can occur with a second-degree burn.
- *Third-degree burn.* A third-degree burn will affect all three layers of the skin. In many instances, the skin will be charred.

Types of burns are summarized in Table 10.6.

TABLE **10.6 Burns**

TYPE	CHARACTERISTIC
First degree	Damage to epidermis
Second degree	Damage to epidermis and dermis
Third degree	Damage to epidermis, dermis, and subcutaneous region of the skin

What Are Examples of Some Common Skin Disorders Caused by a Bacterial Infection?

Common skin disorders caused by bacteria include

- ***Cellulitis.*** Cellulitis is the inflammation of connective tissue, mostly occurring on the legs and face, caused by either a streptococcal or a staphylococcal infection. Cellulitis presents as a painful inflamed red area on the surface of the skin.
- ***Impetigo.*** Impetigo is a very contagious condition caused by either a streptococcal or a staphylococcal infection.

What would be signs and symptoms associated with impetigo?
Impetigo presents as itchy, oozing, crusting lesions that can spread to adjacent skin areas.

- ***Folliculitis.*** Folliculitis, or "swimmer's rash," is caused by either friction on the skin or a bacterial or fungal infection resulting in the inflammation of hair follicles.

What would be signs and symptoms associated with folliculitis?
Folliculitis presents as itchy, inflamed pustules.

- ***Scarlet fever.*** Scarlet fever is caused by *Streptococcus pyogenes.*

What would be signs ansd symptoms associated with scarlet fever?
Scarlet fever presents as a small "gritty" red rash that appears on the trunk of the body 12 hours after the onset of the fever. Chills, vomiting, and abdominal pain may occur, with a "white strawberry"—or "red strawberry"—looking tongue.

- ***Erysipelas.*** Erysipelas is a streptococcal infection of the skin cells.

What would be the signs and symptoms associated with erysipelas?
Erysipelas produces bold red patches on the face and legs that are raised, hot, and tender.

Bacterial skin disorders are summarized in Table 10.7.

TABLE **10.7 Bacterial Skin Disorders**

DISORDER	CHARACTERISTICS
Cellulitis	Inflammation of connective tissue caused by a streptococcal or staphylococcal infection
Impetigo	Itchy, oozing, crusting lesions occurring on the face and around the mouth caused by a staphylococcal or streptococcal infection
Folliculitis	"Swimmer's" rash, caused by a bacterial or fungal infection
Scarlet fever	"Red strawberry" tongue, fever, chills, vomiting, and abdominal pain

What Are Examples of Some Common Skin Disorders Caused by Viral Infections?

Common skin disorders and the viruses that cause them include

- ***Herpes simplex*** virus. Herpes simplex causes cold sores and fever blisters on the face, lips, and mouth. These sores are painful.
- ***Herpes simplex 2*** virus. Herpes simplex 2, or genital herpes, causes painful genital sores. Adequate rest, nutrition, and stress all have an effect on herpes.
- ***Varicella-zoster*** virus. The varicella-zoster virus is a type of herpes virus. This virus causes chickenpox and shingles. In chickenpox, an itchy rash occurs on the face, scalp, trunk, and upper and lower extremities. This disease usually affects children. After a person has had chickenpox, he or she can get shingles because the varicella-zoster virus remains dormant in the spinal nerve roots.

What would be the signs and symptoms associated with varicella-zoster?
When active, the virus presents as a rash along the skin's dermatomes, usually in the trunk, but it can occur anywhere in the body.

- ***Warts.*** Warts, or verrucae, are benign skin growths caused by a virus; they usually occur on the face, hands, and feet, but they can also occur anywhere in the body.

What would be the signs and symptoms of warts?
Warts can be rough or smooth, small or large, and flat or raised.

Viral skin infections are summarized in Table 10.8.

TABLE 10.8 Viral Skin Disorders

VIRUS OR DISORDER	CHARACTERISTICS
Herpes simplex 1 virus	Cold sores, fever blisters
Herpes simplex 2 virus	Genital sores
Varicella-zoster virus	Chickenpox and shingles
Warts	Benign skin growths

What Types of Fungi Can Cause Skin Disorders?

Fungi that invade keratinized tissue are ***dermatophytes***, and the resulting diseases are called ***fungal infections***, or ***dermatomycoses***. Examples of fungi that can cause skin infection are *Epidermopayton floccosum* and *Trichophyton rubrum.* Fungal infections commonly present as red, itchy, scaly patches.

What are common fungal infections of the skin?
Common fungal infections of the skin are

- *Tinea capitis* is ringworm of the scalp.
- *Tinea cruris* occurs in the groin, upper thighs, and buttocks. It is known as "jock itch."
- *Tinea pedis* occurs on the feet and between the toes and is commonly called "athlete's foot."
- *Tinea corporis* is ringworm that occurs all over the body.
- *Tinea versicolor* is a superficial ringworm of the back.
- *Tinea manus* is ringworm of the hands.
- *Tinea barbae* is ringworm of the beard.
- *Tinea unguium* is ringworm of the fingernails, also called *onychomycosis*.

Ringworm in all its forms is caused by fungi and presents as flat circular lesions. These lesions can be scaly, dry, moist, or crusty.

Fungal skin infections are summarized in Table 10.9.

TABLE **10.9 Fungal Skin Infections**

CONDITION	LOCATION
Tinea capitis	Occurs on the scalp
Tinea cruris	Occurs on the groin
Tinea pedis	Occurs on the feet
Tinea corporis	Occurs all over the body
Tinea versicolor	Occurs on the back
Tinea manus	Occurs on the hands
Tinea barbae	Occurs under the beard
Tinea unguium	Occurs on the nails

What Are Some Common Parasite Infections That Cause Skin Disorders?

There are several types of ***parasite infestations*** that can occur. Infestation by *lice*, or *pediculosis*, can occur on the head, body, or pubic region.

- *Pediculosis capitis* is infestation of the head by lice.
- *Pediculosis corporis* is infestation of the body by lice.
- *Pediculosis pubis* is infestation of the pubic area by lice.

All these forms of lice are mostly associated with poor hygiene, overcrowded conditions, and, in the case of *pediculosis pubis*, sexual contact.

What are the signs and symptoms of lice?
Infestation by lice presents as very itchy skin that becomes irritated as a result of scratching.

What does lice look like?
The "nits" (eggs) of *pediculosis capitis* look like dandruff that is stuck to the hair.

Scabies is caused by mites that have burrowed under the skin. Scabies presents as a red pencil-thin line on the skin that is very itchy. Scabies is also very contagious.

Types of parasitic skin infestations are summarized in Table 10.10.

TABLE **10.10 Parasitic Infestations**

PARASITE OR CONDITION	LOCATION
Pediculosis capitis	Head lice
Pediculosis corporis	Body lice
Pediculosis pubis	Pubic lice
Scabies	Pencil-thin skin rash caused by mites

What Is Dermatitis?

Dermatitis is inflammation of the skin. *Eczema* is a chronic form of dermatitis that is seen in both children and adults. Eczema is thought to either be an allergic reaction or an inflammatory condition. This condition can be exacerbated by medications, stress, environmental conditions, and diet.

What are the signs and symptoms of eczema?
Eczema presents as an itchy, red, scaly rash.

Psoriasis is another chronic inflammatory skin condition that may be caused by a genetic autoimmune disorder.

What are the signs and symptoms of psoriasis?
The signs and symptoms of psoriasis include repeated occurrences of silvery, scaly, red, and itchy skin lesions.

10.10 Skin Cancer

What Types of Cancer Can Affect the Skin?

Actinic keratoses or *solar keratoses* are rough precancerous lesions that can develop into squamous cell carcinoma.

What are the signs and symptoms of an actinic keratosis?
An actinic keratosis presents as a red to brownish crusty lesion that may be itchy. These lesions tend to fall off and grow back again.

The skin is our largest organ and endures a lot of wear and tear, injury, infection, and overexposure to ultraviolet radiation. In response, the skin continuously has to repair itself. On occasion, situations can develop where skin cells of the epidermis will replicate uncontrollably, forming tumors. ***Skin cancer*** occurs more frequently in fair-skinned people who have had lots of sun exposure.

What types of cancer affect the skin?
There are three types of skin cancer.

- *Basal cell carcinoma.* Basal cell carcinoma is the most common type of skin cancer, making up around 90 percent of all U.S. skin cancers.

What does basal cell carcinoma look like?
Basal cell carcinomas present as small, rounded, slow-growing lesions that normally do not spread. They usually occur on the face, but they can also be found on the trunk and hands. Basal cell carcinoma presents as a new growth or sore that does not heal. It may look like a "drip of candle wax," and may be red, flat, rounded, or bumpy. These lesions may be crusty and also may bleed.

- *Squamous cell carcinoma.* Squamous cell carcinoma is also found in the epidermis of the skin, but it is more serious because it is more likely to spread to adjacent tissue and lymph.

What does squamous cell carcinoma look like?
Squamous cell carcinoma presents as a hard lump or wart that does not heal. Lesions normally appear on the face, ears, lips, and backs of the hands (places that are most exposed to sunlight).

- *Malignant melanoma.* Malignant melanoma affects melanocytes and is the most aggressive and fastest-growing skin cancer. Malignant melanoma is the least common but is the most often fatal.

What does malignant melanoma look like?
Malignant melanoma usually presents itself on the head, face, neck, trunk, arms, and legs, but it can appear anywhere in the body. Lesions can become lighter or darker, be uneven in color (red, white, blue, black, or brown), be raised or thick, and have uneven borders.

Remember: When assessing any mole or neoplastic lesion on the skin, follow the ABCs:

A Asymmetrical

B Borders (even or uneven)

C Color (even or uneven and multicolored)

D Diameter—malignant melanomas are larger than a pencil eraser (5 mm)

E Elevation

Types of skin cancer are summarized in Table 10.11.

TABLE 10.11 Skin Cancer

TYPE	LOCATION/CHARACTERISTIC
Basal cell carcinoma	Slow growing; normally does not spread; red, flat, or bumpy; occurring on feet, trunk, and back
Squamous cell carcinoma	Found in epidermis of skin and has the ability to spread
Malignant melanoma	Most aggressive and fastest growing; least common; most often fatal

Chapter 10 Review Questions

Fill In the Blank

1. The study of skin, hair, and nails is called ____________________.
2. The middle layer of the skin is called the ____________________.
3. The epidermal cells that produce the "waterproof" protein are ____________________.
4. The cells that protect against ultraviolet radiation are ____________________.
5. The deepest layer of the epidermis is called the ____________________.
6. The superficial region of the dermis is called the ____________________.
7. Sensory receptors for touch in the dermis layer are called ____________________.
8. A yellow/orange pigment is ____________________.
9. An elevated fluid-filled blister is a(n) ____________________.
10. A hive brought on by stress is called a(n) ____________________.

Matching

11. Excoriation
12. Nodule
13. Keloid
14. Pustule
15. Ecchymosis
16. Wheal
17. Scale
18. Papule
19. Petechiae
20. Crust

A. A pus-filled lesion
B. Large growth of scar tissue
C. A scratch
D. Dry patches
E. A bruise

F. A solid elevated mass larger than 6 cm
G. A hive
H. Dried blood or pus
I. A solid elevated mass
J. Small "pinpoint" hemorrhages

True/False

21. The most superficial layer of skin is the dermis.
22. The word *dermis* means "skin."
23. The deep layer of skin is the subcutaneous layer.
24. Melanocytes protect against "wear and tear."
25. Langerhans' cells help fight infection.
26. The stratum spinosum is made up of polyhedral cells.
27. The stratum corneum contains live epithelial cells.
28. The stratum lucidum is found in "hairless skin."
29. Pacinian corpuscles are sensory receptors for pressure.
30. A pigment that carries oxygen is called hemoglobin.
31. A bluish color of the skin occurs when there is a decrease in the amount of oxygen in the blood.
32. A yellowish color of the skin and the sclera of the eyes is called jaundice.
33. Sebaceous glands are oil glands.
34. Apocrine glands are a type of sebaceous gland.
35. Ceruminous glands secrete cerumen.
36. The white region of a nail is called the lunula.
37. Nails are made of hardened epithelial tissue.
38. The nail body is the portion of the nail that cannot be seen.
39. Clogged pores can cause inflammation of follicles and sebaceous glands, causing *acne vulgaris.*
40. Ceruminous glands produce earwax.

Multiple Choice

41. When the base of the nail is greater than 180 degrees, the condition is called __________.
    A. Beau's lines
    B. spoon nails
    C. club nails
    D. leukonychia
    E. nail body

42. The layer of skin composed of 25 to 30 layers of dead cells is the __________.
    A. stratum corneum
    B. stratum lucidum
    C. stratum basale
    D. stratum granulosum
    E. stratum spinosum

43. A flat discoloration in the skin, such as a mole or a freckle, is called a __________.

A. blister
B. bulla
C. vesicle
D. macule
E. pustule

44. These glands are located in the skin of the armpit and groin: __________.

A. eccrine glands
B. sebaceous glands
C. sudoriferous glands
D. ceraminous glands
E. apocrine glands

45. The virus that causes genital sores is __________.

A. herpes simplex 1
B. herpes simplex 2
C. varicella-zoster
D. chickenpox
E. scabies

46. The virus that causes chickenpox is __________.

A. herpes simplex 1
B. herpes simplex 2
C. varicella-zoster
D. shingles
E. scabies

47. Ringworm of the scalp is called __________.

A. tinea cruris
B. tinea pedis
C. tinea corporis
D. tinea versicolor
E. tinea capitis

48. A fungus infection of the foot is called __________.

A. tinea cruris
B. tinea pedis
C. tinea corporis
D. tinea versicolor
E. tinea capitis

49. An infestation of the pubic area by lice is called __________.

A. pediculosis capitis
B. pediculosis corporis
C. pediculosis pubis
D. tinea corporis
E. tinea cruris

50. The most dangerous form of skin cancer is __________.

A. actinic keratosis
B. basal cell carcinoma
C. squamous cell carcinoma
D. malignant melanoma

Chapter 10: Review Questions and Answers

Fill In the Blank Answers

1. Dermatology
2. Dermis
3. Keratinocytes
4. Melanocytes
5. Stratum basale
6. Papillary region
7. Meissner's corpuscles
8. Carotene
9. Bulla
10. Wheal

Matching Answers

11. C
12. F
13. B
14. A
15. E
16. G
17. D
18. I
19. J
20. H

True/False Answers

21. False
22. True
23. True
24. False
25. True
26. True
27. False
28. True
29. True
30. True
31. True
32. True
33. True
34. False
35. True
36. True
37. True
38. False
39. True
40. True

Multiple Choice Answers

41. C
42. A
43. D
44. E
45. B
46. C
47. E
48. B
49. C
50. D

The Skeletal System

Objectives

This chapter will discuss the structures and functions of bone and the diseases associated with bone tissue.

Keywords:

Axial skeleton
Appendicular skeleton
Osteology
Epiphysis
Diaphysis
Metaphysis
Periosteum
Medullary cavity
Endosteum
Osteogenic cells
Osteoblasts
Osteocytes
Osteoclasts
Ossification
Fracture
Fracture hematoma
Procallus
Fibrocartilagenous callus (soft callus)
Bony callus (hard callus)
Synarthroses
Amphiarthroses
Diarthroses
Fibrous joints
Cartilagenous joints
Synovial joints
Osteoporosis
Osteomalacia
Rickets
Osteitis deformans
Osteitis fibrosa cystica
Osteopetrosis
Gout
Osteoid osteoma
Osteoma
Enchondroma
Osteochondroma
Giant cell tumors
Osteosarcoma
Chondrosarcoma
Ewing's sarcoma
Multiple myeloma
Osteoarthritis
Rheumatoid arthritis
Ankylosing spondylitis
Rieter's syndrome
Avascular necrosis
Osteogenesis imperfecta
Charcot's joint
Fractures of the extremities
Vertebral fractures
Lordosis
Kyphosis
Scoliosis

11.1 Overview

How Many Bones Are There in the Human Body?

There are 206 bones in the human body. They are categorized into two groups:

1. The ***axial skeleton***, which includes the skull bones, facial bones, vertebral column, ribs, sternum, and hyoid bone

2. The ***appendicular skeleton***, which includes the bones that form the shoulder girdle, pelvis, upper extremities, and lower extremities

The axial skeleton contains 80 bones, and the appendicular skeleton contains 126 bones. The bones of the skeleton are shown in Figure 11.1.

What Is Osteology?

Osteology is the study of bone structures and functions and the diagnosis and treatment of bone diseases.

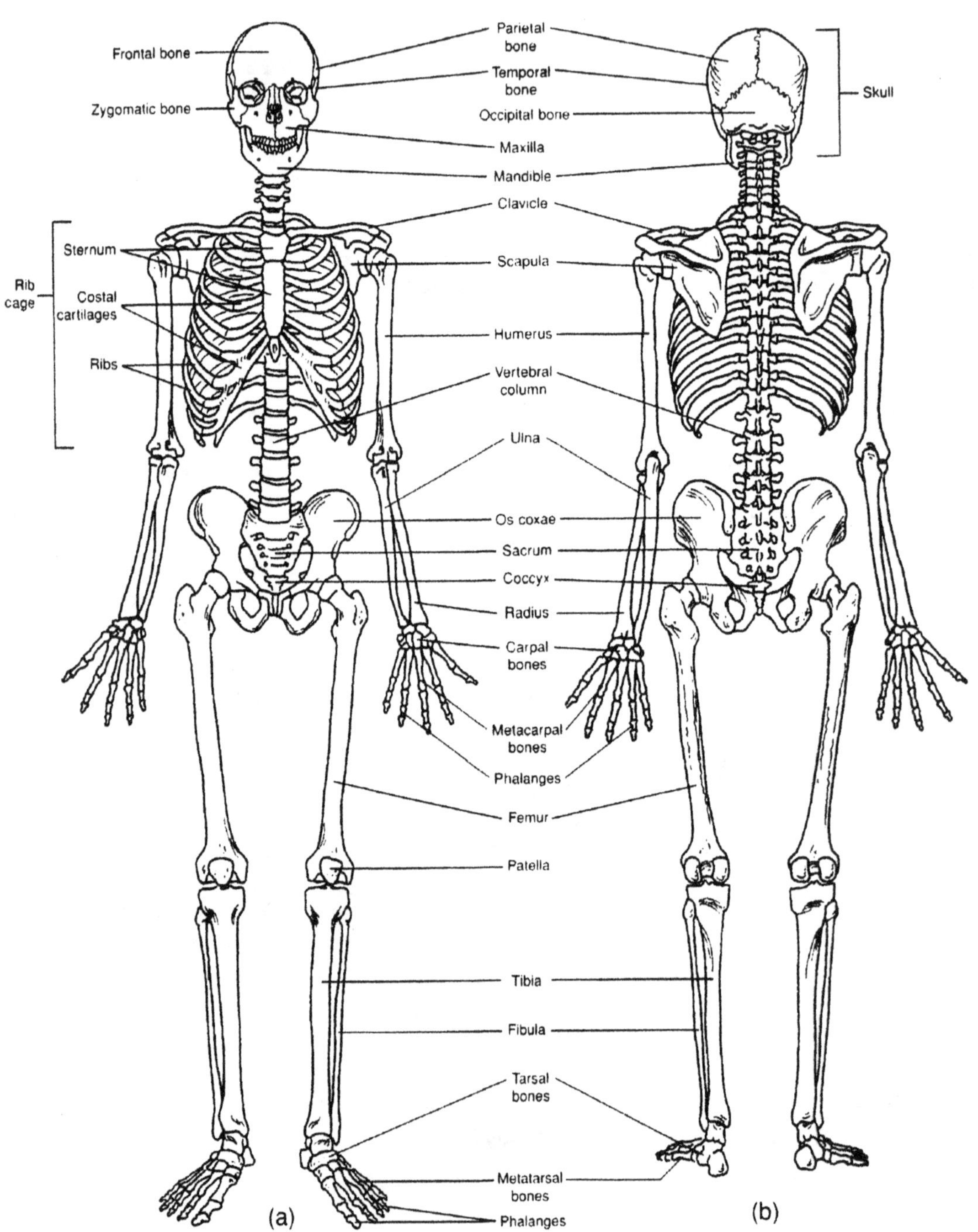

Figure 11.1 The skeleton. (*a*) An anterior view and (*b*) a posterior view.

11.2 Bones

What Are the Functions of Bone?

- Bone supplies structural *support* for the body.
- Bone *protects* the internal organs. Examples include the ribs protecting the heart and lungs and the skull protecting the brain.
- Skeletal muscles are attached to bone. When they contract, they pull on the bone, creating *movement.*
- Bones *store* calcium and phosphorus, which are important in nervous impulses and muscle contractions.
- The red bone marrow, located in the ends of long bones, is where *blood cells are produced.*
- Yellow bone marrow, located in the shaft of long bones, can be used as an *energy reserve*.

What Are the Structures of Bone?

The structures of bone are

- ***Epiphysis.*** The epiphysis is located at the proximal and distal ends of bones.
- ***Diaphysis.*** The diaphysis is the shaft portion of long bone.
- ***Metaphysis.*** The metaphysis is the portion of long bone that connects the epiphysis to the diaphysis. In *growing bone*, this region of the metaphysis is referred to as the *epiphyseal plate* or *growth plate*. In mature bone or bone that has stopped growing, this region is called the *epiphyseal line*.
- ***Periosteum.*** The periosteum is a connective tissue membrane that surrounds the diaphysis. It functions in bone growth in diameter and bone repair, and it is the plate for the attachment of ligaments and tendons. The periosteum consists of two layers:

  1. *Outer fibrous layer.* This layer is composed of irregular connective tissue and contains blood vessels, lymphatic vessels, and nerves.
  2. *Inner osteogenic layer.* This layer is composed of elastic connective tissue fibers, blood vessels, and osteogenic bone cells.

- ***Medullary cavity.*** This is the hollow space of the diaphysis. This cavity or space contains fatty yellow bone marrow.
- ***Endosteum.*** The endosteum lines the medullary cavity and contains osteogenic and osteoclast bone cells.

The structures of the bones are summarized in Table 11.1, and the structure of a long bone is shown in Figure 11.2.

TABLE 11.1 Bone Structure

NAME	LOCATION
Epiphysis	Proximal and distal ends of long bones
Diaphysis	Shaft of long bones
Metaphysis	Portion of bone located between the epiphysis and the diaphysis
Periosteum	Connective tissue surrounding the diaphysis
Medullary cavity	Hollow space in the diaphysis
Endosteum	Lining of the medullary cavity

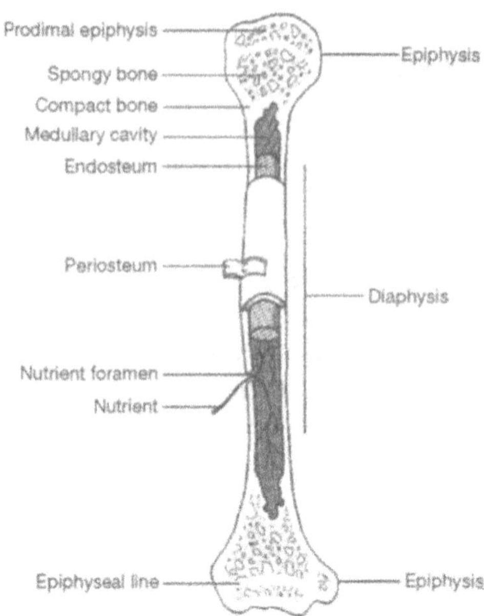

Figure 11.2 The structure of a long bone.

11.3 Bone Tissue

What Types of Cells Make Up Bone Tissue, and What Is Their Function?

The matrix portion of osseous or bone tissue is 25 percent water, 25 percent protein, and around 50 percent calcium phosphate and calcium carbonate. There are four types of bone cells that make up bone tissue:

- ***Osteogenic cells.*** These are bone-producing cells. These cells undergo mitosis and divide into osteoblasts. They can be located in the inner portion of the periosteum and in the endosteum.
- ***Osteoblasts.*** These cells do not divide. They secrete the protein collagen and the chemicals needed to make bone tissue. These cells begin the calcification process, thus building the matrix.
- ***Osteocytes.*** These are mature bone cells and function in maintaining bone tissue. They exchange nutrients and waste products between bone and blood.
- ***Osteoclasts.*** These cells function in the breaking down of the bone matrix and reabsorption. They are important in growth, maintenance, and repair.

The different types of bone cells are summarized in Table 11.2.

TABLE **11.2 Bone Cells**

CELL	FUNCTION
Osteogenic cells	Bone-producing cells that undergo mitosis
Osteoblast cells	Do not divide; secrete the chemicals that produce the matrix
Osteocytes	Function in maintaining bone tissue
Osteoclasts	Function in breaking down bone

How Does Bone Tissue Become Hard?

When osseous tissue becomes bone, this is called ***ossification***. This process begins around the sixth or seventh week of embryonic development and continues until the age of 18 to 25.

How do we form bone?
The formation of bone can happen in one of two ways.

- *Intramembranous ossification.* This refers to the formation of bone within fibrous connective tissue. Osteoblasts turn this fibrous connective tissue into bone. This particular form of ossification does not go through a "classic" cartilaginous stage.
- *Endochondral ossification.* This refers to the formation of bone in hyaline cartilage. In this form of ossification, the matrix of the hyaline cartilage is replaced by bone. This is how bone grows in length.

What Are Examples of Bones That Ossified through Intramembranous Ossification?

The flat bones of the skull, mandible, and fontanels are examples of bones that are formed by intramembranous ossification.

Remember: These two kinds of ossification *do not* create differences in bone structure; they are simply different ways in which the body makes bone from existing fibrous connective tissue.

What Are Examples of Bones That Ossified through Endochondral Ossification?

The long bones of the upper and lower extremities are examples of endochondral ossification.

How Does Bone Grow in Length?

If we want to speak of bone growing in length, we have to explain the epiphyseal plate or growth plate, located in the metaphysis of long bones. There are four stages or zones that lead to bone growth in length.

What are the stages or zones that lead to bone growth in length?

- *Zone of resting cartilage.* In this zone, there is no bone growth.
- *Zone of proliferating cartilage.* In this zone, chondrocytes (cartilage cells) begin to divide and replace cartilage cells that have died and are packed on the diaphysis. Lengthening of the bone takes place in this zone.
- *Zone of hypertrophic cartilage.* In this zone, the chondrocytes arrange themselves in columns.
- *Zone of calcified cartilage.* This zone is a few layers of dead cells thick. Osteoblasts lay down bone matrix, replacing the calcified cartilage.

How Do We Heal a Fractured Bone?

A ***fracture*** is a break in any bone. When a bone is broken, blood vessels are also broken, and bleeding occurs. This bleeding normally will present as a bruising or discoloration of the skin. A clot must be formed in order to stop the bleeding.

This clot is called a ***fracture hematoma***. After the fracture hematoma is formed, granulation tissue begins to form.

This granulation tissue is called a ***procallus***.

The procallus is transformed into a ***fibrocartilagenous callus*** or ***soft callus***, which is composed of cartilage cells.

This soft callus begins to ossify, and the matrix becomes hard. This once-broken area is composed of spongy bone and is called a ***bony callus*** or ***hard callus***.

How Do We Remodel Bone?

Bone remodeling is an ongoing process that occurs throughout our life. Our body continuously replaces old bone tissue with new bone tissue. Old bone is destroyed and reabsorbed by the osteoclasts, and the new bone is constructed by the osteoblasts.

11.4 Naming Bones

What Are the Names of the Bones of the Body?

The Skull

- Frontal bone—the most anterior bone in the skull.
- Occipital bone—the most posterior bone in the skull.
- Two parietal bones on the superior and lateral sides of the skull.
- Two temporal bones on the inferior and lateral sides of the skull; they contain the *external auditory meatus* and mastoid processes.
- Two zygomatic bones, or cheekbones.
- Maxilla, which contains the top teeth.
- Mandible, or "jawbone," which contains the bottom teeth.
- Nasal bone, which forms the bridge of the nose.
- Ethmoid bone, which contains the nasal turbinates.
- Sphenoid—the posterior portion of the eye orbit, which contains the ***sella turcica.***
- Auditory (ear) ossicles—malleus, incus, and stapes, located in the middle ear.
- Palatine bone, which forms the hard palate of the mouth.

Vertebral Column

This consists of

- Seven cervical vertebrae (neck region). The first and second cervical vertebrae are called the *atlas* and the *axis*.
- Twelve thoracic vertebrae (mid-back region).
- Five lumbar vertebrae (lumbar region).
- One sacrum, which is made up of five bones that are fused.
- One coccyx bone, which is made up of three or four bones that are fused.

Rib Cage

- Sternum, or breast bone
- Ribs—twelve pairs of ribs
  - Ribs 1 through 7 are called *true ribs*.
  - Ribs 8, 9, and 10 are called *false ribs*.
  - Ribs 11 and 12 are called *floating ribs*.
- Hyoid bone, located inferior to the mandible. This is the only bone in the body that does not articulate with any other bone.

The bones of the appendicular skeleton include the following.

The Upper Extremities

- Clavicle ("collarbone")—the anterior portion of the shoulder girdle.
- Scapula ("shoulder blade")—the posterior portion of the shoulder girdle.
- Humerus—the arm
- Radius—the lateral bone in the forearm
- Ulna—the medial bone in the forearm
- Carpal bones—eight bones that make up the wrist

- Metacarpal bones—five bones that make up the hand
- Phalanges of the upper extremity—fourteen bones that make up the fingers

The Lower Extremities
The lower extremities begin with the *pelvic girdle*. The pelvic girdle is made up of three bones:

- Ilium—the superior bone of the pelvis.
- Ischium—the inferior bone of the pelvis.
- Pubic bone—the anterior bone of the pelvis; it forms the pubic symphysis.

These three bones make up the *acetabulum*. The acetabulum is the socket that the head or ball of the femur inserts to from the hip joint.

- Femur—the thigh bone.
- Patella—the knee cap.
- Tibia—the shinbone of the leg.
- Fibula—the lateral portion of the leg.
- Tarsal bones—seven bones that make up the ankle.
- Metatarsal bones—five bones that make up the foot.
- Phalanges of the lower extremity—fourteen bones that make up the toes.

11.5 Joints

What Are Joints?

Joints or articulations are any places where two bones, bone and cartilage, or bone and teeth meet or come together.

What Are the Classifications of Joints?

Joints are classified by both structure and function, or how tightly the joint fits together and the degree of motion.

- ***Synarthroses*** are joints that are not movable.
- ***Amphiarthroses*** are joints that are able to move slightly.
- ***Diarthroses*** are joints that can move freely. Diathrosis joints have a space between the bones called a *synovial space*.
- ***Fibrous joints*** are joints that are held together tightly with fibrous connective tissue.

What are examples of fibrous joints?
Examples of fibrous joints include:

1. *Sutures.* Sutures are formed when bones that have a "sawtooth"-like border come together, creating a strong, immovable structure. Sutures are found in the skull and lock the skull bones together. Sutures do not move.
2. *Gomphoses.* Gomphoses are formed when pegs fit into sockets. Gomphoses are found in the teeth. Gomphoses do not move.
3. *Syndesmosis.* In syndesmosis joints, the bones are held together by interosseous ligaments. Syndesmoses are found between the tibia and the fibula and between the ulna and the radius. These joints are slightly movable.

- ***Cartilagenous joints*** are joints that are held together by fibrocartilage and hyaline cartilage.

What are examples of cartilagenous joints?
Examples of cartilaginous joints include:

1. *Synchondroses.* In synchondroses, the joints are held together by hyaline cartilage. Synchondroses are located in the epiphyseal plates (growth plates) in the metaphysis of long bones. These joints do not move.
2. *Symphyses.* In a symphysis, the bones are held together by fibrocartilage. Symphyses are located in the pubic symphysis and the intervertebral joints of the vertebral column. These joints move slightly.

- ***Synovial joints*** are freely movable joints, or diarthroses. These joints have a synovial space and are surrounded by a joint capsule filled with synovial fluid.

What are examples of synovial joints?
Examples of synovial joints include:

1. *Ball-and-socket joints.* This type of joint has a round surface that fits into a cup-shaped socket. Ball-and-socket joints are located at the shoulder joint and the hip joint.
2. *Hinge joint.* In this type of joint, a convex surface of one bone comes together with the concave portion of another bone. Hinge joints are located at the elbow joint, the knee joint, and the phalanges of the upper and lower extremities.
3. *Pivot joint.* This type of joint rotates around an axis. Pivot joints are located at the articulation of the head of the radius and ulna and the atlas-to-axial joint.
4. *Saddle joint.* In this type of joint, the convex portion of one bone "sits in" the concave portion of another bone, like a cowboy sitting in a horse saddle. Saddle joints are located at the carpal and metacarpal joint of the thumb.
5. *Condyloid joint.* In this type of joint, an oval-shaped portion of one bone articulates with a depression of another bone. A location of a condyloid joint would be the radiocarpal joint at the wrist.
6. *Gliding joint.* In this type of joint, flat bones articulate with each other and slide back and forth. Gliding joints are located in the carpal bones (wrist) and the tarsal bones (ankle).

A summary of the different types of joints is given in Table 11.3.

TABLE 11.3 Joints

JOINT TYPE	LOCATION
Fibrous Joints	*Held together by fibrous connective tissue*
1. Suture	Skull bones
2. Gomphosis	Teeth
3. Syndesmosis	Interosseous ligaments between the radius and ulna and the tibia and fibula
Cartilagenous Joints	*Joints held together by fibrocartilage and hyaline cartilage*
1. Synchondrosis	Epiphyseal plates (growth plates in the metaphysis)
2. Symphysis	Pubic symphysis and intervertebral joints
Synovial Joints	*Freely movable joints surrounded by a synovial capsule*
1. Ball-and-socket joint	Hip joint and shoulder joint
2. Hinge joint	Elbow joint, knee joint, phalanges
3. Pivot joint	Proximal portion of radius and ulna, atlantoaxial joint
4. Saddle joint	Thumb (carpal and metacarpal joint)
5. Condyloid joint	Wrist (radiocarpal joint)
6. Glinding joint	Carpal bones of wrist, tarsal bones of ankle

11.6 Disorders and Diseases That Affect Bone Tissue

What Are Some Common Metabolic Disorders and Diseases That Can Affect Bone Tissue?

Metabolic bone disorders include

- ***Osteoporosis.*** This is a decrease in bone mass due to a demineralization of calcium. Osteoporosis is more common in women, especially after menopause. Because of the decrease in bone quantity, the bones may become brittle. This can cause multiple compression fractures of the thoracic vertebrae, resulting in a hyperkyphosis, or "humpback."
- ***Osteomalacia.*** This is the softening of bones as a result of a vitamin D deficiency in adults. Vitamin D is needed for normal calcium absorption. Pseudofractures may result.
- ***Rickets.*** This is the softening of bones as a result of a vitamin D deficiency in children. This condition can result in multiple costochondral bumps called the *rachitic rosary* and also a protrusion of the skin called *pigeon breast* or *pectus carinatum.*
- ***Osteitis deformans.*** This is also known as *Paget's disease* and is an increase in bone density. This disease affects the spine, skull, and pelvis of geriatric patients and is idiopathic (of unknown cause).
- ***Osteitis fibrosa cystica.*** Also known as "*Von Reckinghausen's disease of the bone*," this disease causes osteolytic lesions of the bone.
- ***Osteopetrosis.*** This condition is an increase in bone density that occurs because of the inactivity of osteoclasts.
- ***Gout.*** Also known as the "disease of kings," this is a defect in the way purines are metabolized. This results in uric acid crystals building up in the joints, especially the metatarsophalangeal joint of the big toe. This is called *podagia*.

Metabolic disorders that can affect the bones are summarized in Table 11.4.

TABLE 11.4 Metabolic Disorders

DISORDER	CHARACTERISTICS
Osteoporosis	Decrease in calcium, causing bones to be brittle
Osteomalacia	Vitamin D deficiency, causing softening of bones in adults
Rickets	Vitamin D deficiency, causing softening of bones in children
Osteitis deformans	Paget's disease, abnormal increase in bone density
Osteitis fibrosa cystica	Von Recklinghausen's disease, bone lesions
Osteopetrosis	Increase in bone density because of osteoclast inactivity
Gout	"Disease of kings," inadequate metabolism of purines

What Are Some Benign Bone Tumors?

Some common benign bone tumors include

- ***Osteoid osteoma.*** This is a benign bone tumor that commonly occurs in the neck of the femur, the distal end of the femur, and the proximal tibia. This condition is more common in males between the ages of 10 to 25.
- ***Osteoma.*** This is a benign tumor that occurs in the skull, the bones of the face, and the paranasal sinus.
- ***Enchondroma.*** This type of benign tumor is made of cartilage and is most commonly found on the hands and the feet.

- ***Osteochondroma.*** This type of benign tumor occurs at the distal end of the femur and the proximal end of the tibia, and is most common in males under the age of 25.
- ***Giant cell tumor.*** This type of benign tumor occurs at the distal end of the femur and the proximal tibia. These tumors most commonly occur in women between the ages of 20 and 40. Giant cell tumors look like soap bubbles on an X-ray.

The types of benign bone tumors are summarized in Table 11.5.

TABLE **11.5 Benign Bone Tumors**

TUMOR	CHARACTERISTICS
Osteoid osteoma	Benign tumor of the femur and tibia, ages 10 to 25
Osteoma	Benign tumor of the skull, face, and sinus
Enchondroma	Made of cartilage; found in hands and feet
Osteochrondroma	Found in the femur and tibia, males under the age of 25
Giant cell tumor	Found in the femur and tibia, women between the ages of 20 and 40

What Are Examples of Common Malignant Bone Tumors?

Some common malignant bone tumors include

- ***Osteosarcoma or osteogenic sarcoma.*** This type of malignant bone tumor usually affects the proximal and distal femur, the proximal tibia, and the distal humerus. Osteosarcomas are very malignant, with the capacity to metastasize to lung tissue. These primary bone tumors are the most common and usually affect people between the ages of 20 and 40, although they can occur at any age.
- ***Chondrosarcoma.*** This is a malignant tumor of cartilage. Tumors of this type are most often primary and occur in people who have multiple endochondromas (a benign cartilage tumor). These tumors normally affect the vertebrae, bones of the pelvis, ribs, femur, and tibia.
- ***Ewing's sarcoma.*** This malignant bone tumor is the most common primary lesion between the ages of 10 and 20 and affects males more than females. These tumors affect the diaphysis of the long bones in the lower extremity.
- ***Multiple myeloma.*** This is a malignancy of plasma cells. Multiple myeloma results in hypercalcemia as a result of the destruction of bone tissue. This destruction creates "punched-out lesions" in the axial skeleton. This disease is most common in males ages 50 to 70.

Common types of malignant bone tumors are summarized in Table 11.6.

TABLE **11.6 Malignant Tumors**

TUMOR	CHARACTERISTICS
Osteogenic sarcoma	Osteosarcoma, femur and tibia or humerus, ages 20 to 40
Chondrosarcoma	Malignant tumors of cartilage, found in vertebrae, pelvis, ribs, femur, and tibia
Ewing's sarcoma	Found in diaphysis of long bones of the lower extremities, males between 10 and 20
Multiple myeloma	"Punched-out lesions" of the axial skeleton in males between 50 and 70

What Are Some Common Joint Diseases?

- ***Osteoarthritis*** (O.A. or degenerative joint disease) is a noninflammatory type of joint disease. This condition is most commonly related to or the result of wear and tear on the joint caused by repetitive stress. O.A. presents with a decrease in joint space and bone "lipping and spurring" (called osteophytes). If these osteophytes occur in the distal interphalahgeal joint, they are called *Heberden's nodes*. If they occur in the proximal interphalangeal joints, they are called *Bouchard's nodes*.

What are the signs and symptoms associated with O.A.?
O.A. presents with pain and stiffness in the morning after awakening and after rest, usually relieved by activity.

- ***Rheumatoid arthritis*** (R.A.) is a systemic, chronic inflammatory form of arthritis of autoimmune origin. R.A. starts as an inflammation of the synovial joint linings (synovitis), with edema, hyperplasia, and then hypertrophy of the synovial joint lining. Granulation tissue forms and erodes adjacent bone tissue. This erosion is called *pannus.*

What are the signs and symptoms associated with R.A.?
R.A. presents as pain and swelling, especially in the proximal interphalangeal and metacarpophalangeal joints of the upper and lower extremities and the knees. Ulnar deviation due to joint destruction and ligament laxity is a common sign.

- ***Ankylosing spondylitis*** (A.S.) is also known as Marie-Strumpell disease and is a systemic inflammatory disease affecting mainly males between the ages of 10 and 20.

What are the signs and symptoms associated with A.S.?
A.S. commonly presents as sacroiliac joint and spine pain, especially at night, and pain in the larger joints of the extremities. In untreated patients, kyphosis is common.

- ***Rieter's syndrome*** is an inflammatory condition that is usually the result of a venereal disease or intestinal disease.

What are the signs and symptoms associated with Rieter's syndrome?
Rieter's syndrome presents with inflammation of the urethra, eyes, and joints of the lower extremity (*urethritis, conjunctivitis,* and *arthritis*).

The features of some common joint diseases are summarized in Table 11.7.

TABLE **11.7 Joint Diseases**

DISEASE	CHARACTERISTICS
Osteoarthritis	Wear and tear, decrease in joint space, bone spurs
Rheumatoid arthritis	Chronic systemic inflammatory autoimmune disease; affects the joint lining (pannus)
Ankylosing spondylitis	Sacroiliac joint and spine pain, especially at night
Reiter's syndrome	Arthritis caused by venereal disease or intestinal disease

What Are Other Conditions That Can Destroy Bone?

- ***Avascular necrosis*** is a nonneoplastic disease of bone that is caused by a lack of blood supply to the bone. This condition can be the result of trauma, embolisms, or even sickle cell anemia. In children, if there is avascular necrosis to the femur head, the femur head will not develop properly. Instead of having a normal round ball-shaped femur head, the head will be shallow and flat. This condition is called *Legg-Calvé-Perthes disease.*
- ***Osteogenesis imperfecta***, also known as "*brittle bone disease*," is a congenital abnormality caused by a defect in the production of collagen. When an infant is born with osteogenesis imperfecta

(called congenital in newborns), it is very serious because the baby is born with multiple fractures and may have a soft skull. When the baby is carried, it feels like a bag of bones. Trauma during delivery is common and can cause hemorrhaging within the skull and stillbirth. Children that survive may be deaf or have hearing loss because connective tissue builds up around the auditory ossicles of the inner ear. Also, the sclera (whites of the eyes) may be blue.

- ***Charcot's joint*** is the destruction of a joint as a result of a decrease in sensory proprioception (the awareness of joints, muscle movements, weights of objects, and equilibrium).

What causes Charcot's joints?
Common causes of Charcot's joints are

1. *Tertiary or neurosyphilis.* A disease caused by the *Treponema pallidum* spirochete.
2. *Springomyelia.* A disease affecting the central canal of the spinal cord. This can be the result of a cyst, congenital malformation, infection, tumor, or trauma.
3. *Diabetic neuropathy.* A disease of the nerves caused by diabetes mellitus.

Conditions causing the destruction of bone are summarized in Table 11.8.

TABLE 11.8 Destruction of Bone

CONDITION	CHARACTERISTICS
Avascular necrosis	Caused by lack of blood supply
Osteogenesis imperfecta	"Brittle bone disease," caused by a defect in collagen production
Charcot's joint	Destroyed joints resulting from syphilis, springomyelia, or diabetes mellitus

What Are Some Common Fractures of Bone?

A fracture is a break in any bone. A fracture can be

- *Complete,* or a total break through the bone
- *Incomplete,* or a break that does not go completely through the bone
- *Displaced,* or a situation in which the two broken ends are not aligned
- *Nondisplaced,* or a situation in which the two broken ends stay in alignment
- *Open or compound,.* where the broken part of the bone protrudes through the skin
- *Closed or simple,* where the broken bones do not protrude through the skin
- *Greenstick,* or an incomplete fracture, usually seen in children
- *Avulsion,* or the tearing away of bone from itself. This results from tendinous or ligamentous pulling caused by forceful muscular contractions. In children, this condition is called *Osgood-Schlatter's disease.*

Some common ***fractures of the extremities*** are the following:

- *Colles' fracture* is a fracture of the distal radius bone of the forearm, causing a posterior displacement of the distal fragment.
- *Smith's fracture* is a fracture of the distal radius of the forearm with an anterior displacement of the distal fragment.
- *Chauffeur's fracture,* also known as a "*backfire fracture,*" is an impacted or avulsion fracture of the styloid process of the radius. It is called a "backfire" fracture because, on occasion, the crank to start the engine of an old car would spin when the engine backfired, causing the fracture.

Some common types of ***vertebral fractures*** are the following:

- *Clay shoveler's fracture*, also known as a "*coal miner's fracture*," is an avulsion fracture of the spinous processes of C6 or T1. This fracture is named for the fractures that would occur in workers who had repeated stress on the cervical region caused by shoveling. Trauma will also cause these fractures.
- *Burst fracture*, also known as "*Jefferson's fracture*," is a fracture of C1, or the atlas. These fractures occur when there is a compression-type force placed upon the atlas, causing bilateral fractures in both the posterior and anterior arches of the atlas.
- *Hangman's fracture* is a fracture of axis or C2.These fractures occur with a severe hyperextension injury, causing a traumatic spondylolisthesis (anterior slipping of the vertebra as a result of trauma). These fractures are common in high-speed deceleration injuries seen in car accidents or someone who is hanged.

Some common fractures of bone are summarized in Table 11.9.

TABLE 11.9 Fractures of Bone

TYPE	CHARACTERISTICS
Simple fracture	Closed fracture
Compound fracture	Open fracture
Greenstick fracture	Incomplete fracture, usually seen in children
Avulsion fracture	Tearing away of bone, Osgood-Schlatter's disease
Colles' fracture	Distal radius fracture with posterior displacement
Smith's fracture	Distal radius fracture with anterior displacement
Chauffeur's fracture	"Backfire fracture," avulsion fracture of the styloid process of the radius
Clay shoveler's fracture	Avulsion fracture of the spinous processes of either C6, C7, or T1
Burst fracture	"Jefferson's fracture," or a fracture of C1
Hangman's fracture	High-speed deceleration injury

What Are Abnormal Curvatures of the Spine?

- ***Lordosis*** is also known as a "*swayback*." It is an increase in the normal lumbar curve.
- ***Kyphosis*** is also known as "*humpback*." It is an abnormal increase in the normal thoracic curve.
- ***Scoliosis*** is a lateral curvature of the spine. It can begin between the ages of 3 and 10 (juvenile), although it can also happen after skeletal maturity. It is very important to treat scoliosis early because rapid progression occurs at the ages of 12 to 16.

Abnormal curvatures of the spine are summarized in Table 11.10.

TABLE 11.10 Abnormal Spine Curves

TYPE	CHARACTERISTIC
Lordosis	"Swayback," or an increase in the normal lumbar curve
Kyphosis	"Humpback," or an increase in the normal thoracic curve
Scoliosis	Lateral curvature of the spine

Chapter 11 Review Questions

Fill In the Blank

1. The proximal and distal ends of long bones are called ____________________.
2. The shaft of a long bone is called the ____________________.
3. The portion of a long bone that contains the epiphyseal plate is called the ____________________.
4. Connective tissue that surrounds the diaphysis is called ____________________.
5. The hollow space in the diaphysis is called the ____________________.
6. The lining of the medullary cavity is called the ____________________.
7. Bone-producing cells are called ____________________.
8. The cells that produce the chemicals that form the matrix are called ____________________.
9. The cells that function in maintaining bone tissue are called ____________________.
10. The cells that break down bone are called ____________________.
11. Nonmovable joints are called ____________________.
12. Slightly movable joints are called ____________________.
13. Freely movable joints are called ____________________.
14. The type of joint found in teeth is called ____________________.
15. Joints held together by interosseous ligaments are called ____________________.
16. Freely movable joints have a __________capsule.
17. Softening of bones caused by a vitamin D deficiency is called ____________________.
18. The condition also known as Paget's disease is ____________________.
19. An increase of the thoracic curve is ____________________.
20. A lateral curvature of the spine is ____________________.

True/False

21. The skull and ethmoid bone are part of the appendicular skeleton.
22. The ribs and sternum are part of the axial skeleton.
23. In growing bone, the region of the metaphysis is referred to as the epiphyseal plate.
24. In mature bone, the region of the metaphysis is referred to as the epiphyseal line.
25. The medullary cavity contains red bone marrow.
26. Osteoblasts begin the calcification process, thus building the matrix.
27. Rheumatoid arthritis is a noninflammatory "wear and tear" disease.
28. Rotation around an axis is called a gliding joint.
29. A burst fracture is also known as a Smith's fracture.
30. The study of bones is called hematology.

Matching

31. Hangman's fracture

32. Jefferson's fracture

33. Clay shoveler's fracture

34. Chauffeur's fracture

35. Smith's fracture

36. Colles' fracture

37. Avulsion fracture

38. Greenstick fracture

39. Closed fracture

40. Open fracture

A. Broken bone protrudes through the skin
B. Broken bone does not protrude through the skin
C. Usually seen in children
D. Tearing away from bone
E. Distal radius fracture with posterior displacement
F. Distal radius fracture with anterior displacement
G. Also called a "backfire fracture"
H. Also called a "coal miner's fracture"
I. A fracture of the atlas
J. A fracture of the axis

Multiple Choice

41. A disease affecting the spinal cord that is a result of a cyst, malformation, tumor, or trauma would be __________.

A. neurosyphilis
B. diabetes
C. springomyelia
D. diabetic neuropathy
E. Charcot's joint

42. A condition in which the entire joint is destroyed is called __________.

A. neurosyphilis
B. diabetes
C. springomyelia
D. diabetic neuropathy
E. Charcot's joint

43. A "brittle bone" disease that may present with a blue sclera is __________.

A. avascular necrosis
B. ankylosing spondylitis
C. Reiter's syndrome

D. osteogenesis imperfecta
E. rheumatoid arthritis

44. The condition that is also known as Marie-Strumpell disease is __________.
A. ankylosing spondylitis
B. Reiter's syndrome
C. rheumatoid arthritis
D. osteogenesis imperfecta
E. multiple myeloma

45. __________ is a malignant tumor of cartilage.
A. Multiple myeloma
B. Chondrosarcoma
C. Ewing's sarcoma
D. Osteosarcoma
E. Osteochondroma

46. A benign tumor of cartilage that is commonly found on the hands and feet is __________.
A. multiple myeloma
B. chondrosarcoma
C. osteosarcoma
D. osteochondroma
E. enchondroma

47. A benign tumor that appears as "soap bubbles" on the femur and tibia is a(n) __________.
A. osteochondroma
B. enchondroma
C. giant cell tumor
D. osteoid osteoma
E. gout

48. The disease that causes osteolytic lesions of the bone and is referred to as "Von Recklinghausen's disease" is __________.
A. osteochondroma
B. osteoid osteoma
C. osteitis fibrosa cystica
D. osteopetrosis
E. osteoporosis

49. Osteomalcia in children is called __________.
A. Ewing's sarcoma
B. Paget's disease
C. Marie-Strumpell disease
D. rickets
E. Von Recklinghausen's disease

50. A decrease in bone mass caused by a demineralization of calcium is called __________.
A. osteomalacia
B. osteopetrosis

C. osteoma
D. osteoporosis
E. osteochondroma

Chapter 11: Review Questions and Answers

Fill In the Blank Answers

1. Epiphyses
2. Diaphysis
3. Metaphysis
4. Periosteum
5. Medullary cavity
6. Endosteum
7. Osteogenic cells
8. Osteoblasts
9. Osteocytes
10. Osteoclasts
11. Synarthroses
12. Amphiarthroses
13. Diarthroses
14. Gomphosis
15. Syndesmoses
16. Synovial
17. Osteomalacia
18. Osteitis deformans
19. Kyphosis
20. Scoliosis

True/False Answers

21. False
22. True
23. True
24. True
25. False
26. True
27. False
28. False
29. False
30. False

Matching Answers

31. J
32. I
33. H
34. G
35. F
36. E
37. D
38. C
39. B
40. A

Multiple Choice Answers

41. C
42. E
43. D
44. A
45. B
46. E
47. C
48. C
49. D
50. D

The Muscular System

Objectives

This chapter will discuss the structures and functions of the muscular system and diseases associated with muscular tissue.

Keywords:

Myology	Fascia	Dupuytren's contracture
Kinesiology	Tendon	Shin splints
Skeletal muscle	Strain	
Cardiac muscle		
Smooth muscle		
Sarcolemma	Ligament	Lateral epicondylitis
	Sprain	
Sarcoplasm	Aponeurosis	Medial epicondylitis
Myofibrils	Motor neuron	Anterior compartment syndrome
Sarcoplasmic reticulum	Myositis ossificans	
	Isotonic contraction	Myositis ossificans circumscripta
Actin		
Myosin	Isometric contraction	Myositis ossificans progressiva
Sarcomere	Botulism	Fibromyalgia
Endomysium	Tetanus	Muscular dystrophy
	Spasticity	
	Flaccidity	
Perimysium	Atrophy	Duchenne's muscular dystrophy
Fascicle	Cramp (muscle spasm)	Myasthenia gravis
Epimysium	Volkmann's contracture	

12.1 Overview

The study of muscles is called ***myology***, and the study of movement is called ***kinesiology***.

The movement of bones, and thus the movement of the body, is caused by muscles.

How Do Muscles Cause Bones to Move?

The contraction (shortening) and relaxation (lengthening) of muscles cause bone to move. When muscles contract, there is a change of *chemical energy* in the form of ATP (adenosine triphosphate) into *mechanical energy*. This mechanical energy generates the force needed to perform work and produce movement.

What Types of Muscles Do We Have?

There are three types of muscles in the human body.

- ***Skeletal muscle.*** Skeletal muscle is striated, meaning that it contains contractile proteins. Skeletal muscle is voluntary, meaning that it is under conscious control.
- ***Cardiac muscle.*** Cardiac muscle is heart muscle. It is striated and is under unconscious or involuntary control.
- ***Smooth muscle.*** Smooth muscle is found in blood vessels and organs of the gastrointestinal tract. These muscles are nonstriated and involuntary.

How Do Muscles Function?

- Muscles function in *motion*. For example, skeletal muscles move bones, causing the movements of the upper and lower extremities.
- Muscles *move* substances. For example, cardiac muscle (in the heart) pumps blood to all the cells of the body, and smooth muscles move food through the gastrointestinal tract.
- Muscles *stabilize* body positions and regulate organ volume. For example, certain muscles are responsible for maintaining posture.
- Muscles *generate heat* (thermogenesis). When muscles contract to perform work, the by-product that they produce is heat. For example, you shiver when you are cold.

What Are the Characteristics of Muscles?

The characteristics of muscle include the following:

- Muscles are *excitable*, meaning that they must respond to stimuli. This includes chemical neurotransmitters from nerves or hormones through the blood.
- Muscles have *conductivity*, meaning that they must be able to carry an action potential (electrical impulse) along their plasma membrane.
- Muscles can *contract*, meaning that they shorten and thicken in response to an action potential from a nerve.
- Muscles can relax and stretch without damage after contracting. This is called *extensibility*.
- Muscles can return to normal after they contract, relax, or extend. This is called *elasticity*.

12.2 Muscle Anatomy

What Is the Anatomy of Muscle Cells?

- *Sarcolemma.* The ***sarcolemma*** is the plasma membrane of the muscle cell. This structure separates the cell's external environment from its internal environment.
- *Sarcoplasm.* The ***sarcoplasm*** contains the internal structures of the cell. The sarcoplasm is the "cytoplasm" of muscle cells. It contains glucose, glycogen, and myoglobin.

- *Myofibrils.* ***Myofibrils*** are the contractile units of muscle cells. These organelles are located in the sarcoplasm and give the skeletal muscle its striated appearance.
- *Sarcoplasmic reticulum.* The ***sarcoplasmic reticulum*** of muscle cells is a fluid-filled sac system that surrounds the myofibrils. This structure stores calcium (Ca^{2+}), which is needed in contracting the muscle.
- *Filaments.* Filaments are very small, thin structures located in myofibrils. There are two types:
  1. ***Actin*** is called the thin filament.
  2. ***Myosin*** is called the thick filament.
- *Sarcomere.* Each myofibril is split into sections or ***sarcomeres***. These sarcomeres contain
  1. *Contractile proteins:* myosin and actin
  2. *Structural proteins:* titin, nebulin, myomesin, and dystrophin
  3. *Regulatory proteins:* tropomyosin and troponin

What Is the Anatomy of Muscle?

Each individual muscle cell is surrounded by areolar connective tissue called an ***endomysium***. Between 10 and 100 of these structures are wrapped by dense irregular connective tissue called a ***perimysium.*** This whole structure is called a ***fascicle.*** Fascicles are wrapped by another layer of dense irregular connective tissue called an ***epimysium.*** These structures make up the muscle. The entire muscle is supported by a wrapping or "bandage" of dense irregular connective tissue called ***fascia***. The structures of a skeletal muscle are shown in Figure 12.1.

What Is the Function of Fascia?

Fascia holds the muscle together, protects the muscle, stores water and fat, reduces heat loss, and is a framework for blood vessels, nerves, and lymphatic vessels.

What Is a Tendon?

Tendons are made up of dense regular connective tissue. Tendons attach muscle to bone. If a tendon is overstretched or torn, it is called a ***strain***.

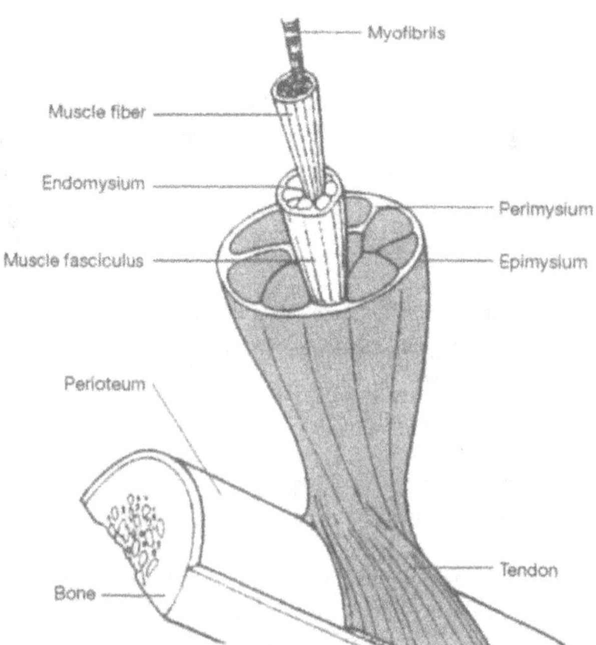

Figure 12.1 The associated connective tissues of a skeletal muscle.

What Is a Ligament?

Ligaments are made up of dense regular connective tissue and attach bone to bone. If a ligament is overstretched or torn, it is called a ***sprain***.

Remember: Tendon and strain both have a T in their spelling. This will help you remember the difference between a strain and a sprain.

What Is an Aponeurosis?

An ***aponeurosis*** is a broad, flat tendon.

What would be an example of where an aponeurosis would be located?
An example of where an aponeurosis is found is the *epicranial aponeurosis or galea aponeurotica*. This is a broad, flat tendon that connects the belly of the occipitalis muscle to the belly of the frontalis muscle, forming the occipitofrontalis muscle. This muscle is located on top of the skull.

What Stimulates a Muscle to Contract?

A ***motor neuron*** is a type of nerve cell that stimulates muscle cells in order for them to contract. A motor neuron and the muscle cell it stimulates are called a *motor unit*.

12.3 Muscle Physiology

How Does a Muscle Contract?

A muscle contraction starts with a stimulus from a motor neuron. The synaptic end bulbs from a nerve release acetylcholine from their vesicles. Acetylcholine is a neurotransmitter. Once released, acetylcholine will cross the synaptic gap and adhere to its receptor sites on the muscle's motor end plate. Acetylcholine is like a key opening up a lock. The gates of the sarcolemma open, letting the cation (positively charged ion) Na^+ (sodium) rush into the cell. Remember, the cell, prior to this, is in a negative state or "resting state." *The cell is polarized.* When Na^+ ions rush into the cell, the cell becomes positively charged. *The cell is now depolarized.* The action potential travels along the sarcolemma (plasma membrane). This action potential (electrical impulse) opens the gates of the sarcoplasmic reticulum, causing Ca^{2+} (calcium) to flow into the cytosol of the cell. Calcium removes the troponin/tropomyosin complex from the thin filament, which is actin. With the troponin and tropomyosin removed, the "heads" of the thick filament, myosin, can swivel up and contact actin. When the myosin heads touch actin, ATP located in the heads is broken down into ADP + energy. This makes myosin pull actin toward the myomesin line of the sarcomere, causing the sarcomere to shorten. When all of the sarcomeres shorten, the myofibril shortens; when the myofibrils shorten, the muscle fiber (cell) shortens; when all the cells that make up the fascicle shorten and all the fascicles shorten, the muscle shortens, and we call this a muscle contraction. The sliding effect of myosin pulling on actin is called a *power stroke*.

What Are the Parts of the Sarcomere?

- *Z disks* separate the sarcomeres along the myofibril.
- *A bands* extend along the entire length of the filament. A bands mostly contain myosin filaments, with fewer actin filaments.
- *I bands* are areas that contain only actin filaments.
- The *H zone* is located in the middle of each A band.
- The *M line* (myomesin) is connected to the thick filament and divides the H zone.

The structure of the sarcomere is shown in Figure 12.2.

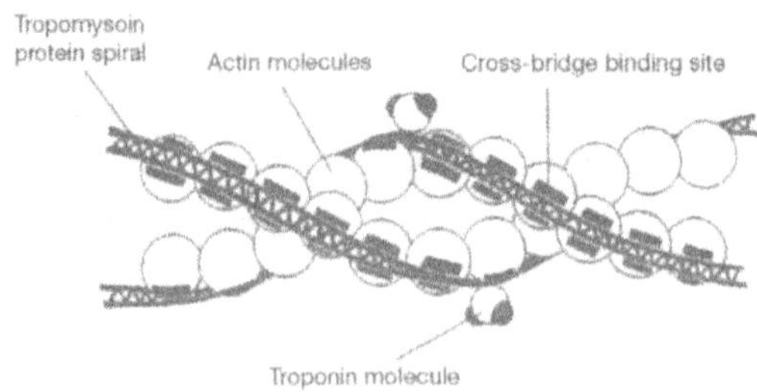

Figure 12.2 A sarcomere.

What Are the Functions of the Proteins Located in Muscle Tissue?

- *Actin* is the thin filament contractile protein. The structure of thin filaments is shown in Figure 12.3.

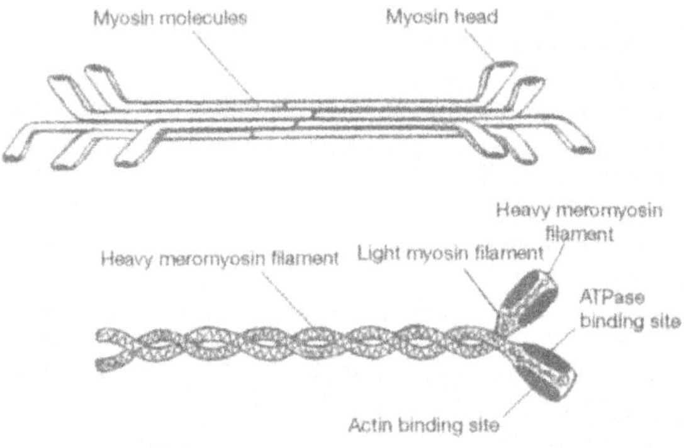

Figure 12.3 The structure of thin myofilaments.

- *Myosin* is the thick filament contractile protein. The structure of thick filaments is shown in Figure 12.4.

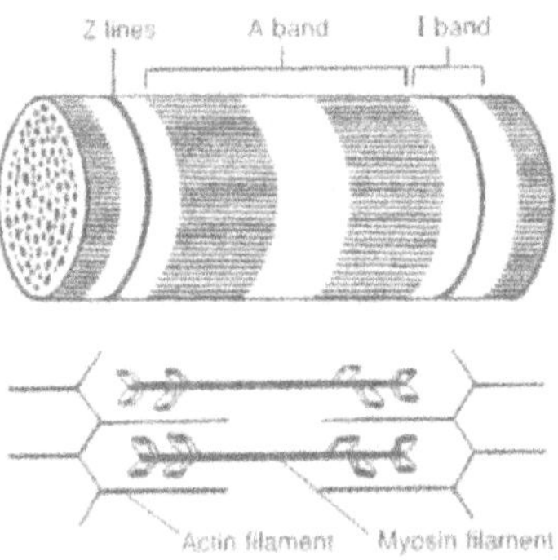

Figure 12.4 The structure of thick myofilaments.

- *Troponin* is a regulatory protein that attaches the tropomyosin protein to actin.
- *Tropomyosin* is a regulatory protein that covers the myosin binding sites of actin, preventing myosin from touching actin.
- *Titin* is a structural protein that attaches the Z disks to the M line. This protein is responsible for much of the muscle's elasticity and extensibility because it can be stretched and can recoil back into position.
- *Myomesin* forms the sarcomere's M line and attaches myosin filaments to one another.
- *Nebulin* is a structural protein that wraps around actin filaments and attaches them to Z disks.
- *Dystrophin* is a structural protein that attaches actin to the integral proteins of the sarcolemma.

How Does a Muscle Relax?

After a contraction, the enzyme *acetylcholinesterase* is released into the synaptic gap and quickly breaks down acetylcholine. The Na^+ gates will close, and the muscle cell will *repolarize*. Ca^{2+} active transport pumps will pump the Ca^{2+} in the sarcoplasm back into the sarcoplasmic reticulum. Here the protein *calsequestrin* will bind to the Ca^{2+} to allow it to be stored. Myosin detaches from actin, and the troponin-tropomyosin complex returns to block the myosin binding sites on actin. This process enables the muscle to relax. Another contraction will not occur unless the muscle is stimulated by the nerve.

How Are Muscle Contractions Classified?

There are two classifications of muscle contractions.

What happens in an isotonic contraction?

1. *Isotonic contraction.* In an ***isotonic contraction***, there is constant motion. There are two types of motion seen in isotonic contractions:
   - *Concentric motion.* In this type of motion, the muscle shortens and the angle of the joint decreases.
   - *Eccentric motion.* In this type of motion, the muscle lengthens and the angle of the joint increases.

What happens in an isometric contraction?

2. *Isometric contraction.* In an ***isometric contraction***, the muscle does not or cannot shorten or move, although tension is placed on the muscle.

What Types of Fibers Do Muscles Have?

Skeletal muscles are classified by how rapidly they split ATP. Skeletal muscles are classified into three types:

1. *Slow twitch* or *slow oxidative fibers*
   - These fibers are small in diameter compared to the other two types.
   - They have many capillaries.
   - They have large amounts of myoglobin and hemoglobin.
   - They have many mitochondria.
   - They have a high capacity to generate ATP by aerobic cellular respiration.
   - They split ATP at a very slow rate, thus resisting fatigue.
   - These muscle fibers are very red in color.

   Slow twitch muscle fibers are found in postural muscles, are used during aerobic or endurance-type exercises, and are not very powerful.
2. *Fast twitch A* or *fast oxidative–glycolytic fibers*
   - These fibers are intermediate in diameter compared to the other two types.
   - They possess many capillaries.
   - They have many mitochondria.
   - They have large amounts of myoglobin and hemoglobin.
   - Fast twitch A fibers have a high capacity to generate ATP by oxidation and the breakdown of glucose (glycolysis).
   - These fibers split ATP three times faster than slow twitch fibers.

   Fast twitch A muscle fibers have some resistance to fatigue.
3. *Fast twitch B* or *fast glycolytic fibers*
   - These fibers are the largest of the three types.
   - They have few blood capillaries.

- They are low in myoglobin and hemoglobin.
- They have very few mitochondria.
- These fibers generate ATP by glycolysis.
- These fibers are very fatigable.
- These muscle fibers are white in color.

Fast twitch B fibers contract quickly and strongly.

Remember: Red muscle fibers are red in color because they are high in myoglobin and hemoglobin and have many capillaries.

White muscle fibers are white in color because they are low in myoglobin and hemoglobin and have few capillaries.

12.4 Muscular Diseases, Conditions, and Disorders

What Are Some Common Muscular Diseases Caused by Infectious Organisms?

Some common muscular diseases caused by organisms are

- ***Botulism*** is caused by *Clostridium botulinum. Clostridium botulinum* is a bacterium that is commonly found in soil and water, but it can get into food, especially into food that is not properly canned. The toxin blocks the synaptic cleft, preventing the neurotransmitter from reaching the motor end plate of the muscle.

What are the signs and symptoms of botulism?
The signs and symptoms of botulism include abdominal cramps, muscle weakness, muscle paralysis, nausea, vomiting, difficulty swallowing, and difficulty breathing. These signs and symptoms appear around 8 to 40 hours after infection.

- ***Tetanus*** is caused by the bacterium *Clostridium tetani. Clostridium tetani* is commonly found in soil and water, especially in soils containing manure from horses, cattle, and even humans. Once inside the body, the organism releases exotoxins.

What are the signs and symptoms of tetanus?
The signs and symptoms include severe muscle spasms, especially in the face, neck, and jaw. These spasms can become very violent and can break bones. Symptoms of tetanus, also called "lockjaw," appear around 5 to 10 days after infection. Infection can occur with deep tissue wounds caused by an object that is contaminated with the *C. tetani* spores.

What Are Some General Muscular Conditions?

- *Spasticity.* ***Spasticity***, or a muscle spasm, is an increase in stiffness and tone.
- *Flaccidity.* ***Flaccidity*** is a loss of muscle tone. Flaccidity is commonly the beginning of atrophy.
- *Atrophy.* ***Atrophy*** is the wasting away of muscle tissue. This can be the result of nonuse, lack of nervous impulses, or poor nutrition.
- *Cramps* or *muscle spasms.* ***Cramps*** or ***muscle spasms*** are involuntary muscle contractions that will not relax. This "hypertonicity" of muscles most often results in trigger points or "knots." Cramps are commonly caused by injury, muscle splinting at an injured joint, ischemia, or mineral deficiency.
- *Myofascial trigger points* or *pressure points.* These spots within a tight, taut band of muscle or fascia are very tender, hyperirritable, and painful upon compression. A "twitch response" is commonly seen, where the tight, taut muscles contract or twitch uncontrollably.
- *Contractures.* Contractures are muscles that are permanently shortened and have become hard and immovable. The contracted muscle will be surrounded by thickened fascia, commonly the result of nonmovement or damage to the nerve supply.

What would be examples of contracture syndromes?
Two examples of contracture syndromes are:

1. ***Volkmann's contracture*** is an ischemic contracture of the wrist and fingers. This is the result of an injury that alters arterial flow to the muscles. The wrist, proximal interphalangeal joints, and distal interphalangeal joints are affected. These structures will be in a flexed position, with stiffness and atrophy to the muscle.
2. ***Dupuytren's contracture*** is a condition affecting the palmar fascia, causing it to shorten and thicken. The result is a flexion deformity with loss of finger function, especially to the fourth and fifth phalanges.

What Are Some Common Muscular Conditions Caused by Injuries?

- A *strain* is an overstretching or tearing of a muscle tendon. The severity of a strain is indicated by its degree:
  1. *First-degree strain.* In a first-degree strain, the tendon fibers are overstretched but not torn. Pain will be present, with possible inflammation.
  2. *Second-degree strain.* In a second-degree strain, the tendon fibers are partially torn. This strain injury will present with pain, swelling, and muscle splinting in the surrounding muscles.
  3. *Third-degree strain.* In a third-degree strain, the tendon is completely ruptured.

  Remember: Strain injuries can be very serious. Proper healing of a strain is very important because scar tissue or adhesions can form, affecting the proper elasticity of the fiber.
- ***Shin splints*** are a very painful condition involving a strain injury to either the *tibialis anterior muscle* or the *tibialis posterior muscle* or both. This condition is caused by jumping or running on hard or uneven surfaces, causing a tear in the muscles or the interosseous membrane between the tibia and fibula bones of the leg. The periosteum surrounding the bone can be affected and become inflamed (periostitis). If the stress continues or worsens, the tearing of these muscles can occur.
- ***Lateral epicondylitis***, or *tennis elbow*, is an overuse or strain injury of the extensor carpi radialis brevis and extensor carpi radialis longus muscle tendons.
- ***Medial epicondylitis***, or golfer's elbow, also known as Little Leaguer's elbow, is an overuse or strain injury of the pronator teres, flexor carpi radialis, and flexor carpi ulnaris muscle tendons.
- ***Anterior compartment syndrome*** is an injury caused by repetitive stress, overuse, or trauma resulting in a buildup of excess fluid in the anterior compartment of the leg. Edema and bleeding in the compartment cause pressure, which impedes blood flow and can cause nerve damage and muscle death. This condition is extremely painful and very dangerous. The muscles of the anterior compartment of the tibia include the tibialis anterior, extensor hallucis longus, and extensor digitorum longus.
- ***Myositis ossificans*** is a disease that deposits bone into muscle, causing pain and swelling. Trauma, such as a contusion, fracture, or dislocation, can cause myositis ossificans. The trauma causes a hematoma that can pool blood within soft tissue. The iron and calcium in the blood harden and resemble bone. There are two types of myositis ossificans:
  1. ***Myositis ossificans circumscripta.*** This is a localized deposit of calcium, commonly occurring in the quadriceps muscles of the anterior thigh, usually following a trauma.
  2. ***Myositis ossificans progressiva.*** This is a rare and frequently fatal form of myositis ossificans. This condition is characterized by the progressive ossification of the muscles of mastication (chewing). The affected person cannot chew, and this results in death by starvation.
- ***Fibromyalgia*** is a chronic inflammatory disorder that affects connective tissue and muscle tissue.

What are the signs and symptoms of fibromyalgia?
The signs and symptoms of fibromyalgia include chronic muscle pain all over the body, with tender trigger points and difficulty sleeping. The condition can be caused by emotional problems, stress, gastrointestinal problems, insomnia, chronic fatigue, and sleep disorders.

What Other Conditions Cause Disorders and Diseases of Muscle?

- ***Muscular dystrophy.*** Muscular dystrophy is a group of genetic X-linked disorders that cause the muscles to become weak, atrophy, and waste away. The structural protein *dystrophin* in muscle cells is affected. There are many types of muscular dystrophy, distinguished by age of onset, types of symptoms, and muscle groups affected.

What are the signs and symptoms of muscular dystrophy?
The signs and symptoms of muscular dystrophy include muscle weakness, uncoordinated movements, falls, and difficulty breathing and swallowing.

- ***Duchenne's muscular dystrophy.*** Duchenne's muscular dystrophy is the most common and most severe type, usually occurring in male children and presenting during the first year of life. This form of muscular dystrophy is steadily progressive and is eventually fatal. The most common sign is hypertrophy of the gastrocnemius and soleus muscles (the muscles that make up the calf).
- ***Myasthenia gravis.*** Myasthenia gravis is an autoimmune disorder in which antibodies in the neuromuscular junction prevent neurotransmitters (acetylcholine) from reaching the muscle motor end plate. This disorder usually affects women between the ages of 20 and 40 and men over 60.

What are the signs and symptoms of myasthenia gravis?
The signs and symptoms of myasthenia gravis include double vision and difficulty in talking, chewing, swallowing, walking, and breathing. The person may often have problems with drooling. These signs and symptoms usually get better with rest and are exacerbated with activity.

TABLE 12.1 Review of the Major Muscles of the Body

This table will review the major muscles of the body and their primary actions.

MUSCLE	ACTION
Muscles of the Head and Face	
Occipitofrontalis	
Frontal portion	Pulls the scalp to the front and wrinkles the forehead
Occipital portion	Pulls the scalp posterior
Orbicularis oculi	Closes the eye
Orbicularis oris	Closes the mouth around the teeth
Levator palpebrae superioris	Elevates (opens) the eye
Corrugator supercilii	Wrinkles the eyebrow
Zygomaticus major	Makes you smile
Zygomaticus minor	Raises the top lip
Levator labii superioris	Raises the top lip
Depressor labii inferioris	Lowers (depresses) the lower lip
Buccinator	Lets you kiss, whistle, or blow
Platysma	Makes you pout
Mentalis	Makes you pout
Muscles of the Arm, Forearm, Wrist, and Hand	
Pectoralis major	Horizontally adducts the arm, medially adducts the arm
Latissimus dorsi	Extends, medially rotates, and adducts the arm
Deltoid	Abducts the arm
Subscapularis	Medially rotates the arm

Supraspinatus	Externally (laterally) rotates and abducts the arm
Infraspinatus	Externally (laterally) rotates the arm
Teres major	Internally (medially) rotates the arm
Teres minor	Externally (laterally) rotates and adducts the arm
Coracobrachialis	Flexes and adducts the arm
Brachialis	Flexes the forearm at the elbow
Biceps brachii	Flexes and supinates the forearm
Brachioradialis	Flexes, supinates, and pronates forearm
Triceps brachii	Extends the arm and the forearm
Anconeus	Extends the arm
Flexor carpi radialis	Flexes the wrist, radial deviation of the wrist
Flexor carpi ulnaris	Flexes the wrist, ulnar deviation of the wrist
Palmaris longus	Flexes the hand at the wrist
Flexor digitorum superficialis	Flexes the fingers (superficial muscle)
Flexor digitorum profundus	Flexes the fingers (deep muscle)
Extensor carpi radialis longus	Extends the wrist, radially deviates the wrist
Extensor carpi ulnaris	Extends the wrist, deviates the wrist to the ulnar side
Extensor digitorum	Extends the phalanges
Extensor digiti minimi	Extends the little finger
Extensor indicis	Extends the index finger
Extensor pollicis longus	Extends the thumb
Extensor pollicis brevis	Extends the thumb
Abductor pollicis longus	Abducts and extends the thumb
Abductor pollicis brevis	Abducts the thumb
Flexor pollicis brevis	Flexes the thumb
Adductor pollicis	Adducts the thumb
Opponens pollicis	Opposes the thumb toward the little finger
Muscles of the Abdominal Wall	
Rectus abdominis	Flexes the trunk, compresses the abdomen
Internal Oblique	Compresses the abdomen, flexes the trunk, laterally flexes and rotates the vertebral column
External Oblique	Compresses the abdomen, flexes the trunk, laterally flexes and rotates the vertebral column
Transversus abdominis	Compresses the abdomen
Quadratus lumborum	Extends the trunk, laterally flexes the vertebral column
Muscles of Breathing	
Diaphragm	Contraction of the diaphragm causes inhalation. Relaxation of the diaphragm causes exhalation.
Intercostales externi	Contraction causes inhalation
Intercostales interni	Contraction causes exhalation

(*Continued*)

TABLE 12.1 **Review of the Major Muscles of the Body (*Continued*)**

MUSCLE	ACTION
Muscles of the Hips, Thighs, and Legs	
Iliacus	All flex the thigh at the hip joint
Psoas major	
Psoas minor	
Tensor fasciae latae	All abduct the thigh at the hip joint
Gluteus medius	
Gluteus minimus	
Gluteus maximus	Extends the thigh at the hip joint
Adductor longus	All adduct the thigh at the hip
Adductor brevis	
Adductor magnus	
Gracilis	
Pectineus	
Rectus femoris	All extend the leg at the knee
Vastus lateralis	
Vastus intermedius	
Vastus medialis	
Biceps femoris	All flex the leg at the knee
Semimembranosus	
Semitendinosus	
Gastrocnemius	Plantar flexes the foot
Soleus	
Tibialis anterior	Dorsiflexes and inverts the foot
Peroneus (fibularis) longus Peroneus (fibularis) brevis	Both evert the foot

Chapter 12 Review Questions

Fill In the Blank

1. The study of muscles is called ____________________.
2. The study of body movement is called ____________________.
3. When a muscle shortens, it is called ____________________.
4. When a muscle lengthens, it is called ____________________.
5. Muscles of the gastrointestinal tract are which type of muscle? ________________
6. If a muscle responds to stimuli, it is said to be ____________________.
7. Muscles ____________ in response to stimuli.
8. The plasma membrane of a muscle cell is called the ____________________.

9. The contractile units of muscle cells are called ________________________.

10. The thick filament is called ____________________.

11. The thin filament is called ____________________.

12. Troponin and tropomyosin are ________________ proteins.

13. A broad, flat tendon is called a(n) ________________.

14. When a ligament is overstretched or torn, it is called a(n) ________________.

15. When a tendon is overstretched or torn, it is called a(n) ________________.

16. In a(n) ______________ contraction, the muscle does not or cannot move.

17. In a(n) ______________ contraction, there is constant motion.

18. The muscle fibers that resist fatigue are ______________________.

19. Muscle fibers that are high in myoglobin and hemoglobin are what color? ______________

20. Titin is a(n) ______________ protein.

Matching

21. Actin
22. Myosin
23. Troponin
24. Tropomyosin
25. Titin
26. Myomesin
27. Nebulin
28. Dystrophin
29. Sprain
30. Strain

    A. Attaches tropomyosin to actin
    B. Forms the M line
    C. Tear in a tendon
    D. Covers the myosin binding sites
    E. Attaches actin to Z disks
    F. Thin filament
    G. Tear in a ligament
    H. Attaches actin to internal proteins
    I. Attaches the Z disks to the M line
    J. Thick filament

Matching

31. Botulism
32. Tetanus
33. Flaccidity

34. Atrophy

35. Tennis elbow

36. Golfer's elbow

37. Myositis ossificans

38. Myasthenia gravis

39. Myositis ossificans progressiva

40. Fibromyalgia

A. Bone deposits in a muscle
B. Loss of muscle tone
C. Rare fatal form of myositis ossificans
D. Chronic inflammatory disorder
E. Caused by *Clostridium botulinum*
F. Medial epicondylitis
G. Antibodies in the neuromuscular junction
H. Lateral epicondylitis
I. Wasting away of muscle
J. Caused by *Clostridium tetani*

Multiple Choice

41. This muscle lets you kiss.

A. Orbicularis oculi
B. Buccinator
C. Levator labii superioris
D. Zygomaticus minor
E. Corrugator supercilii

42. This muscle wrinkles the eyebrow.

A. Orbicularis oculi
B. Buccinator
C. Levator labii superioris
D. Zygomaticus minor
E. Corrugator supercilii

43. This muscle raises the top lip.

A. Orbicularis oculi
B. Buccinator
C. Levator labii superioris
D. Zygomaticus minor
E. Corrugator supercilii

44. This muscle flexes the forearm at the elbow.

A. Biceps brachii
B. Teres minor
C. Brachialis
D. Coracobrachialis
E. Infraspinatus

45. This muscle abducts the arm.
   A. Latissimus dorsi
   B. Teres major
   C. Infraspinatus
   D. Brachialis
   E. Deltoid

46. This is an extensor muscle of the leg.
   A. Adductor longus
   B. Rectus femoris
   C. Deltoid
   D. Pronator teres
   E. Biceps brachii

47. This muscle flexes the leg.
   A. Biceps femoris
   B. Vastus lateralis
   C. Deltoideus
   D. Teres major
   E. Infraspinatus

True/False

48. When the diaphragm contracts, it causes exhalation.
49. *Clostridium tetani* causes "lockjaw."
50. A disease that deposits bone into muscle is called myositis ossificans.

Chapter 12: Review Questions and Answers

Fill In the Blank Answers

1. Myology
2. Kinesiology
3. Contraction
4. Relaxation
5. Smooth muscle
6. Excitable
7. Shorten
8. Sarcolemma
9. Myofibrils
10. Myosin
11. Actin
12. Regulatory
13. Aponeurosis
14. Sprain
15. Strain
16. Isometric
17. Isotonic
18. Slow twitch or slow oxidative
19. Red
20. Structural

Matching Answers

21. F

22. J

23. A

24. D

25. I

26. B

27. E

28. H

29. G

30. C

Matching Answers

31. E

32. J

33. B

34. I

35. H

36. F

37. A

38. G

39. C

40. D

Multiple Choice Answers

41. B

42. E

43. C

44. C

45. E

46. B

47. A

True/False Answers

48. False

49. True

50. True

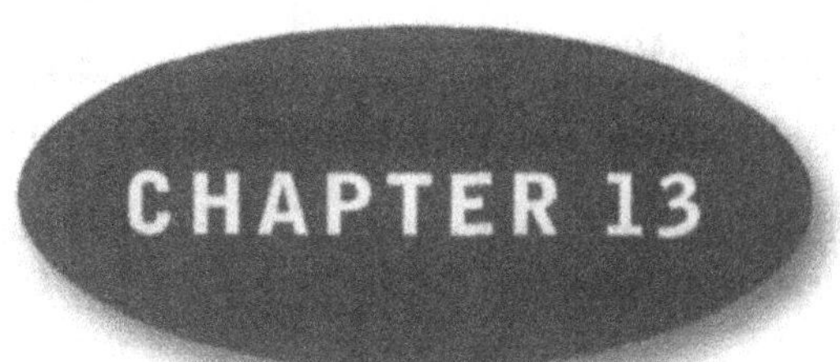

The Lymphatic System and Immunity

Objectives

This chapter will introduce the structures of the lymphatic system and how these structures protect us against invading microorganisms. It will also discuss the inflammatory responses, immunodeficiency disorders, autoimmune disorders, and hypersensitivity disorders.

Keywords:

Lymphatic fluid (lymph)
Lymphatic vessels
Red bone marrow
Thymus gland
Lymph nodules
Lymph nodes
Spleen
Resistance
Phagocytosis
Phagocyte
Chemotaxis
Inflammation
Fever
Immunity

Antigens
Antibodies
Naturally acquired active immunity
Artificially acquired active immunity
Naturally acquired passive immunity
Artificially acquired passive immunity
Acquired immunodeficiency syndrome (AIDS)
Human immunodeficiency virus (HIV)
Bruton's agammaglobulinemia
Chronic fatigue syndrome

DiGeorge syndrome
Hashimoto's thyroiditis
Lymphedema
Mononucleosis
Cytomegalovirus
Epstein-Barr virus
Myasthenia gravis
Systemic lupus erythematosus

13.1 Overview

What Does the Lymphatic System Consist Of?

The lymphatic system consists of fluid called ***lymphatic fluid*** or ***lymph.*** This fluid flows through vessels called ***lymphatic vessels.***

What Is the Function of the Lymphatic System?

The lymphatic system *drains* our interstitial spaces (extracellular spaces), *transports* our fat- or lipid-soluble vitamins (vitamins A, D, E, and K), transports the lipids or fats that we eat, and protects our bodies from invasion of microorganisms by *carrying out immune responses*.

How Does Lymph Flow through Our Body?

Lymphatic vessels begin as lymph capillaries located in between the cells that make up tissues. These capillaries are said to be "blind-ended," meaning that they have little slits at their ends. The interstitial fluid drains or flows into these little slits. Once inside, the capillary fluid is called *lymph fluid* or *lymphatic fluid*. These lymph capillaries drain into larger *lymphatic vessels*. These lymphatic vessels contain *valves* that prevent the backflow of lymphatic fluid. Lymphatic vessels drain or flow into larger lymphatic vessels called *lymphatic trunks*. Lymphatic trunks, in turn, drain into *lymphatic ducts*. The lymphatic ducts drain the fluid into the *right and left subclavian veins*.

What Are the Lymphatic Trunks?

The lymphatic trunks include the following:

- Lumbar trunk
- Intestinal trunk
- Right bronchomediastinal trunk
- Left bronchomediastinal trunk
- Right subclavian trunk
- Left subclavian trunk
- Right jugular trunk
- Left jugular trunk

What drains into the thoracic duct?
The lumbar trunk, intestinal trunk, left bronchomediastinal trunk, left subclavian trunk, and left jugular trunk drain their lymph fluid into the *thoracic duct*.

What drains into the right lymphatic duct?
The right bronchomediastinal trunk, the right subclavian trunk, and the right jugular trunk drain their lymph fluid into the *right lymphatic duct*.

- *Lumbar trunk.* The lumbar trunk receives lymph fluid from the lymphatic vessels of the lower extremities, kidneys, adrenal glands, abdominal wall, and pelvis.
- *Intestinal trunk.* The intestinal trunk receives lymph fluid from the stomach, intestines, pancreas, liver, and spleen.
- *Left bronchomediastinal trunk.* The left bronchomediastinal trunk receives lymph fluid from the left thoracic wall, the left side of the abdominal wall, the diaphragm, the left lung, and the left side of the heart.
- *Left subclavian trunk.* The left subclavian trunk receives lymph fluid from the left upper extremity.

- *Left jugular trunk.* The left jugular trunk receives lymph fluid from the left side of the head and neck.
- *Right bronchomediastinal trunk.* The right bronchomediastinal trunk receives lymph fluid from the right side of the thoracic region, the right and anterior portions of the abdominal wall, the right side of the heart, the right lung, and the liver.
- *Right subclavian trunk.* The right subclavian trunk receives lymph fluid from the right upper extremity.
- *Right jugular trunk.* The right jugular trunk receives lymph from the right side of the head and neck.

Remember: The whole bottom half of the body and the left upper part of the body drain lymphatic fluid into the *thoracic duct*. The right upper portion of the body drains lymphatic fluid into the *right lymphatic duct*.

How Does Lymphatic Fluid Actually Move through the Lymph Vessels?

Lymphatic fluid is actually pushed or "squished" through the vessels every time your muscles contract.
Remember: Blood gets pumped (under pressure) through arteries.
Blood flows through veins.
Blood oozes through capillaries.
Lymphatic fluid gets "squished" or contracted through lymph vessels.

13.2 Lymphatic Tissue

What Is Lymphatic Tissue?

There are two types of lymphatic or lymphoid tissue:

- Primary lymphatic or lymphoid tissue
- Secondary lymphatic or lymphoid tissue

Primary lymphoid tissue includes

1. ***Red bone marrow***, located at the ends of long bones, called the epiphyses, and in the flat bones of the skeleton. The red bone marrow is the place where we make (pre) T lymphocytes and B lymphocytes.
2. ***Thymus gland***, located posterior to (in back of) the sternum and anterior to (in front of) the heart. The thymus gland is the organ where (pre) T lymphocytes mature into T lymphocytes (T cells) and is a site that plays an important role in our immune responses.

Secondary lymphoid tissue includes

1. *Lymph nodules.* **Lymph nodules** are small, oval-shaped clusters of lymphoid tissue. Lymph nodules are located in the mucous membranes and are known as *mucosa-associated lymphoid tissue*, or *MALT*. Lymph nodes fight against foreign substances by being involved in the immune response.

What would be examples of lymph nodules?
Examples of lymph nodules include the *tonsils* and the *adenoids*. These lymph nodules provide protection against invaders that are ingested or inhaled.

2. *Lymph nodes.* **Lymph nodes** are larger bean-shaped structures. These structures are located along the lymphatic vessels. Lymph nodes are located throughout the lymphatic system, although the areas of the axilla, groin, and mammary glands contain large quantities of lymph nodes.
   - *Afferent lymphatic vessels.* Lymphatic fluid travels *into* the lymph nodes through afferent lymphatic vessels.
   - *Efferent lymphatic vessels.* Lymphatic fluid travels *out of* the lymph nodes through efferent lymphatic vessels.

Remember: E for exit, E for efferent.

3. *Spleen.* The ***spleen*** is the largest kind of lymph tissue, although it is still secondary. The spleen is one of our largest organs and is referred to as "the lymph node of the blood." It is located lateral and inferior to the stomach. The spleen contains two types of tissue or pulp.
   - *Red pulp* is a place where bacteria and worn-out or dead red blood cells (erythrocytes) get phagocytosed.
   - *White pulp* is the place where B lymphocytes (B cells) become plasma cells. White pulp functions in immunity.

13.3 Resistance and Immunity

What Is Resistance?

Resistance is our body's ability to defend itself against disease processes or pathogens. There are two forms of resistance:

- *Nonspecific resistance*, which deals with a wide variety of responses against pathogens
- *Specific resistance*, which deals with immunity

How Does Nonspecific Resistance Work?

Nonspecific resistance plays a role in our *first line of defense*. Our first line of defense is to prevent microorganisms from entering the body.

There are two types: mechanical protection and chemical protection.

What is mechanical protection?

1. *Mechanical protection* would include the following:
   - *Skin* (with no cuts, burns, or cracks) creates a barrier to the external environment.
   - *Lacrimal apparatus* (tear ducts and tears) flushes the eyes.
   - *Saliva* has a slightly acidic pH.
   - *Mucus and cilia* trap dust and foreign debris.
   - *Urine flow* flushes out the bladder and urethra.
   - *Defecation* (diarrhea) removes microorganisms from the lower digestive tract.
   - *Vomiting* removes microorganisms from the upper digestive tract.

What is chemical protection?

2. *Chemical protection* would include
   - *Sebum* is the oil secreted from sebaceous glands in the skin. This sebum has a low pH.
   - *Lysozyme* is one of the components of sweat. Lysozyme has antimicrobial properties.
   - *Gastric juice* contains hydrochloric acid (secreted by parietal cells in the stomach). Gastric juice has a pH of 1 to 3. This helps kill many microorganisms that are ingested with food and drink.
   - *Vaginal secretions* have a low pH (are acidic). This helps to kill many microorganisms.

What Is Phagocytosis and How Does It Occur?

Phagocytosis is the condition of a cell eating. ***Phagocytes*** fight infection by engulfing foreign cells and microorganisms that have evaded the body's first line of defense. Phagocytes include neutrophils and monocytes, which are the most active in our blood. These phagocytes have the ability to leave the blood and fight invading pathogens in surrounding tissue.

Phagocytosis occurs in four stages:

1. *Chemotaxis.* ***Chemotaxis*** is the chemical attraction of the phagocytes to the area of infection or colonization of pathogen.
2. *Adherence.* In this phase, the phagocyte attaches itself to the microorganisms.
3. *Ingestion.* In this phase, the phagocyte's plasma membrane encircles the microorganism (pseudopods), engulfs it, and pulls the microorganism into its cytosol, creating a phagosome.
4. *Killing.* In the cytosol, the phagosome merges with a lysosome. This lysosome contains enzymes that will kill the microorganisms.

What Is Inflammation?

Inflammation occurs when the cells of a particular area of the body become damaged, injured, or infected by microorganisms, chemical agents, or physical agents.

What are the signs and symptoms of inflammation?
The signs and symptoms of inflammation include

- *Redness.* Blood vessels dilate, allowing more blood containing white blood cells into the area so that they can begin fighting the infections. Platelets in blood help to stop bleeding by forming clots and proteins to start replacing the damaged tissue.
- *Swelling.* This can result because of vasodilation and an increase in the permeability of the blood vessels.
- *Pain.* The increase in fluid irritates pain receptors.
- *Heat.* Because there is an increase in blood supply to the area, the area will feel hot.
- *Loss of function.* A joint in the inflamed area will feel stiff and painful. It will be unable to move properly. Loss of function will also prevent the spreading of infection.

What Is a Fever?

A ***fever*** is an increase in body temperature. When a person has a fever, he or she is called *febrile*. Fevers can be the result of infections caused by bacteria or viruses. Fevers will speed up the body's ability to heal itself, and in some cases will inhibit the growth of microorganisms and activate phagocytes to attack and kill microorganisms.

What Is Immunity?

Immunity is the specific resistance to disease. This process involves the production of lymphocytes (B lymphocytes and T lymphocytes) and antibodies in order to combat specific antigens.

What Are Immune Responses?

Immune responses include cell-mediated immunity and antibody-mediated immunity.

- *Cell-mediated immunity* is the destruction of antigens by T cells (T lymphocytes). Cell-mediated immunity fights against parasites, fungi, and some forms of cancer and attacks foreign tissue transplants. *Remember:* Cell-mediated immunity always involves cells attacking cells.
- *Antibody-mediated immunity* is the destruction of antigens by antibodies. Antibody-mediated immunity (also called humoral immunity) fights extracellular pathogens, such as bacteria. *Remember:* Antibody-mediated immunity involves the antibody binding to the antigens, making them clump together so that phagocytes can destroy them.

What Are Antigens?

Antigens are chemicals that our antibodies recognize when they enter the body. *Epitopes*, or *antigen determinants*, are parts of an antigen molecule that trigger an immune response.

What Are Antibodies?

Antibodies (also called immunoglobulins) are proteins that combine with the antigens. Antibodies are categorized based on their chemical structure.

- *IgG* is the most abundant and can pass from mother to fetus. IgG recognizes viruses and bacteria.
- *IgA* provides localized protection on mucous membranes and in breast milk, sweat, tears, and saliva, preventing pathogens from entering the body.
- *IgM* is a large antibody that binds to bacteria and incompatible blood cells. It is found in blood and lymph and is secreted by plasma cells after the initial infection by the antigen.
- *IgD* is found on the plasma membranes of B lymphocytes and activates the activity of the B lymphocytes.
- *IgE* is found in mucous membranes and is involved in allergic reactions and infections by parasitic worms.

What Is Acquired Immunity?

Acquired immunity is immunity that we can gain throughout our lives. There are four types:

1. *Naturally acquired active immunity* develops when a person is naturally exposed to a pathogen, becomes sick, and actively makes antibodies against the pathogen.
2. *Artificially acquired active immunity* develops when a person receives a vaccine. The person is injected with the pathogen. Thus, the person acquires the pathogen artificially, but will make antibodies against it.
3. *Naturally acquired passive immunity* develops when a person gets immunity from his or her mother, either through the placenta or through breast milk. The person acquires the pathogen naturally but fights it with the antibodies that he or she passively received from his or her mother.
4. *Artificially acquired passive immunity* develops when a person gets an injection of antibodies.

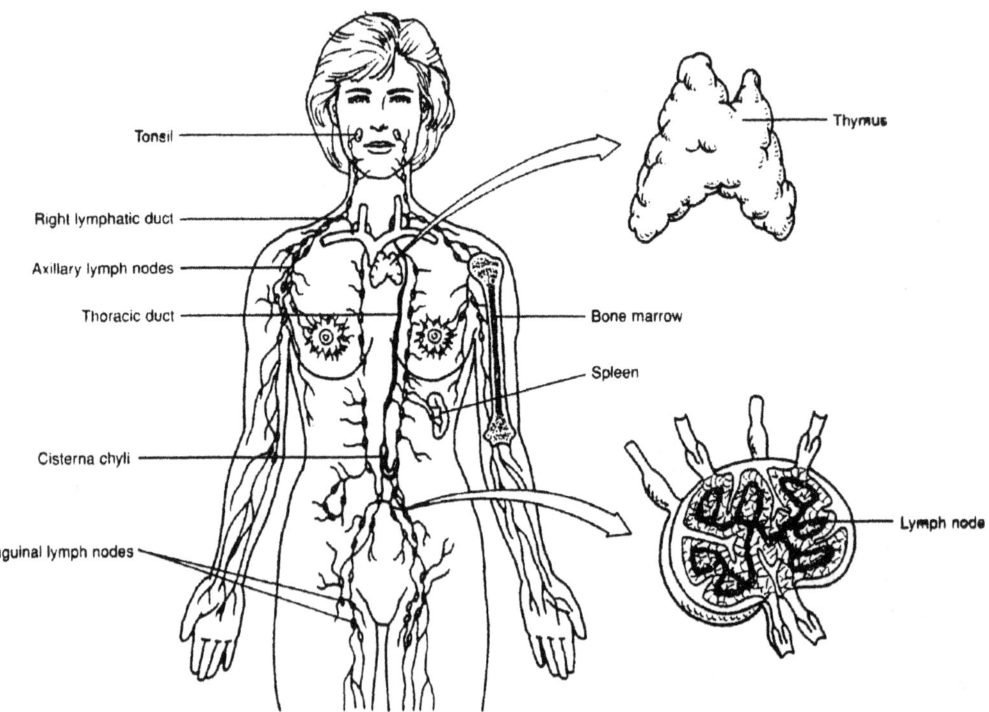

Figure 13.1 Representation of the immune system as a whole.

13.4 Disorders That Affect the Immune System

What Are Some Disorders That Affect the Immune System?

Acquired Immunodeficiency Syndrome

Acquired immunodeficiency syndrome, or ***AIDS***, is caused by the ***human immunodeficiency virus,*** or ***HIV***. This retrovirus targets T cells and kills the T cells, weakening the immune system and making the body more susceptible to a secondary infection. Secondary opportunistic infections include Pneumocystis carinii pneumonia, cytomegalovirus, *Candida albicans* (a fungal infection), toxoplasmosis, histoplasmosis, Kaposi's sarcoma, and non-Hodgkin's lymphoma (two forms of cancer).

What are the signs and symptoms associated with acquired immunodeficiency syndrome?
The signs and symptoms include a T cell count below 200 (400 would be normal); fever; weight loss; herpetic ulcers of the mouth, skin, and genitals; yeast infections of the mouth, vagina, and esophagus; meningitis; and encephalitis.

Bruton's Agammaglobulinemia

Bruton's agammaglobulinemia is more dominant in males. This X-linked chromosome disorder is characterized by the absence of plasma cells (B cells). Because of the absence of immunoglobulins resulting from the lack of B cells, the individual can have recurrent bacterial infections.

Chronic Fatigue Syndrome

With ***chronic fatigue syndrome***, the individual feels tired constantly. This tiredness cannot be relieved by rest. The cause of chronic fatigue syndrome is unknown. The Epstein-Barr virus (which causes mononucleosis) may be a possible cause.

What are the signs and symptoms associated with chronic fatigue syndrome?
The signs and symptoms of chronic fatigue syndrome include severe fatigue and tiredness, fever, body aches, joint pain, loss of or disrupted sleep, tender lymph nodes, and depression.

DiGeorge Syndrome

DiGeorge syndrome is a congenital condition that causes hypoplasia of the thymus gland, resulting in T-lymphocyte deficiency (lymphopenia). Because of the deficiency of T cells, the individual can have recurrent fungal and viral infections.

Hashimoto's Thyroiditis

Hashimoto's thyroiditis is an autoimmune condition affecting the thyroid gland. This condition is caused by antithyroglobulin antibodies. These antibodies affect the thyroid follicles, resulting in hypothyroidism or myxedema.

Lymphedema

Lymphedema is a condition in which lymph nodes become blocked. Lymphedema can be caused by trauma to the vessels, tumors, infections caused by parasites, cellulitis caused by skin infections, radiation therapy, or surgical removal and biopsies of lymph nodes and lymphatic vessels.

What are the signs and symptoms associated with lymphedema?
The signs and symptoms of lymphedema include swelling, especially in the upper and lower extremities.

Mononucleosis

Also known as the "kissing disease," ***mononucleosis*** is spread by saliva, sneezing, and coughing. ***Cytomegalovirus*** (CMV) and the ***Epstein-Barr virus*** cause mononucleosis.

What are the signs and symptoms associated with mononucleosis?
Signs and symptoms include sore throat; swollen, tender lymph nodes; severe fatigue; weakness; and cephalgia (headache).

Myasthenia Gravis

Myasthenia gravis is an autoimmune disease affecting the acetylcholine receptors at the neuromuscular junction. This disease normally affects women between the ages of 20 and 40 and men over the age of 60.

What are the signs and symptoms associated with myasthenia gravis?
The signs and symptoms of myasthenia gravis include weakness of skeletal muscles, especially muscles innervated by cranial nerves and muscles of the extremities.

Systemic Lupus Erythematosus

Systemic lupus erythematosus, or SLE, is commonly called just *lupus*. This autoimmune disease can affect many organs of the body. These individuals will produce antibodies that attack their own cells and tissues. Women are affected more than men. The cause of lupus is unknown, although some drugs or bacterial infections can be the cause.

What are the signs and symptoms associated with systemic lupus erythematosus?

The signs and symptoms of systemic lupus erythematosus include nausea, loss of weight, anemia, fatigue, aches, fever, arthritis, paresthesia of the upper and lower phalanges, cephalgia, seizures, chest pain, shortness of breath, and a rash that looks like a "butterfly on the face."

Chapter 13 Review Questions

Fill In the Blank

1. Lymphatic fluid is located in ____________________.
2. Lymphatic vessels begin as blind-ended lymph ________________.
3. Lymphatic vessels drain into lymphatic ______________________.
4. Lymphatic trunks drain into _______________________.
5. Ducts drain into the _____________________________.
6. Red bone marrow is a form of _________________ lymphoid tissue.
7. The lymphatic tissue where T cells mature is called the ___________________.
8. Lymph nodules that are located in the mucous membranes are also known as _________.
9. Large "bean-shaped" structures are known as ___________________.
10. Clusters of lymphoid tissue are called ___________________.
11. Lymphatic fluid travels into the lymph nodes by ___________________.
12. Lymphatic fluid travels out of the lymph nodes by ___________________.
13. The largest lymph organ is the _________________.
14. In the spleen, white pulp is the place where B cells become _________________.
15. In the spleen, red pulp is the place where dead or worn-out ______________ are phagocytosed.
16. The body's ability to defend itself against pathogens is called ____________.
17. Gastric juice is a form of _________________ resistance.
18. The condition of a cell eating is called ___________________.
19. Neutrophils and monocytes are examples of _________________.
20. A disease-causing organism is called a(n) ___________________.

True/False

21. The chemical attraction of phagocytes to an area of infection is called attraction.
22. When pseudopods engulf a microorganism, it is called ingestion.
23. Redness is a sign of inflammation.

24. An immune response would include cell-mediated immunity.

25. Lymphatic fluid is actually pushed or "squished" through the lymphatic vessels.

26. Swelling is not a symptom of inflammation.

27. Antibodies are chemicals that our antigens recognize when they enter the body.

28. IgG is an antibody that can be passed from mother to fetus.

29. T cells are T lymphocytes.

30. Our first line of defense includes our skin and mucous membranes.

Multiple Choice

31. The chemical attraction of phagocytes to the area of infection is called __________.
    A. chemotaxis
    B. adherence
    C. ingestion
    D. killing
    E. pseudopods

32. When the digestive enzymes contained in the lysosomes cause the death of the pathogen, __________ occur(s).
    A. chemotaxis
    B. adherence
    C. ingestion
    D. killing
    E. pseudopods

33. When the plasma membrane of the cell encircles the microorganism, __________ occur(s).
    A. chemotaxis
    B. adherence
    C. ingestion
    D. killing
    E. pseudopods

34. When the phagocyte attaches to the microbe, __________ occurs.
    A. chemotaxis
    B. adherence
    C. ingestion
    D. killing
    E. pseudopods

35. What are "false feet"?
    A. pseudopods
    B. adherence
    C. ingestion
    D. killing
    E. chemotaxis

Matching

36. Epstein-Barr
37. Artificially acquired active immunity
38. Naturally acquired passive immunity
39. Artificially acquired passive immunity
40. Mononucleosis
41. Lupus
42. Bruton's agammaglobulinemia
43. Hashimoto's thyroiditis
44. DiGeorge syndrome
45. Chronic fatigue syndrome
46. Lymphedema
47. AIDS
48. Myasthenia gravis
49. HIV
50. Naturally acquired active immunity

    A. Virus that causes mononucleosis
    B. Autoimmune disease that affects many organs
    C. Affects acetylcholine receptors
    D. Kissing disease
    E. Blocked lymph nodes
    F. Affects the thyroid gland
    G. Hypoplasia of the thymus gland
    H. Severe tiredness and fatigue
    I. Absence of B cells because of an X-linked disorder
    J. Virus that causes AIDS
    K. Syndrome caused by the human immunodeficiency virus
    L. Develops with an injection of antibodies
    M. Immunity from mother
    N. Immunity caused by a vaccine
    O. Person gets sick and produces antibodies against the pathogen

Chapter 13: Review Questions and Answers

Fill In the Blank Answers

1. Lymphatic vessels
2. Capillaries
3. Trunks
4. Lymphatic ducts
5. Subclavian veins
6. Primary
7. Thymus gland
8. Mucosa-associated lymphoid tissue

9. Lymph nodes
10. Lymph nodules
11. Afferent lymphatic vessels
12. Efferent lymphatic vessels
13. Spleen
14. Plasma cells
15. Red blood cells
16. Resistance
17. Nonspecific
18. Phagocytosis
19. Phagocytes
20. Pathogen

True/False Answers

21. False
22. True
23. True
24. True
25. True
26. False
27. False
28. True
29. True
30. True

Multiple Choice Answers

31. A
32. D
33. C
34. B
35. A

Matching Answers

36. A
37. N
38. M
39. L
40. D
41. B
42. I
43. F
44. G
45. H
46. E
47. K
48. C
49. J
50. O

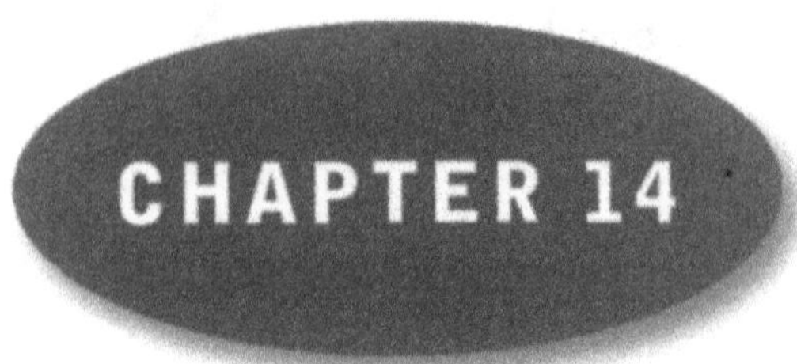

The Respiratory System

Objectives

This chapter introduces the structures and functions of the respiratory system. It also discusses pathologies and disorders of these structures.

Keywords:

Nose
Pharynx
Larynx
Epiglottis
Trachea
Bronchi
Bronchioles
Alveoli
Otorhinolaryngology
Rhinoplasty
Tracheostomy
Intubation
Allergic rhinitis
Asthma
Atelectasis
Bronchitis
Chronic obstructive pulmonary disease (COPD)
Hypoxia
Emphysema
Pneumoconiosis
Silicosis
Asbestosis
Anthracosis
Pneumonia
Lobar pneumonia
Bronchopneumonia
Interstitial pneumonia
Pneumocystis pneumonia
Aspiration pneumonia
Pneumothorax
Severe acute respiratory syndrome (SARS)
Tuberculosis

14.1 Overview

How Do the Cardiovascular System and the Respiratory System Work Together?

The cardiovascular system and the respiratory system work together in order to supply needed oxygen to the various cells of the body and to eliminate harmful carbon dioxide from these cells.

How do the cardiovascular system and respiratory system work together?
The cardiovascular system and the respiratory system work together by

- Providing the gaseous exchange of CO_2 (carbon dioxide) when we exhale and O_2 (oxygen) when we inhale (respiratory system).
- Transporting or carrying these respiratory gases throughout the body (cardiovascular system).

Remember: Failure of either will drastically disrupt homeostasis and cause necrosis (cell death) by either oxygen starvation or carbon dioxide intoxication.

The exchange of respiratory gases takes place between the atmosphere (the air we breathe), the blood, and the cells of the body.

How Does This Exchange Take Place?

Respiratory exchange occurs through

- Breathing or ventilation
- External or pulmonary respiration
- Internal or tissue respiration

What Structures Make Up the Respiratory System?

The respiratory system is composed of the nose, the pharynx (throat), the larynx (voice box), the trachea (windpipe), the three types of bronchi, and the two lungs. These structures are divided into two categories:

1. The *upper respiratory system*, which includes the nose and pharynx
2. The *lower respiratory system*, which includes the larynx, trachea, bronchi, and structures of the lungs

What Is the Nose Constructed Of?

The ***nose*** is constructed of cartilage lined with mucous membranes on the inside and covered with skin on the outside. These structures moisten and warm the incoming air that is inhaled. This area also filters dust and debris out of the air and receives stimuli for the olfactory (cranial nerve I) receptors. The frontal bone, maxilla, and nasal bone make up the framework of the nose. The nose is also a resonating chamber that modifies sound for speaking.

What Is the Pharynx?

The ***pharynx*** is also called the *throat*. This muscular tube is lined with mucous membranes. The pharynx has three sections:

1. Nasopharynx
2. Oropharynx
3. Laryngopharynx

What Is the Larynx?

The ***larynx*** is also called the *voice box*. This structure connects the pharynx to the trachea. It is composed of thyroid cartilage and is called the *"Adam's apple."* The larynx contains the ***epiglottis***. The epiglottis is a structure that prevents food, drink, and saliva from entering the larynx every time we swallow. Also contained in the larynx are the *vocal cords*.

What Is the Trachea?

The ***trachea***, which is also called the windpipe, connects the larynx to the bronchi.

What Is the Trachea Composed Of?

The trachea is composed of *cricoid cartilage* and lined with ciliated epithelial cells that move debris and mucus up to the pharynx, where they are coughed up and spit out or swallowed. As the individual inhales, the mucus will trap potentially harmful viruses and bacteria. When the mucus is swallowed, the stomach acid contained in digestive juice will destroy these harmful organisms.

How Would Smoking Affect These Structures?

Smoking for many years can destroy the cilia or the epithelium. People who do so will have to cough to move the mucus to the pharynx, thus causing the "smoker's cough."

What Are the Bronchi?

The trachea splits into primary ***bronchi***. The right and left primary bronchi split into secondary bronchi and then tertiary bronchi. The bronchi consist of rings of cartilage.

What Are Bronchioles?

Bronchioles are structures that branch off from the tertiary bronchi. Bronchioles are composed of smooth muscle.
Remember: Bronchi are made of cartilage. Bronchioles are made of smooth muscle.

What Are the Lungs and Where Are They Located?

The ***lungs*** are located in the thoracic cavity and are surrounded and protected by a pleural membrane.

- The right lung has three lobes, the superior, middle, and inferior lobes.
- The left lung has two lobes, the superior and inferior lobes, and a cardiac notch (a depression for the heart).

The tertiary bronchi supply sections of the lungs called *bronchopulmonary segments*. Each of these segments contains small spaces called *lobules*. These lobules contain arterioles, venules, lymphatic vessels, terminal bronchioles, alveolar ducts, alveolar sacs, and alveoli. Figure 14.1 shows the entire respiratory system, and Figure 14.2 gives a more detailed view of the trachea, lungs, and bronchial tree.

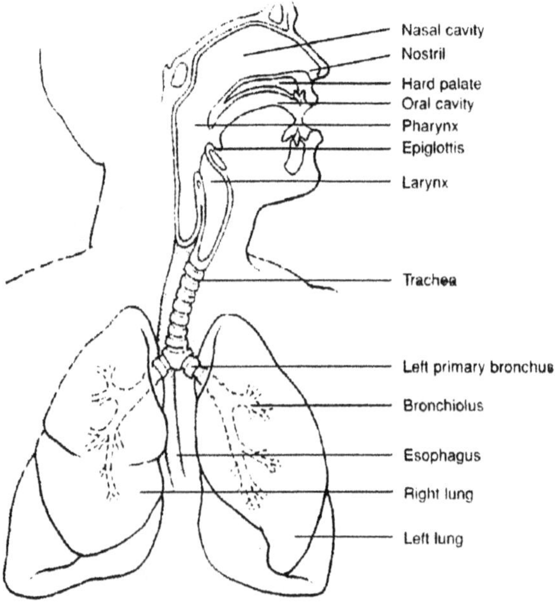

Figure 14.1 The respiratory system.

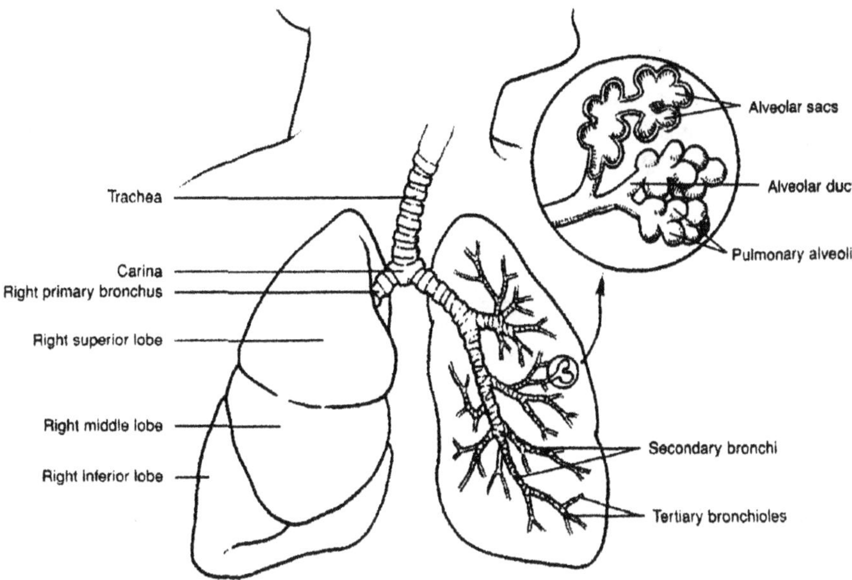

Figure 14.2 The trachea, lungs, and bronchial tree.

What Are the Alveoli?

The ***alveoli*** are very small structures made up of squamous pulmonary epithelial cells, septal cells, and macrophages. The alveoli are the places where the atmospheric gas exchange (CO_2 and O_2) across the alveolar-capillary membrane takes place. The *septal cells* secrete *surfactant*, which prevents the lungs from collapsing during expiration.

What Is the Path That Air Travels When It Is Inhaled?

The air follows this path:

1. Nose and mouth
2. Pharynx
3. Larynx
4. Trachea
5. Primary bronchi
6. Secondary bronchi
7. Tertiary bronchi
8. Bronchioles
9. Terminal bronchioles
10. Respiratory bronchioles
11. Alveolar ducts
12. Alveolar sacs
13. Alveoli

What Are the Mechanisms of Breathing?

The process of breathing occurs when there is an exchange between the atmosphere and the alveoli of the lungs.

What Is Inspiration?

Inspiration, or inhalation, is bringing air into the lungs. This occurs when there are contractions of inspiratory muscles, such as the diaphragm and the external intercostal muscles of the ribs. As these muscles contract, the size of the thoracic cavity increases, thus decreasing intrathoracic pressure. This allows the air to move along the gradient from the atmosphere to the lungs and into the alveoli.

What Is Expiration?

Expiration, or exhalation, occurs when alveolar pressure is greater than atmospheric pressure. This process occurs when the diaphragm relaxes and the internal intercostal muscles of the ribs contract. This increase in alveolar pressure moves air out of the lungs and respiratory system into the atmosphere.

What Is the Function of Surfactant?

Surfactant is a combination of phospholipids and lipoproteins synthesized by alveolar septal cells. Lung surfactant prevents the lungs from collapsing with each exhalation.

What Is the Branch of Medicine That Deals with the Diagnosis and Treatment of Diseases of the Ear, Nose, and Throat?

The branch of medicine that deals with the diagnosis and treatment of diseases associated with the ear, nose, and throat is called ***otorhinolaryngology***, or ENT (for ears, nose, and throat).

What is Rhinoplasty?

A ***rhinoplasty*** is the surgical alteration of the external structures of the nose for cosmetic or functional reasons. Rhinoplasty is also called a "nose job."

How Can We Bypass an Obstruction of the Trachea?

Two ways of bypassing an obstruction to open the respiratory passageway are a ***tracheostomy*** and ***intubation.***

What is a tracheostomy?
A tracheostomy is an incision into the trachea.

What is intubation?
Intubation is the insertion of a tube into the trachea in order to maintain the airway.

14.2 Respiratory Disorders and Infections

What Are Common Disorders That Can Affect the Respiratory System?

- *Allergies.* A hypersensitivity reaction to many allergens is called ***allergic rhinitis.*** Allergies can be caused by dust, dust mites, and animal dander; seasonal allergies (such as "hay fever") are caused by plant pollen.

What are the signs and symptoms associated with allergies?
The signs and symptoms of allergies include itchy, watery, inflamed red eyes and congestion of the nasal passageways with mucus discharge.

- *Asthma.* ***Asthma***, also known as bronchial asthma, occurs when the bronchioles become inflamed, obstructed, and narrowed. The causes of asthma include allergies to pet dander, dust, cigarette smoke, cold temperatures, and cleaning products.

What are the signs and symptoms associated with asthma?
The signs and symptoms of asthma include wheezing upon expiration, difficulty breathing (dyspnea), coughing, and tightness in the chest.

- *Atelectasis.* ***Atelectasis*** is a collapsed lung. This can be caused by an accumulation of fluid (hydrothorax), blood (hemothorax), air (pneumothorax), or pus (pyothorax) in the pleural cavity. Atelectasis can be caused by tumors, cystic fibrosis, trauma to the thoracic cavity and/or ribs, and chronic obstructive pulmonary disease (COPD).

What are the signs and symptoms associated with atelectasis?
The signs and symptoms of atelectasis are chest pain, anxiety, excessive perspiration (diaphoresis), difficulty breathing (dyspnea), rapid resting heart rate (tachycardia), and bluish discoloration of the skin (cyanosis).

- *Bronchitis.* ***Bronchitis*** is inflammation of the bronchi. It is frequently the result of a cold. Frequent bronchitis can be caused by asthma, emphysema, or smoking. Bronchitis can also be caused by viruses, gastroesophageal reflux disease (GERD), cigarette smoking, and pollutants.

What are the signs and symptoms associated with bronchitis?
The signs and symptoms of bronchitis include difficulty breathing, coughing up yellowish or greenish mucus, fever, chills, wheezing, and rales or crackles (bubbling noises heard when auscultating the lungs).

- *Chronic obstructive pulmonary disease.* ***Chronic obstructive pulmonary disease***, or ***COPD***, is a group of diseases or disorders that obstruct the flow of air into the lungs. These disorders include asthma, bronchitis, and emphysema. The causes of COPD include smoking and environmental irritants, such as pollutants in the air.

What are the signs and symptoms associated with COPD?
The signs and symptoms of COPD include difficulty breathing, tiredness, coughing (frequently), and hypoxia. *Remember:* ***Hypoxia*** is a decrease in oxygen to the cells.

- *Emphysema.* ***Emphysema*** is a chronic condition in which the walls of the alveoli are damaged and the air spaces become dilated. Causes of emphysema include smoking cigarettes, secondhand cigarette smoke, environmental pollutants, and industrial or occupational pollutants, such as coal dust, wood dust, and grain dust.

What are the signs and symptoms associated with emphysema?
The signs and symptoms of emphysema include frequent, chronic coughing, tiredness, shortness of breath, and weight loss.

- *Pneumoconiosis.* ***Pneumoconiosis*** is caused by inhaling environmental and industrial or occupational airborne dust particles.

What are examples of conditions that can cause pneumoconiosis?
Examples include silicosis, asbestosis, and anthracosis. The causes of these forms of pneumoconiosis are

1. ***Silicosis*** is caused by prolonged exposure to and inhalation of silica dust from sandblasting, cement work, and/or ceramic work.
2. ***Asbestosis*** is caused by prolonged exposure to and inhalation of asbestos fibers. This can lead to bronchogenic carcinoma and mesothelioma (pleural cancer).
3. ***Anthracosis***, also called "coal miner's pneumoconiosis" or "black lung," is caused by the inhalation of coal dust.

What are the signs and symptoms associated with pneumoconiosis?
The signs and symptoms of pneumoconiosis include difficulty breathing, rapid breathing, and continued respiratory infection. The types of pneumoconiosis discussed here are summarized in Table 14.1.

TABLE 14.1 Types of Pneumoconiosis— Examples

Silicosis	Inhalation of silica from sandblasting, cement work, and ceramic work
Asbestosis	Inhalation of asbestos fibers
Anthracosis	Coal miner's lung; occurs with the inhalation of coal dust

Remember: In pneumoconiosis, scar tissue replaces the normal tissue in the alveoli of the lungs.

- *Pneumonia.* ***Pneumonia*** is inflammation of the lungs as a result of an infection. These infections can be caused by bacteria, viruses, or fungi. There are different types of pneumonia:
  1. ***Lobar pneumonia*** is normally caused by a streptococcus infection and affects part of or the entire lobe.
  2. ***Bronchopneumonia*** can be caused by a variety of microorganisms and affects the bronchioles and alveoli.
  3. ***Interstitial pneumonia*** is the result of a viral infection (influenza).
  4. ***Pneumocystis pneumonia*** is the result of infection with *Pneumocystis carinii.* This opportunistic infection usually occurs in individuals who have AIDS.
  5. ***Aspiration pneumonia*** occurs when the contents of the stomach are vomited and aspirated into the lungs.

What are the signs and symptoms associated with a pneumonia?
The signs and symptoms of pneumonia include fever, chills, tiredness, fatigue, difficulty breathing, chest myalgia (muscle pain), and yellowish, green, or rust-colored sputum.

The types of pneumonia discussed here are summarized in Table 14.2.

TABLE 14.2 Types of Pneumonia

Pneumonia	Inflammation of the lungs caused by an infection
Lobar pneumonia	Caused by a strep infection
Bronchopneumonia	Caused by an infection of the bronchioles and alveoli
Interstitial pneumonia	Caused by influenza
Pneumocystis pneumonia	Opportunistic infection, usually occurring in AIDS patients
Aspiration pneumonia	Occurs when stomach contents are vomited into the lungs

- *Pneumothorax.* ***Pneumothorax*** occurs when air enters the thoracic cavity and causes the lung to collapse. Trauma (stabbing or gunshot wounds) and diseases of the respiratory tract can cause a pneumothorax.

What are the signs and symptoms associated with a pneumothorax?
The signs and symptoms of a pneumothorax include sharp pain in the chest, difficulty breathing, and shortness of breath.

- *Severe acute respiratory syndrome.* ***Severe acute respiratory syndrome***, or ***SARS***, is a respiratory condition caused by the coronavirus. This condition is very contagious and can cause severe sickness and even death. The lungs are the target organ of this pathogen.

What are the signs and symptoms associated with SARS?
Signs and symptoms include body aches, fever, chills, cephalgia (headache), and cough.

- *Tuberculosis.* ***Tuberculosis***, or TB, affects the lungs but can spread to other parts of the body. TB is caused and spread by the inhalation of droplets containing *Mycobacterium tuberculosis*. Infection with *M. tuberculosis* begins as a granulomatous inflammatory area called a *Ghon complex*. These granulomas affect the lungs and lymph nodes and are characterized by caseous necrosis. Tuberculosis can spread from the lungs to other parts of the body through the blood (circulatory system). An example of this is Pott's disease, or tuberculosis of the spine.

What are the signs and symptoms associated with TB?
The signs and symptoms of tuberculosis include fever, cough, chills, night sweats, wasting away, and difficulty breathing.

TABLE 14.3 Types of Breathing

Dyspnea	Difficulty breathing (respiration)
Tachypnea	Abnormally fast breathing (respiration)
Bradypnea	Abnormally slow breathing (respiration)
Apnea	Temporary loss of breathing
Eupnea	Normal breathing
Kussmaul respiration	Slow, deep aspirations caused by diabetes
Cheyne-Stokes respiration	Alternating periods of apnea due to disorders of the respiratory centers in the medulla oblongata of the brain or cardiac disorders

Chapter 14 Review Questions

Fill In the Blank

1. The respiratory system provides the gaseous exchange between ______ and ______.
2. The throat is called the ________________.
3. The voice box is called the ________________.
4. The windpipe is called the ________________.
5. The larynx contains ___________, which produce sound.
6. The trachea is composed of ____________________.
7. The larynx is composed of ____________________.
8. Bronchi are composed of ____________________.
9. Bronchioles are composed of ____________________.
10. Alveolar septal cells secrete ________________.

True/False

11. The cardiovascular system and the respiratory system work together.
12. The respiratory system takes in oxygen and eliminates carbon dioxide.
13. Respiration does not take place at the cellular level.
14. The upper respiratory tract consists of the larynx, trachea, and bronchi.
15. The upper respiratory tract consists of the nose and pharynx.
16. The occipital bone forms the framework of the nose.
17. The larynx contains the epiglottis.

18. The larynx contains the vocal cords.
19. The trachea splits into primary bronchi.
20. The bronchi consist of rings of smooth muscle.

Matching

21. Surfactant
22. Rhinoplasty
23. Dyspnea
24. Atelectasis
25. Pneumothorax
26. Pyothorax
27. Hemothorax
28. Cyanosis
29. Bronchitis
30. Diaphoresis
    A. A collapsed lung
    B. Pus in the pleural cavity
    C. Inflammation of the bronchi
    D. Blood in the pleural cavity
    E. Difficulty breathing
    F. Excessive perspiration
    G. Prevents the collapsing of the lung with expiration
    H. Bluish color of the skin
    I. Air in the pleural cavity
    J. Surgical alteration of the nose

Matching

31. Tachypnea
32. Hydrothorax
33. Bradypnea
34. GERD
35. Hypoxia
36. Pneumoconiosis
37. Pneumonia
38. Anthracosis
39. Tuberculosis

40. Asbestosis

A. Fluid in the pleural cavity
B. A decrease in the amount of oxygen going to the cells
C. Abnormally fast breathing
D. A condition caused by the inhalation of airborne dust particles
E. Black lung
F. Abnormally slow breathing
G. A condition caused by *Mycobacterium tuberculosis*
H. A condition caused by prolonged exposure to asbestos fibers
I. Inflammation of the lungs caused by an infection
J. Gastroesophageal reflux disease

Multiple Choice

41. The condition that occurs with prolonged exposure to sandblasting, cement work, and ceramic work is __________.

A. asbestosis
B. anthracosis
C. silicosis
D. pneumonia
E. emphysema

42. Coal miner's pneumoconiosis is __________.

A. asbestosis
B. anthracosis
C. silicosis
D. pneumonia
E. emphysema

43. A chronic condition in which the walls of the alveoli are damaged and the air spaces become dilated is __________.

A. silicosis
B. emphysema
C. asbestosis
D. anthracosis
E. pneumonia

44. The condition that occurs when air enters the thoracic cavity and causes the lung to collapse is __________.

A. emphysema
B. pneumonia
C. asbestosis
D. silicosis
E. pneumothorax

45. The form of pneumonia that is normally caused by a strep infection and affects part of or the entire lobe is __________.

A. bronchopneumonia

B. interstitial pneumonia

C. pneumocystis pneumonia

D. lobar pneumonia

E. aspiration pneumonia

46. The form of pneumonia that is normally caused when the contents of the stomach are vomited into the lungs is __________.

A. aspiration pneumonia

B. interstitial pneumonia

C. pneumocystis pneumonia

D. lobar pneumonia

E. bronchopneumonia

47. The form of pneumonia that is caused by an opportunistic infection and usually occurs in individuals who have AIDS is __________.

A. aspiration pneumonia

B. interstitial pneumonia

C. pneumocystis pneumonia

D. lobar pneumonia

E. bronchopneumonia

48. The form of pneumonia that is the result of a variety of microorganisms affecting the bronchioles and alveoli is __________.

A. aspiration pneumonia

B. pneumocystis pneumonia

C. interstitial pneumonia

D. bronchopneumonia

E. lobar pneumonia

49. *Mycobacterium tuberculosis* causes the disease __________.

A. pneumonia

B. SARS

C. silicosis

D. pneumothorax

E. tuberculosis

50. There is a group of diseases or conditions that obstruct the flow of air into the lungs. These disorders include __________.

A. bronchitis

B. emphysema

C. asthma

D. smoking

E. all of the above

Chapter 14: Review Questions and Answers

Fill In the Blank Answers

1. O_2; CO_2
2. Pharynx
3. Larynx
4. Trachea
5. Vocal cords
6. Cricoid cartilage
7. Thyroid cartilage
8. Cartilage
9. Smooth muscle
10. Surfactant

True/False Answers

11. True
12. True
13. False
14. False
15. True
16. False
17. True
18. True
19. True
20. False

Matching Answers

21. G
22. J
23. E
24. A
25. I
26. B
27. D
28. H
29. C
30. F

Matching Answers

31. C
32. A
33. F
34. J
35. B
36. D
37. I
38. E
39. G
40. H

Multiple Choice Answers

41. C
42. B
43. B
44. E
45. D
46. A
47. C
48. D
49. E
50. E

The Urinary System

Objectives

This chapter will introduce the structures and functions of the urinary system and discuss pathologies and disorders of these structures.

Keywords:

Nephrology

Urology
Kidney
Ureter
Urinary bladder
Urethra
Renal capsule
Adipose capsule
Renal fascia
Hilum
Renal cortex
Renal medulla
Renal pyramids
Renal columns
Renal papillae
Minor calyx
Major calyx
Renal pelvis
Micturition
Renal calculi (kidney stones)
Hematuria
Acute renal failure
Chronic renal failure
Glomerulonephritis
Polycystic kidney disease (PKD)
Pyelonephritis
Urinary tract infection
Nephrotic syndrome
Proteinuria
Hypoalbuminemia

Nephritic syndrome
Oliguria
Azotemia
Goodpasture's syndrome

Cystitis

Nocturia

Polyuria

Uremia

15.1 Overview

What Is the Study of the Anatomy and Physiology of the Kidney and the Diagnosis and Treatment of Pathologies That Can Affect These Structures Called?

The branch of science that deals with the structures associated with the kidney and their functions and pathologies is called ***nephrology.***

What Is the Study of the Anatomy and Physiology of the Urinary System and the Reproductive System Called?

The branch of science that studies the male and female urinary systems and the male reproductive system is called ***urology***.

The branch of science that is associated with the female reproductive system is called *gynecology*.

What Are the Structures That Make Up the Urinary System?

The urinary system consists of

- *Two kidneys.* The two ***kidneys*** are located in the posterior portion of the abdominopelvic cavity. The kidneys filter wastes out of the blood and return needed chemicals and water back to the blood.
- *Two ureters.* The two ***ureters*** send the waste products (urine) to the urinary bladder, where they are stored.
- *Urinary bladder.* The ***urinary bladder*** is located in the pelvic cavity and stores urine until it is ready to be passed out of the body.
- *Urethra.* The ***urethra*** is a tube that eliminates urine from the body. This process is called *urination, voiding*, or *micturation*.

Figure 15.1 shows the structures of the urinary system.

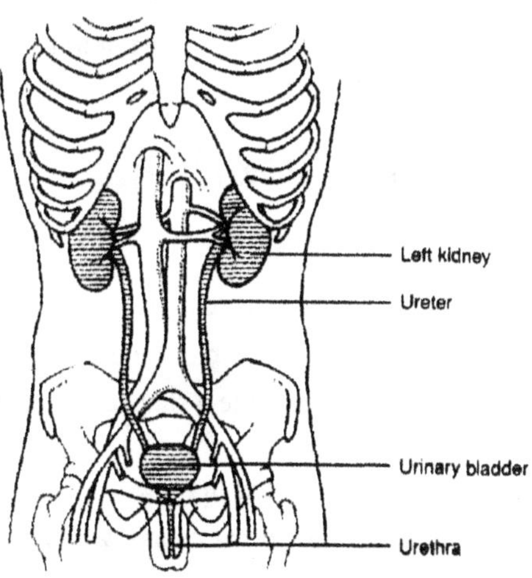

Figure 15.1 The urinary system.

What Are Examples of Waste Products That Are Eliminated or Excreted from the Kidney?

The toxic substances excreted from the kidneys are wastes from the metabolism of foods and excess chemicals in blood. Examples of these chemicals include ammonia, urea, and uric acid.

What Is the Function of the Urinary System?

The urinary system functions by

- Regulating blood volume and blood pressure.
- Stimulating the production of red blood cells by secreting *erythropoietin*.
- Helping in the making of vitamin D. Vitamin D aids in the regulation of calcium homeostasis. It aids in the absorption of calcium in the ileum of the small intestine.

What Happens if There Is a Deficiency of Vitamin D in Children?

If there is a deficiency of vitamin D, the bones will become soft and bend. This condition is called *rickets* in children.

What Happens When There Is a Deficiency of Vitamin D in Adults?

If there is a deficiency of vitamin D in adults, the bones will also become soft. This condition is called *osteomalacia*.

15.2 The Kidneys

What Are the Layers of the Kidneys?

There are three layers that surround each kidney.

- The innermost layer is called the ***renal capsule***. This layer maintains the shape of the kidney.
- The middle layer is called the ***adipose capsule***. This layer provides protection to the kidney.
- The outermost layer is called the ***renal fascia***. This layer anchors the kidney to the abdomen.

What Are the External Structures of the Kidney?

The external medial portion of the kidney has a concave shape. This region is called the ***hilum***. The hilum region is important because the two ureters, the nerves of the kidney, the blood vessels of the kidney, and the lymphatic vessels of the kidney all enter and exit at this region.

What Are the Internal Structures of the Kidney?

The internal structures that make up the kidney include the

- ***Renal cortex.*** This is the outer portion of the kidney.
- ***Renal medulla.*** This is the middle or inner portion of the kidney.
- ***Renal pyramids.*** These are the pyramid- (triangle-) shaped structures located in the middle portion of the kidney.
- ***Renal columns.*** These are the structures located in between the renal pyramids, separating them.
- ***Renal papillae.*** The papillae project into the renal pelvis, which projects into the minor calyx.
- ***Minor calyx.*** The minor calyx or calyces (if there are many) enters the major calyx.
- ***Major calyx.*** The major calyces, in turn, come together and form the renal pelvis.
- ***Renal pelvis.*** This structure collects all the urine from the major calyces and funnels it into the ureters.

How Does Blood Enter and Exit the Kidneys?

Blood enters the kidneys through the *renal artery* and exits through the *renal vein*.

What Is the Nervous Innervation of the Kidneys?

The kidneys are innervated by the *renal plexus* division of the autonomic nervous system.

The structures of the kidney are shown in Figure 15.2.

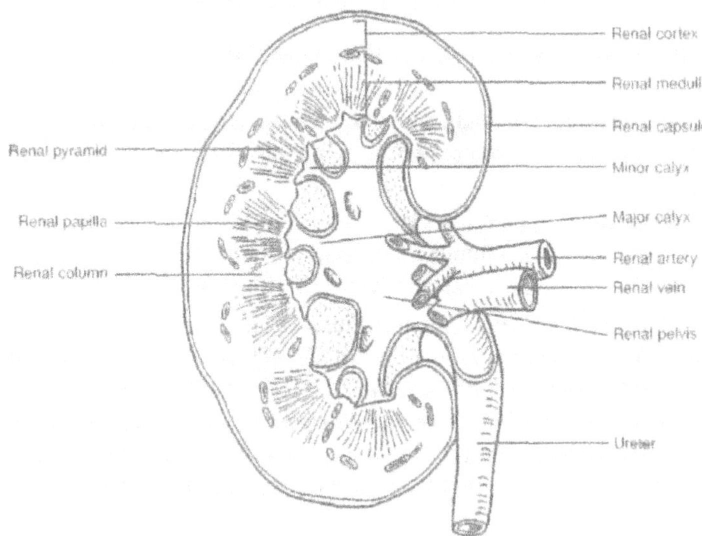

Figure 15.2 The kidney viewed in coronal section.

What Is a Nephron?

The *nephron* is the structural and functional unit of the kidney. There are approximately 1 million nephrons per kidney. The nephrons are located in the pyramids of the renal cortex.

What Structures Make Up the Nephrons?

Nephrons consist of two structures:

1. *Glomerulus.* The glomerulus is a network of capillaries that contain both afferent and efferent arterioles surrounded by the glomerular (Bowman's) capsule.
2. *Glomerular (Bowman's) capsule.* Bowman's capsule is a double-walled cup containing epithelial cells. This cup collects the filtrate from the glomerulus (capillary network). Bowman's capsule is the place where the kidneys filter the blood. This filtering process takes place because of hydrostatic pressure and blood pressure.

Remember: This filtration process enables the nephrons to regulate the chemistry and fluid volume of blood and produce urine.

How Do the Nephrons Filter the Blood?

The walls of the glomerular capsule (Bowman's capsule) contain simple squamous epithelial cells called *podocytes*. These podocytes, along with the endothelial cells of the glomerular capillaries, form a filtration membrane or *endothelial capsular membrane*. The endothelial capsular membrane consists of

- *Endothelial fenestrations (pores) of the glomerulus.* These large pores prevent the passing of blood cells (i.e., red blood cells, white blood cells, and platelets). This layer is composed of a single layer of endothelial cells.

- *Basal lamina.* These structures prevent the passing of large proteins.
- *Slit membranes.* These structures prevent the passing of medium-sized proteins. What is filtered is called *glomerular filtrate* and consists of H_2O, glucose, amino acids, ions, urea, and uric acid.

What Happens after the Filtrate Leaves Bowman's Capsule?

After the filtrate leaves Bowman's capsule, it passes through the following parts:

- *Proximal convoluted tubules.* Proximal convoluted tubules are coiled tubules in the renal cortex. These coils begin at Bowman's capsule, where *reabsorption* and *secretion* of certain ions and molecules occur.
- *Loop of Henle (also called the nephron loop).* The loop of Henle is a loop-shaped tubule that connects the proximal and distal convoluted tubules. The loop of Henle consists of both an ascending limb and a descending limb. These structures reabsorb certain ions and water and secrete urea.
- *Distal convoluted tubules.* The distal convoluted tubules are coiled extensions of the ascending limb of the loop of Henle. These structures are involved in the reabsorption of certain ions and molecules. The distal convoluted tubules converge into *collecting ducts* located in the renal medulla. Collecting ducts travel through the renal pyramids into large *papillary ducts* in the *renal papilla*. Papillary ducts drain into the *minor calyces*. The minor calyces drain urine into the *major calyces*. The major calyces drain into the *renal pelvis*, where the urine leaves the kidney through the *ureters*.

What Are the Ureters, and What Is Their Function?

The ureters are located in the posterior abdominal cavity (retroperitoneal). There are two ureters, one for each kidney. The ureters transport urine from the urinary pelvis of the kidney to the urinary bladder. The action of transporting the urine from the renal pelvis to the urinary bladder occurs mainly by peristalsis, but also by hydrostatic pressure and gravity.

What Is the Urinary Bladder, Where Is It Located, and What Is Its Function?

The urinary bladder is located in the pelvic cavity. Its function is storing urine until *urination (micturation)* occurs. The bottom portion of the urinary bladder contains an area called the *trigone*. This trigone region is a triangular area where the ureters enter the urinary bladder. The urinary bladder is composed of mucosa (with rugae), lamina propria, muscularis (made up of a detrusor muscle), and a serosa. The structure of the urinary bladder is shown in Figure 15.3.

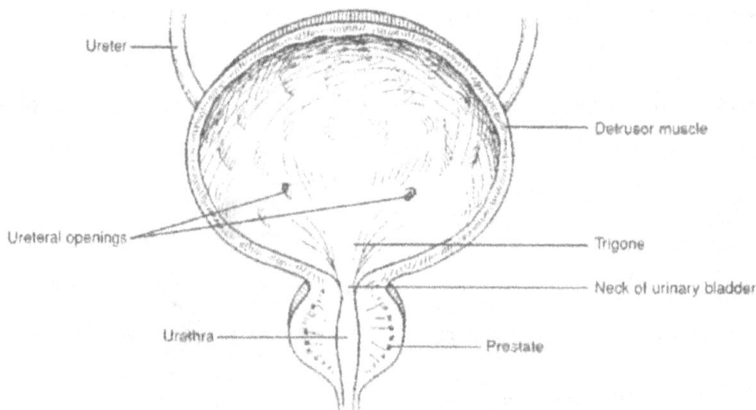

Figure 15.3 The urinary bladder.

What Is the Process of Urination, and How Does It Occur?

The *urethra* is a tube that expels urine from the body. It contains an internal urethral sphincter (it is like a muscular door) and an external urethral sphincter. The *internal urethral sphincter* is located around the opening of the urethra and is made of smooth muscle. The *external urethral sphincter* constricts to close the lumen of the urethra, enabling the urinary bladder to fill up. The external urethral sphincter is made of skeletal muscle.

Urination, also called *voiding*, is the process by which urine leaves the urinary bladder. The physiological process of expelling urine from the urinary bladder, which includes electrical nerve impulses from the nervous system and muscular contractions, is called ***micturation***.

In males, the urethra also serves as a duct for the ejaculation of semen and sperm. (This will be explained in Chapter 16, "The Reproductive System").

What Is Urine Made Up Of?

Urine is mostly made up of water (95 percent) and solutes, both organic and inorganic material (such as certain drugs) (about 5 percent).

15.3 Pathophysiology of the Urinary System—Some Common Diseases and Disorders of the Urinary System

What Are Kidney Stones?

Kidney stones, also called ***renal calculi***, can be the result of gout, a defect in one or both ureters, frequent urinary tract infections, urine that is very concentrated, or not drinking enough water. Many times the crystals of salts in the urine solidify or turn hard, causing a stone. Lytic metastases, hyperparathyroidism (which can cause hypercalcemia), and even a person's diet can cause a kidney stone.

Kidney stones are more common in males than in females. Kidney stones are mostly acid stones, being made of either *calcium oxalate* or *calcium phosphate crystals*. However, some kidney stones are alkaline stones, being made of *ammonium magnesium phosphate*.

What are the signs and symptoms of kidney stones?

The signs and symptoms of kidney stones include back pain and abdominal pain, which can be very severe, nausea, fever, urgency to void, and blood in the urine (***hematuria***).

What Is Acute Renal Failure?

Acute renal failure is the sudden, immediate loss of kidney function.

Acute renal failure can be caused by low blood pressure (hypotension), trauma to the kidneys, burns, bleeding, dehydration, infections, allergies, poison, kidney stones, an enlarged prostate, childbirth, and alcoholism.

What are the signs and symptoms of acute renal failure?

Acute renal failure presents with a decrease in the output of urine, no urine, an increase in the output of urine, inflammation (edema) of the extremities, back or abdominal pain, high blood pressure (hypertension), and an increase in potassium levels during urinalysis.

What Is Chronic Renal Failure?

Chronic renal failure occurs over a large period of time. The kidneys will slowly stop functioning. In some cases, the patient will have no symptoms (be *asymptomatic*).

Chronic renal failure can be caused by high blood pressure (hypertension), diabetes, obstructed ureters, renal calculi (kidney stones), glomerulonephritis, and polycystic kidney disease.

What Is Glomerulonephritis?

Glomerulonephritis is the inflammation of the glomerulus of the nephron. This inflammation is commonly the result of a streptococcal infection, most commonly *Streptococcus pyogenes*.

S. pyogenes gives off a toxin causing an antigen-antibody response, resulting in the inflammation of the glomerulus. If it is severe and untreated, scar tissue can form, causing chronic renal failure.

What are the signs and symptoms of glomerulonephritis?
Glomerulonephritis will present with bloody urine (hematuria), high blood pressure (hypertension), nausea, anemia, tiredness, seizures, and even a coma.

Table 15.1 lists the different types of glomerulonephritis.

TABLE 15.1 Types of Glomerulonephritis

CONDITION	CHARACTERISTIC
Acute glomerulonephritis	Is benign and resolves quickly
Rapid progressive glomerulonephritis	Is quick to advance and can lead to death
Chronic glomerulonephritis	Is long term, taking years or even decades to cause damage
Diffuse glomerulonephritis	Affects most or all of the glomeruli
Focal glomerulonephritis	Affects only some of the glomeruli
Segmental glomerulonephritis	Affects some of the capillaries in a given glomerulus

What Is Polycystic Kidney Disease?

Polycystic kidney disease, or ***PKD***, is a genetic disorder that is inherited from one parent. This disease occurs between the ages of 15 and 30 years. In polycystic kidney disease, the kidneys become enlarged, and the tissue is partially replaced by cysts. This condition develops rather slowly. Signs and symptoms become more severe over time.

What are the signs and symptoms of PKD?
Polycystic kidney disease presents with hypertension (high blood pressure), blood in the urine (hematuria), anemia, back and abdominal pain, fatigue and tiredness, the formation of renal calculi, and even liver disease.

What Is Pyelonephritis?

Pyelonephritis is a bacterial infection of the kidney tissue (parenchyma). It can be either acute or chronic. Pyelonephritis is a type of *urinary tract infection* that starts in the urinary bladder and spreads to either one or both kidneys.

Pyelonephritis is caused by a bacterial infection, a clogged duct in the urinary tract, or renal calculi (stones). Bacteria that are blood-borne can travel through the blood into the kidney from another infected area of the body. This can cause an abscess and lead to necrosis of the renal cortex. Pyelonephritis, which starts in the urinary bladder, is commonly caused by feces containing *Escherichia coli*, *Proteus* species, *or Enterococcus* species.

What are the signs and symptoms of pyelonephritis?
The signs and symptoms of pyelonephritis include white blood cell casts in the urine; pain in the back, flank, and abdomen; fever; fatigue and tiredness; and blood and pus in the urine (the urine will appear either dark brown or cloudy).

What Is a Urinary Tract Infection?

A ***urinary tract infection***, also called a ***UTI***, is more frequent in females because of the shortness of the urethra. In addition, males will have fewer urinary tract infections because of the acidity of prostate secretions. However, after the age of about 40, enlargement of the prostate gland can occur, limiting the complete emptying of the bladder, and this can lead to an increase in urinary tract infections.

Urinary tract infections are commonly caused by bacterial infections, *E. coli* being the most common.

What are the signs and symptom of UTIs?
The signs and symptoms of urinary tract infections include an increase in urinary frequency, pain during urination, and urine that contains blood or pus.

What Is Nephrotic Syndrome?

Nephrotic syndrome is a group of kidney diseases that cause an increase in basement membrane permeability, which leads to urinary protein loss. The protein that is most affected is *albumin*.

Nephrotic syndrome can be caused by diabetic kidney disease, systemic lupus erythematosus (SLE), or glomerulonephritis.

What are the signs and symptoms of nephrotic syndrome?
The signs and symptoms of nephrotic syndrome include ***proteinuria*** (protein in the urine), ***hypoalbuminemia*** (a decrease in albumin as a result of urinary loss), and generalized systemic edema (because of the loss of protein). After glomerular damage and hypoalbuminemia occur, blood osmotic pressure decreases dramatically. The interstitial fluid that would normally be drawn into the blood stays in the tissue spaces, causing edema. Hyperlipidemia also occurs. The liver tries to compensate and makes lipoproteins to replace the low plasma proteins.

What Is Nephritic Syndrome?

Nephritic syndrome is a condition in which inflammatory damage to the glomerulus (glomerulonephritis) causes a restriction of glomerular filtration and enables red blood cells to pass into the urine (hematuria). The restriction of filtration causes a reduction in the quantity of urine (***oliguria***), high blood pressure (hypertension), and an accumulation of nitrogen waste in the blood (***azotemia***).

Another condition is called ***Goodpasture's syndrome.*** This is a defect in the immune system. The immune system makes antibodies against the glomerular basement membrane, also causing glomerulonephritis. The antibodies in Goodpasture's syndrome also attack the pulmonary basement membrane in the lungs, causing bloody sputum (hemoptysis).

What are the signs and symptoms of nephritic syndrome?
The signs and symptoms of nephritic syndrome include glomerulonephritis, hematuria, oliguria, hypertension, and azotemia (failure of the kidney to remove urea and nitrogen coumpounds from the blood).

What Is Cystitis?

Cystitis is an infection of the urinary bladder. Cystitis is more frequent in females than in males because of the shorter urethra and the proximity of the urethral orifice to the anus. This allows bacteria from the anus easy access to the urinary tract.

Cystitis can be caused by bacteria, the placement of a catheter into the urinary bladder, improper hygiene (women should always wipe anterior to posterior to prevent infection), and holding urination and not voiding when the urgency first occurs.

What are the signs and symptoms of cystitis?
The signs and symptoms of cystitis present with the frequent urge to urinate, pain during urination, fatigue, fever, and chills. The urine can be cloudy because of the presence of pus and smoky or reddish/brown because of the presence of blood.

TABLE 15.2 Key Terms of the Urinary System

TERM	DEFINITION
Anuria	Absence of urine formation
Azotemia	Excess blood nitrogen levels
Cystitis	Inflammation of the urinary bladder
Diuresis	Producing unusually large amounts of urine
Glomerulonephritis	Inflammation of the glomerulus
Hematuria	Blood in the urine
Hypoalbuminemia	Decrease in albumin as a result of urinary loss

(*Continued*)

TABLE 15.2 Key Terms of the Urinary System (*Continued*)

TERM	DEFINITION
Hypertension	High blood pressure
Hypotension	Low blood pressure
Micturition	The physiological process of urination
Nocturia	Urination during sleep
Oliguria	Decrease in the quantity of urine
Polyuria	Excessive urine output
Proteinuria	Protein in the urine
Uremia	Kidney dysfunction that causes constituents of urine to go into the blood
Urination	The act of voiding urine from the body
Urethritis	Inflammation of the urethra

Chapter 15 Review Questions

Fill In the Blank

1. The study of the kidney is called ___________________.
2. The study of the male reproductive system and urinary system is called __________.
3. The study of the female urinary system is called __________.
4. The study of the female reproductive system is called __________.
5. How many ureters are there?
6. How many urethras are there?
7. Where is the urinary bladder located?
8. A deficiency of vitamin D in children can cause ________________.
9. A deficiency of vitamin D in adults is called ___________________.
10. The outermost layer of the kidney is called the ________________.
11. The innermost layer of the kidney is called the ________________.
12. The middle layer of the kidney is called the ________________.
13. The layer of the kidney that maintains the shape of the kidney is the ________________.
14. The layer of the kidney that provides protection is the ___________________.
15. The "concave-shaped" region of the kidney is called the _________________.
16. The triangle-shaped structures in the kidney are called the __________________.
17. The structures that separate the pyramids are the ____________________.
18. The structure that collects all the urine from the major calyces is the __________________.
19. Blood enters the kidneys through the _______________.
20. Blood exits the kidneys through the ________________.
21. The sudden loss of kidney function is called ________________.
22. The loss of kidney failure over time is called ___________________.

23. Inflammation of the glomerulus of a nephron is called ________________.

24. A genetic kidney disorder is called ________________.

25. A bacterial infection of the urinary bladder that spreads to one or both kidneys is called ___________.

26. A UTI is a(n) ______________.

27. The bacterium that most commonly causes urinary tract infections is ____________.

28. The protein that is most affected by nephrotic syndrome is ________________.

29. An infection of the urinary bladder is called ________________.

30. Renal calculi are ________________.

True/False

31. The branch of medicine that deals with the male reproductive system is called gynecology.

32. An example of a waste product in urine is ammonia.

33. Most of the substances filtered from the kidney are reabsorbed.

34. A function of the urinary system is the regulation of blood volume and blood pressure.

35. The kidneys absorb calcium.

36. A decrease in vitamin D in children is called osteomalacia.

37. Papillary ducts drain into the major calyces.

38. Kidney stones can be made of calcium oxalate.

39. Kidney stones can be made of ammonium magnesium phosphate.

40. Acute renal failure can be caused by trauma or burns.

Matching

41. Nephrotic syndrome
42. UTI
43. Cystitis
44. Glomerulonephritis
45. Calcium phosphate
46. Acute renal failure
47. Urethra
48. Adipose capsule
49. Renal pelvis
50. Polycystic kidney disease
    - A. An infection of the urinary bladder
    - B. Kidney tissue becomes replaced by cysts
    - C. Inflammation of the glomerulus
    - D. A group of kidney diseases that cause an increase in basement membrane permeability
    - E. Immediate loss of kidney function
    - F. Urinary tract infection
    - G. Expels urine from the urinary bladder

H. Middle protective layer around the kidney
I. Collects urine from the major calyces
J. Kidney stones

Chapter 15: Review Questions and Answers

Fill In the Blank Answers

1. Nephrology
2. Urology
3. Urology
4. Gynecology
5. Two
6. One
7. Pelvic cavity
8. Rickets
9. Osteomalacia
10. Renal fascia
11. Renal capsule
12. Adipose capsule
13. Renal capsule
14. Adipose capsule
15. Hilum
16. Renal pyramids
17. Renal columns
18. Renal pelvis
19. Renal artery
20. Renal vein
21. Acute renal failure
22. Chronic renal failure
23. Glomerulonephritis
24. Polycystic kidney disease
25. Pyelonephritis
26. Urinary tract infection
27. *Escherichia coli*
28. Albumin
29. Cystitis
30. Kidney stones

True/False Answers

31. False
32. True
33. True
34. True
35. False
36. False
37. False
38. True
39. True
40. True

Matching Answers

41. D
42. F
43. A
44. C
45. J
46. E
47. G
48. H
49. I
50. B

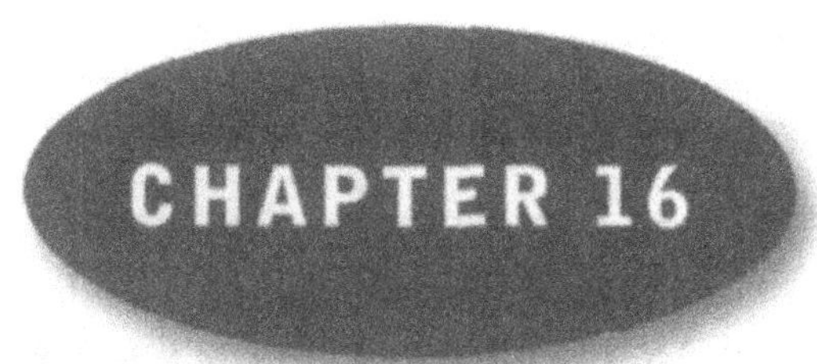

The Reproductive System

Objectives

This chapter will discuss the structures and functions of the male and female reproductive systems. It will also discuss the major diseases and disorders that can affect these structures.

Keywords:

Gonads
Gametes
Scrotum
Testes
Ductus (vas) deferens
Ejaculation

Urethra
Seminal vesicles
Prostate gland
Cowper's gland

Semen
Penis
Sperm
Cryptorchidism

Seminoma
Torsion
Benign prostatic hypertrophy (BPH)
Prostate cancer
Epididymitis
Erectile dysfunction (ED)
Ovaries
Uterine tubes (fallopian tubes)
Uterus

Vagina
Mammary glands

Secondary oocyte

Fibrocystic breast disease

Breast cancer
Pelvic inflammatory disease (PID)
Cervicitis
Cervical cancer

Endometriosis

Endometrial carcinoma
Fibroid tumor (uterine leiomyoma)
Ovarian cancer
Sexually transmitted diseases (STDs)
Acquired immunodeficiency syndrome (AIDS)

Chlamydia

Condyloma acuminatum
Gonorrhea
Syphilis
Herpes simplex type 1
Herpes simplex type 2
Trichomoniasis

16.1 Overview

What Are the Organs of Reproduction?

The organs of reproduction are called ***gonads.***

What Are the Male and Female Gonads Called?

The male gonads are called *testes*. The female gonads are called *ovaries*.

What Do These Gonads Produce?

Gonads produce ***gametes.***

What Are Gametes?

Male gametes are *sperm*. Female gametes are *secondary oocytes*.

16.2 The Male Reproductive System

What Are the Male Reproductive Structures?

The male reproductive structures are the

- Scrotum
- Testes
- Ductus (vas) deferens
- Ejaculatory duct
- Urethra
- Seminal vesicles
- Prostate gland
- Cowper's gland
- Penis

What Is the Scrotum and What Is Its Function?

The ***scrotum*** is a sac that hangs from the base of the penis inferior to the pubic bone and outside of the body. The scrotum contains the two testes, which are surrounded by a *dartos* and separated by a *septum*. Heat will lower the production of sperm; this is why the testes hang outside of the body in the scrotum. The temperature in the scrotum is three degrees cooler than that inside the body.

What Are the Testes?

The ***testes*** are the male gonads. During fetal life, the testes develop high in the abdominal wall. During the seventh month of fetal life, the testes descend into the scrotum through the inguinal canal.

What Are the Ducts Inside the Testes Called?

The ducts inside the testes are called *seminiferous tubules*. These tubules make sperm cells. This process is called *spermatogenesis*. The cells of the seminiferous tubules that function in spermatogenesis are called *spermatogenic cells*. After the sperm cells are produced, they travel from the *seminiferous tubules* into the *straight tubules* into the *rete testis* and out of the testes through the *efferent ducts*. From the efferent ducts, the sperm enter the *ductus epididymis* or *epididymis*.

What Is the Function of the Epididymis?

The *epididymis* is the area where sperm mature and are stored. The epididymis is located on the superior portion of each testis.

What Is the Ductus Deferens?

The ***ductus deferens*** is also called the ***vas deferens.*** This structure is a tube that stores the sperm. It propels them from the epididymis to the urethra located in the pelvic cavity in a process called ***ejaculation.***

What Is the Urethra?

The male ***urethra*** is a tube that begins in the pelvic cavity and travels through the penis. The urethra is responsible for both eliminating urine from the urinary bladder and propelling sperm and semen from the vas deferens through the penis. The male urethra has three parts: the

1. Prostatic urethra
2. Membranous urethra
3. Spongy urethra

What Are the Accessory Structures of Male Reproduction, and What Are Their Functions?

The accessory structures of male reproduction include the

- *Seminal vesicles.* The ***seminal vesicles*** secrete an alkaline fluid. The seminal vesicles secrete 60 percent of the volume of semen.
- *Prostate gland.* The ***prostate gland*** secretes a slightly acidic solution to help eliminate any bacteria located in the male urethra.
- *Cowper's gland.* ***Cowper's gland*** is also called the *bulbourethral gland.* This gland secretes an alkaline substance that neutralizes the acid and also secretes mucus for lubrication.

What Is Semen?

Semen is a combined mixture of the accessory structures' secretions.

What Is the Function of Semen?

The function of semen is to

1. Provide nutrients for sperm.
2. Neutralize acid.

What Are the Structure and Function of the Penis?

The ***penis*** is located anterior and superior to the scrotum sac and is attached to the pubis. The penis is made up of a *root, body*, and *glans penis*. The function of the penis is to expel urine, semen, and sperm from the body, and it is the organ used during *sexual intercourse* or *coitus*.

The structure of the male reproductive system is shown in Figure 16.1.

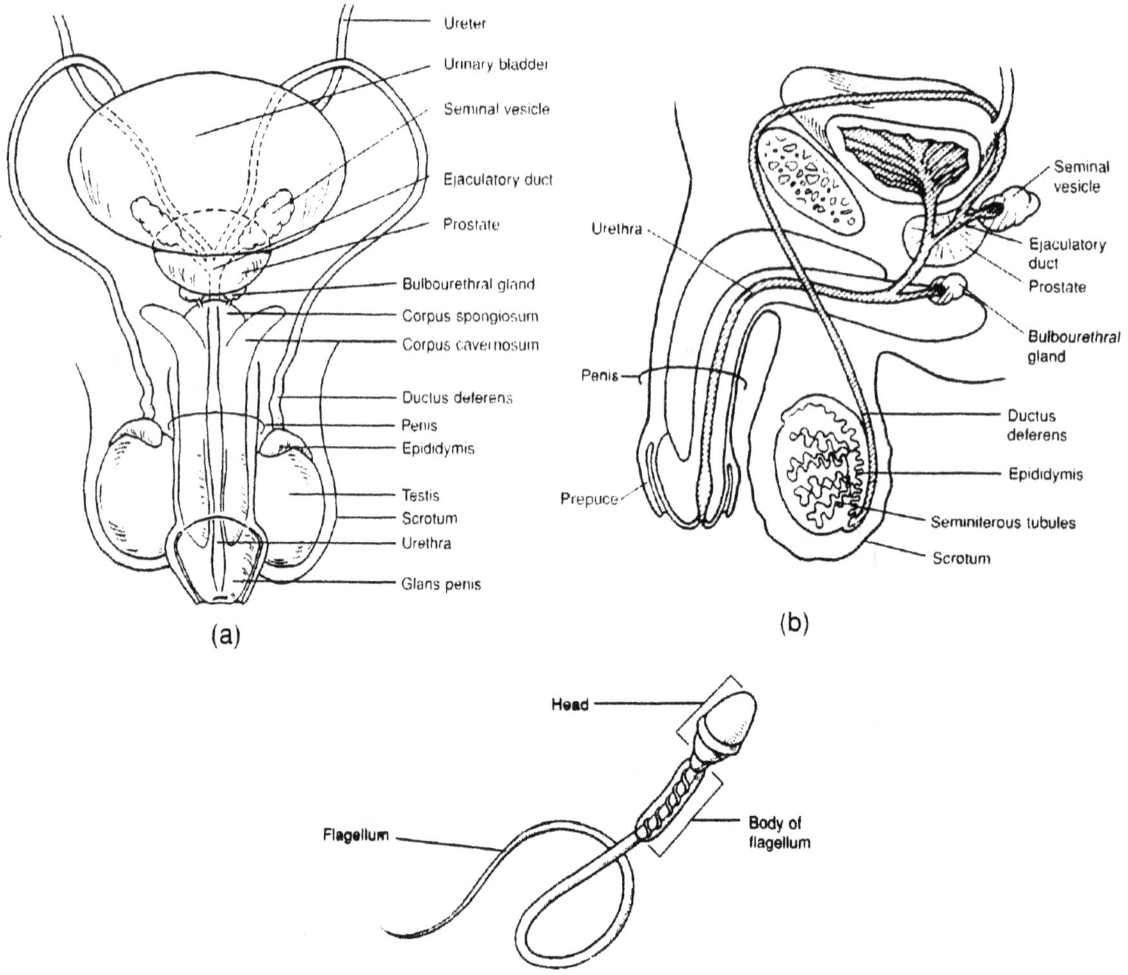

Figure 16.1 The male reproductive system. (*a*) An anterior view and (*b*) a sagittal view.

16.3 Physiology of the Male Reproductive System

What Is the Function of Sperm?

The function of ***sperm*** is to fertilize the female gamete (*secondary oocyte* or *egg cell*).

How Does a Sperm Cell Develop?

At Puberty

- Gonadotropin releasing hormone, or GnRH, is secreted from the hypothalamus (which is located in the diencephalon portion of the brain).
- GnRH stimulates the anterior portion of the pituitary gland (also called the master gland) to secrete follicle stimulating hormone (FSH) and luteinizing hormone (LH). Luteinizing hormone stimulates the production of testosterone. Follicle stimulating hormone stimulates the production of sperm.

What Is Testosterone Responsible For?

Testosterone is responsible for the growth, maintenance, and development of the male sex organs; helps sperm mature; stimulates the growing of bone; and stimulates the making of protein. Testosterone is also responsible for the secondary sexual characteristics of males.

What Are the Secondary Sexual Characteristics of Males?

Male secondary sexual characteristics include

1. Muscle growth
2. Voice change
3. Body and facial hair

What Is Spermatogenesis?

Spermatogenesis is the process that makes sperm. This process takes place in the *seminiferous tubules* located inside the testes.

What Are Sustentacular Cells?

Sustentacular cells are also called *Sertoli cells*. These cells are located in the testes among the sperm cells.

What Is the Function of Sustentacular Cells?

Sustentacular cells support and protect sperm cells.

What Are Leydig Cells and What Is Their Function?

Leydig cells are also called *interstitial cells* and are located between the seminiferous tubules. Leydig cells produce and secrete male sex hormones.

What Are the Parts of a Sperm Cell, and What Are Their Functions?

The function of sperm is to fertilize the female secondary oocyte, or egg cell. The parts of the sperm include

- *Head.* The head portion of a sperm cell contains 23 chromosomes.
- *Acrosome.* The acrosome is located on the top of the head. It helps the sperm enter or penetrate into the ovum, or egg cell.
- *Midpiece or body of the tail.* The midpiece contains the mitochondria of the cell. The mitochondria provide the adenosine triphosphate (ATP) or energy for movement.
- *Tail or flagellum.* The tail provides the movement of the sperm.

The entire process of the production of sperm to maturation takes around 8 weeks. Sperm cells mature at a rate of approximately 300 million per day.

16.4 Pathophysiology of the Male Reproductive System

What Are Some Common Disorders and Diseases Associated with the Male Reproductive System?

We will first look at disorders that can affect the testes. Disorders of the testes can be caused by congenital defects, acquired abnormalities or trauma, infections, circulation problems, or neoplasms. We will then look at disorders that can affect other structures in the male reproductive system.

What Congenital Defect Can Involve the Testes?

The most common congenital defect that involves the testes is ***cryptorchidism.*** Around the seventh month of fetal life, the testes (which develop in the pelvic cavity) descend through the inguinal canal into the scrotum. When the testes do not descend, this is called cryptorchidism. Testes that do not descend can still produce and secrete testosterone; however, they stop producing sperm. This happens as a result of the warmer temperature in the pelvic cavity. The seminiferous tubules will atrophy, and infertility will follow. Because of the increase in temperature, undescended testes, especially after the age of five years, have an increased tumor and cancer risk. The medical procedure used to descend the testes into the scrotum is called *orchiopexy*.

What Is the Most Common Type of Testicular Tumor?

The most common type of testicular tumor is called a ***seminoma.*** A seminoma is a malignant *germ cell tumor*, meaning that it arises from precursor cells that have not differentiated. These types of tumors are associated with undescended testes (cryptorchidism) in males between the ages of 15 and 35.

With the initial tumor, the sign may be swelling because of the growing tumor. Pain is variable until the swelling creates pressure. Metastases can cause urinary tract obstructions and produces abdominal and low back pain. The individual tends to lose weight, and breast enlargement may result in *gynecomastia*.

What Can Cause a Blood Circulation Problem within the Testes?

Compromised testicular circulation can be caused by a ***torsion*** of the spermatic cord. A torsion is a twisting of the spermatic cord, causing compression of the testicular blood vessels. The result is reduced blood flow to the testes and restricted drainage of the veins.

Torsions are commonly caused by trauma, vigorous exercise or activity, and a scrotum that is loosely suspended. As a result of a decrease in venous drainage, inflammation and congestion occur which causes pain.

What Is Benign Prostatic Hypertrophy?

Common diseases and disorders of the prostate gland include ***benign prostatic hypertrophy***. Benign prostatic hypertrophy, also called BPH, is actually the production of new prostate cells (hyperplasia). This is a benign condition that occurs in about 90 percent of all males over the age of 70.

BPH is caused by hormonal changes associated with normal aging.

What are the signs and symptoms associated with benign prostatic hypertrophy?

The signs and symptoms associated with benign prostatic hypertrophy (hyperplasia) include frequent urination and urinary obstruction or difficulty in starting or stopping urination. Obstruction can lead to infections and pyelonephritis.

What Is Prostate Cancer?

Prostate cancer is one of the most common types of cancers in males over the age of 40. Signs and symptoms of prostate tumors usually occur after the age of 50. There is a higher incidence of prostate cancer in men over 70.

It is possible that prostate cancer may have a genetic component, although testosterone supports prostate tumor growth.

What are the signs and symptoms associated with prostate cancer?

The signs and symptoms of prostate cancer include difficulty starting and stopping urine flow, pain during urination, low back pain, abdominal pain, blood in the urine, weight loss, anemia, and an increased secretion of *prostate-specific antigen*, or PSA, into the blood by prostate tissue. Prostate cancer can spread to area lymph nodes, lungs, and bone.

What Is Epididymitis?

Epididymitis involves the inflammation of the epididymis.

Epididymitis can be caused by a urinary tract infection that has spread to the epididymis. These infections can be the result of a catheter being placed into the urethra. Epididymitis can also be caused by sexually transmitted diseases (STDs), such as chlamydia and gonorrhea. (STDs will be discussed later in this chapter.)

What are the signs and symptoms associated with epididymitis?
The signs and symptoms of epididymitis include pain and swelling of the testes and scrotum, pain during urination and/or ejaculation, urethral discharge, blood in semen, testicular lumps, enlarged pelvic lymph nodes, and a fever.

What Is Erectile Dysfunction?

Erectile dysfunction, or ED, is also called *impotence*, the inability of a male to achieve and/or maintain an erection of the penis. This disorder is commonly the result of a physical condition rather than a psychological one.

The causes of erectile dysfunction include hypertension; diabetes; vascular disease; heart disease; anemia; certain medications; cigarette smoking; drinking excessive amounts of alcohol; cocaine, heroin, and marijuana use; emotional stress; depression; and anxiety.

What are signs and symptoms associated with erectile dysfunction?
The signs and symptoms of erectile dysfunction are the inability to achieve or maintain an erection.

16.5 The Female Reproductive System

What Are the Female Reproductive Structures?

The reproductive structures of the female include

- Ovaries
- Uterine tube (fallopian tubes)
- Uterus
- Vagina
- Mammary glands

What Are the Ovaries?

The ***ovaries*** are the female gonads. They are located in the superior portion of the female pelvic cavity. The ovaries produce and discharge secondary oocytes in a process called *ovulation*. They also produce and secrete the hormones estrogen, progesterone, relaxin, and inhibin.

What Are the Uterine Tubes?

The ***uterine tubes*** are also called the ***fallopian tubes*** and *oviducts*. The secondary oocyte is transported along the fallopian tubes by ciliated epithelial cells and peristaltic contractions. The distal portions of the fallopian tubes are the normal site of fertilization.

What Is the Uterus?

The ***uterus*** is about the size and shape of a pear and is located in the female pelvis. The lining of the uterus is called the *endometrium*, and the muscular portion (which contracts during labor) is called the *myometrium*.

The uterus functions in

1. Implantation of the fertilized oocyte
2. Development of the embryo and fetus
3. Labor
4. Menstruation

What is the Cervix?

The ***cervix*** is the lower narrow portion of the uterus. The cervix extends into the vagina.

What Is the Vagina?

The ***vagina*** is the orifice and passageway for menstrual flow and for sperm during intercourse, and also receives the penis during intercourse.

What Are the Mammary Glands?

The ***mammary glands*** are actually sweat glands that are modified to produce and eject milk in the process called *lactation*. Milk production is stimulated by the hormones prolactin, estrogen, and progesterone. Milk ejection is stimulated by the hormone oxytocin.

Figure 16.2 shows the structures of the female reproductive system, excluding the mammary glands.

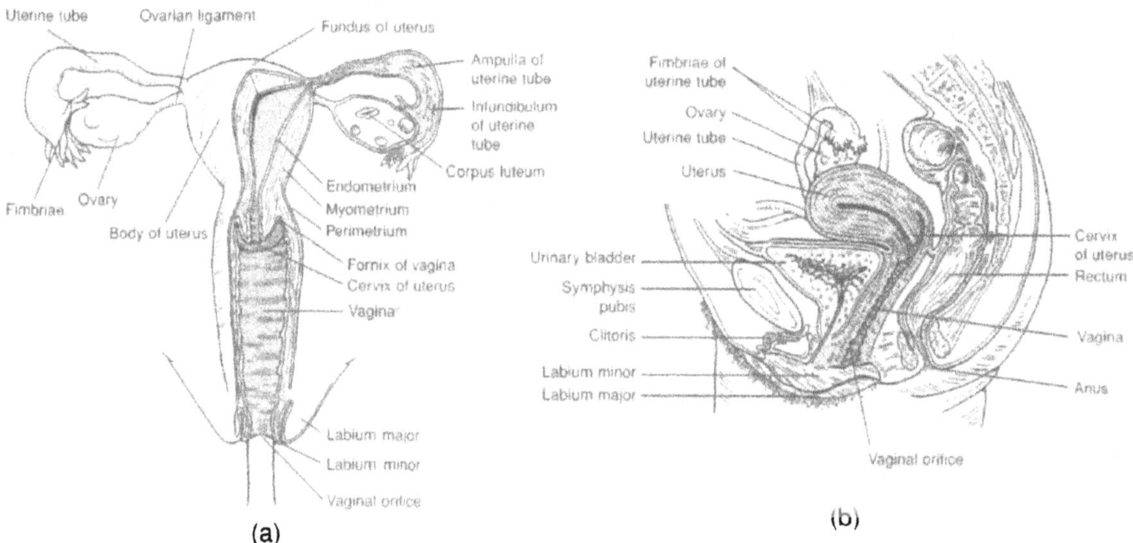

Figure 16.2 The female reproductive system. (*a*) An anterior view and (*b*) a sagittal view.

16.6 Physiology of the Female Reproductive System

What Is the Function of the Menstrual Cycle?

The menstrual cycle prepares the endometrial lining of the uterus to receive the fertilized ***secondary oocyte***.

What Is the Control Mechanism of the Female Reproductive System?

The female reproductive system is controlled by gonadotropin releasing hormone (GnRh), which is released by the hypothalamus. GnRh stimulates the anterior pituitary gland to release follicle stimulating hormone (FSH) and luteinizing hormone (LH). FSH will stimulate the development of the secondary oocyte and start the secretion of estrogen. Both of these events take place in the ovaries. LH will continue to stimulate the development of the ovarian follicles and the secretion of estrogen. LH will cause the dominant follicle in the ovary to rupture. This is the start of *ovulation* and forms the corpus luteum. LH will stimulate the newly formed corpus luteum to secrete the hormones estrogen, progesterone, relaxin, and inhibin.

What Are the Functions of These Hormones?

The functions of the female reproductive hormones during the reproductive cycle are given in Table 16.1.

TABLE 16.1 **Hormones of Female Reproduction**

HORMONE	FUNCTION
Estrogen	Growth, development, and maintenance of the female reproductive cycle. Responsible for secondary sexual characteristics.
Progesterone	With estrogen, gets the endometrium (lining of the uterus) ready for implantation.
Relaxin	Relaxes the pubic symphysis and aids in dilating the uterine cervix.
Inhibin	A regulatory hormone; inhibits the secretion of FSH and LH.

16.7 Pathophysiology of the Female Reproductive System

What Is Fibrocystic Breast Disease?

Fibrocystic breast disease presents as abnormal cysts within the tissues of the breasts. This condition is common in women between 25 and 50 years of age. Fibrocystic breast disease is directly related to hormonal changes. This is why the condition is rare in postmenopausal women and why the size of the cysts will vary, especially during the menstrual cycle.

The cause of fibrocystic breast disease is hormonal changes and the ingestion of certain drugs or other substances, such as nicotine, caffeine, birth control pills, and sugar.

What are the signs and symptoms associated with fibrocystic breast disease?
The signs and symptoms of fibrocystic breast disease include mid-menstrual cycle tender lumps found in the breasts. These lumps vary in size during different phases of the menstrual cycle.

What Is Breast Cancer?

Breast cancer is the second leading cause of cancer deaths in women (lung cancer is the first). Early diagnosis increases the success of treatment.

Breast cancer can be caused by changes in hormones or be predisposed by family history, a diet high in animal fats, or increase in age; it is more common among nulliparous women (those with no children).

What are the signs and symptoms associated with breast cancer?
The signs and symptoms of breast cancer include hard or firm, usually painless, lumps in the breast and/or armpit (axillary region). There may be a discharge from the nipples, dimples in the skin of the breasts, pain in the breast, and swelling in the breast and arm.

What Is Pelvic Inflammatory Disease?

Pelvic inflammatory disease is also called ***PID*** and *salpingitis*. PID is commonly caused by a vaginal infection that spreads to the uterus and up the uterine tubes to the ovaries. If the infection is severe enough, it can spread to the ligament of the uterus, peritoneum, liver, colon, and appendix.

Pelvic inflammatory disease is commonly caused by the bacteria *Chlamydia trachomatis* and *Neisseria gonorrhoeae.*

What are the signs and symptoms associated with pelvic inflammatory disease?
The signs and symptoms of pelvic inflammatory disease include abdominal pain (which can be very severe with progression), irregular bleeding, low-grade to high fever, and cervical discharge.

What Is Cervicitis?

Cervicitis is inflammation of the cervix, commonly as the result of an infection.

Cervicitis is most commonly caused by the sexually transmitted microorganisms *Chlamydia trachomatis* and *Ureaplasma urealyticum* and the use of spermicidal creams.

What are the signs and symptoms associated with cervicitis?
Many women are asymptomatic (have no symptoms). When signs and symptoms do occur, they normally present as vaginal pain (dyspareunia) and bleeding (especially after intercourse), dysuria (difficulty or painful urination), and vaginal discharge.

What Is Cervical Cancer?

Cervical cancer is the second most common form of cancer of the female reproductive system. Cervical cancer normally affects women between the ages of 40 and 50 years.

Women who have had early and frequent sex or have had multiple partners are more susceptible to getting cervical cancer. The *human papillomavirus*, or *HPV*, increases the risk and can cause cervical cancer. The strains or subtypes of HPV that increase the risk of cancer are HPV 16, 18, 31, 33, and 35. These viruses and having multiple sexual partners, along with age, hormonal changes, changes in pH, and childbirth, can cause the normal stratified squamous epithelium located at the entrance of the uterus (cervix) to thicken. This is called *metaplasia*.

These cells can also become dysplastic. Dysplasia of these cells is also adaptive and, if minimal, can also reverse to normal. If severe dysplasia occurs, these cells can change to cancer. In cervical dysplasia, one-third of the epithelial cells become abnormal. If these cells become cancer cells, they may proliferate abnormally and can affect the entire thickness of the epithelial tissue. This is called *carcinoma in situ*. Cervical dysplasia and carcinoma in situ are considered *preinvasive cancer*. When cancer cells (which are usually squamous cell carcinoma) go through the basement membrane and invade the underlying connective tissue, it is called *invasive carcinoma*. Invasive carcinoma can spread to the organs located in the pelvis directly or through the lymphatic system.

What are the signs and symptoms associated with cervical cancer?
Signs and symptoms of cervical cancer include abnormal sporadic bleeding from the vagina, bleeding after intercourse, pain after intercourse, and vaginal discharge (which is yellow in color, can contain blood, and is foul-smelling). Later stages of cervical cancer can present with lower extremity bone pain and pelvic pain.

What Is Endometriosis?

Endometriosis is a condition that occurs when the lining of the uterine wall (the endometrium) grows outside of the uterus. The endometrial tissue can proliferate and grow on the ovaries, ligaments, and even other structures located in the pelvic region.

In endometriosis, the tissue proliferates and bleeds. Following the menstrual cycle, the formation of cysts occurs. These blood-filled cysts are referred to as "chocolate cysts."

What are the signs and symptoms associated with endometriosis?
The signs and symptoms of endometriosis include pain during the menstrual cycle, heavy bleeding, bleeding between periods (spotting), pain during intercourse, and infertility.

What Is Endometrial Carcinoma?

Endometrial carcinoma is one of the most common gynecological malignancies of the uterus, commonly occurring in older women after menopause.

Women who have had prolonged or high levels of estrogen therapy and women who are diabetic, are obese, have had no children, have high blood pressure, and have had delayed menopause are at a higher risk of developing endometrial carcinoma. Endometrial carcinoma can invade the myometrium of the uterus and spread to the lungs. Tumors can also spread along the uterine tubes (Fallopian tubes) to the ovaries.

What are the signs and symptoms associated with endometrial carcinoma?
Endometrial carcinoma commonly presents as postmenopausal bleeding, a white, watery mucoid discharge that follows the bleeding, and pelvic pain.

What Is a Fibroid Tumor?

Fibroid tumors, also called ***uterine leiomyomas***, are the most common uterine tumors and the most common of all tumors associated with women. These benign tumors are common in women between the ages of 30 and 50.

Fibroid tumors are affected by estrogen levels. They increase in size during pregnancy and decrease during menopause.

What are the signs and symptoms associated with fibroid tumors?
Fibroid tumors present with abdominal pressure, heavy menstrual bleeding, severe menstrual pain and cramping, bleeding between periods, lower extremity pain, and low back pain.

What Is Ovarian Cancer?

Although ***ovarian cancer*** has a rather low incidence rate, it is the fourth deadliest form of cancer in women. This is probably due to the lack of or only mild signs and symptoms associated with this form of cancer. By the time the symptoms occur, the tumor has usually grown and invaded surrounding tissue, and metastasis has occurred. The cause of ovarian cancer is unknown, although there appears to be a genetic component.

What are the signs and symptoms associated with ovarian cancer?
Ovarian tumors commonly present as abdominopelvic distention; abdominopelvic discomfort, such as pain, nausea, and indigestion; and dysfunction of normal intestinal or urinary functions. Tumor growth will cause the ovaries to grow incredibly large. This can be mistaken for obesity. As the tumor grows, it can also compress and block the surrounding lymphatic vessels. This will result in fluid accumulation in the peritoneal cavity. This accumulation of fluid will also cause distention of the abdominopelvic region.

16.8 Sexually Transmitted Diseases

What Are Sexually Transmitted Diseases?

Sexually transmitted diseases, also known as ***STDs***, are transmitted by direct sexual contact with an individual who is infected with the disease. These diseases can be viral or bacterial or caused by fungi, protozoa, or parasites.

Some of the most common sexually transmitted diseases are listed in Table 16.2.

TABLE 16.2 **Pathophysiology of Sexually Transmitted Diseases**

DISEASE	CAUSE/ORGANISM	SIGNS AND SYMPTOMS
Acquired immunodeficiency Syndrome (AIDS)	Human immunodeficiency virus (HIV)	Flulike symptoms, low-grade fever, night sweats, decrease in T lymphocyte count
Chlamydia	*Chlamydia trachomatis* bacterium	Urethritis, pain during intercourse, vaginal discharge, pain during urination; can cause infertility
Condyloma acuminatum	Human papillomavirus (HPV)	In women, the warts appear in the vulva, vagina, and cervix. In men, the warts appear on the penis and scrotum
Gonorrhea	*Neisseria gonorrhoeae* bacterium	Males present with a burning pain upon urination and a white, yellow, or green discharge from the penis. Can lead to epididymitis. Females present with pus in the urine, vaginal discharge, and bleeding between periods. Can lead to pelvic inflammatory disease
Syphilis	*Treponema pallidum* bacterium	*Primary syphilis* presents with a painless sore called a *chancre. Secondary syphilis* presents as lesions around mucous membranes and "flulike" systems. *Tertiary syphilis* can spread (usually after the person has been infected and untreated for years) to the brain, heart and blood vessels, liver, eyes, and bone. The damage caused by this bacterial infection can include dementia, paralysis, blindness, and death.

(*Continued*)

TABLE 16.2 Pathophysiology of Sexually Transmitted Diseases (*Continued*)

DISEASE	CAUSE/ORGANISM	SIGNS AND SYMPTOMS
Herpes simplex type 1	Herpes simplex type 1 and herpes simplex type 2 are caused by the Herpesviridae	Herpes simplex type 1 presents with sores around the mouth and lips.
Herpes simplex type 2		Herpes simplex type 2 presents with sores around the genital region. Remember, the type 1 virus can cause type 2 or genital herpes because infection is caused by direct contact with an active lesion. Infection sites include the mucous membranes around the mouth and in the oral cavity, genital orifices, and anus.
Trichomoniasis	*Trichomonas vaginalis*, a protozoan parasite	Affecting the male urethra, this parasitic infection causes mild irritation to the penis, pus in the urine, and urethral discharge. Affecting the female vagina, this parasitic infection causes irritation and itch to the vulva and a foul-smelling, greenish-yellow vaginal discharge.

Chapter 16 Review Questions

Fill In the Blank

1. The male gonads are called ___________________.
2. The female gonads are called ___________________.
3. Gonads produce ___________________.
4. The male gamete is the _________________.
5. The female gamete is the _________________.
6. The process of making sperm is called ____________________.
7. The sperm is made in the ______________________ tubules.
8. The area where sperm mature and are stored is the __________________.
9. The ductus deferens is also called the ___________________.
10. The process in which the sperm are propelled from the epididymis to the urethra is called _________________.
11. The tube in males that begins in the pelvic cavity and travels through the penis is the ________.
12. A mixture of accessory organ secretions is called ___________________.
13. GnRH is secreted by the _________________.
14. GnRH stimulates the ___________________.
15. The hormone responsible for the growth, maintenance, and development of the male sex organs is ___________________.
16. Sustentacular cells are also called ___________________.
17. The cells located in between the seminiferous tubules are called _________________.
18. The portion of a sperm cell that contains the chromosomes is the ________________.

19. The portion of a sperm cell that functions in movement is the ________________.

20. Sperm mature at a rate of ________________ million per day.

21. When a secondary oocyte is discharged from an ovary, this is called ___________.

22. The lining of the uterus is called the ________________.

23. The muscular portion of the uterus is called the ________________.

24. The production and ejection of milk is called ________________.

25. The ejection of milk is stimulated by the hormone _____________.

True/False

26. During fetal life, the testes develop high in the abdominal wall.

27. The testes descend into the scrotum at the age of seven years.

28. Gynecomastia can occur with a testicular tumor.

29. BPH is a form of prostate cancer.

30. High blood pressure can cause erectile dysfunction.

31. Estrogen is responsible for female secondary sexual characteristics.

32. Fibrocystic breast disease is directly related to hormonal changes.

33. Salpingitis is pelvic inflammatory disease.

34. The human papillomavirus has no relation to cervical cancer.

35. Fibroid tumors can be affected by estrogen levels.

Matching

36. Cryptorchidism

37. Seminoma

38. BPH

39. ED

40. Fibrocystic breast disease

41. Pelvic inflammatory disease

42. Endometriosis

43. Fibroid tumor

44. Relaxin

45. Inhibin

   A. Most common type of testicular cancer
   B. Relaxes the pubic symphysis and aids in dilating the cervix
   C. The production of new prostate cells
   D. Impotence
   E. Uterine lining growing outside of the uterus
   F. Salpingitis
   G. Uterine leiomyoma

H. Abnormal cysts within the tissues of the breasts
I. Testes fail to descend into the scrotum
J. Inhibits the secretion of FSH and LH

Multiple Choice

46. This virus can cause cervical cancer.
A. HIV
B. AIDS
C. HPV
D. Epstein-Barr
E. Herpes simplex 1

47. The organism that is the cause of syphilis is __________.
A. *Neisseria gonorrhoeae*
B. *Treponema pallidum*
C. *Chlamydia trachomatis*
D. *Trichomonas vaginalis*
E. Herpes-zoster

48. A parasite that can affect the female vagina and male urethra is __________.
A. *Neisseria gonorrhoeae*
B. *Trichomonas vaginalis*
C. *Chlamydia trachomatis*
D. *Treponema pallidum*
E. Condyloma acuminatum

49. The virus that causes genital warts is __________.
A. Human papillomavirus
B. *Neisseria gonorrhoeae*
C. *Treponema pallidum*
D. Herpes simplex 2
E. Herpes simplex 1

50. The hormone that works with estrogen in preparing the endometrial lining of the uterus for implantation is __________.
A. Relaxin
B. Testosterone
C. Oxytocin
D. Inhibin
E. Progesterone

Chapter 16: Review Questions and Answers

Fill In the Blank Answers

1. Testes
2. Ovaries
3. Gametes
4. Sperm

5. Secondary oocyte

6. Spermatogenesis

7. Seminiferous

8. Epididymis

9. Vas deferens

10. Ejaculation

11. Urethra

12. Semen

13. Hypothalamus

14. Anterior pituitary gland

15. Testosterone

16. Sertoli cells

17. Leydig cells

18. Head

19. Tail

20. 300

21. Ovulation

22. Endometrium

23. Myometrium

24. Lactation

25. Oxytocin

True/False Answers

26. True

27. False

28. True

29. False

30. True

31. True

32. True

33. True

34. False

35. True

Matching Answers

36. I

37. A

38. C

39. D

40. H

41. F

42. E

43. G

44. B

45. J

Multiple Choice Answers

46. C

47. B

48. B

49. A

50. E

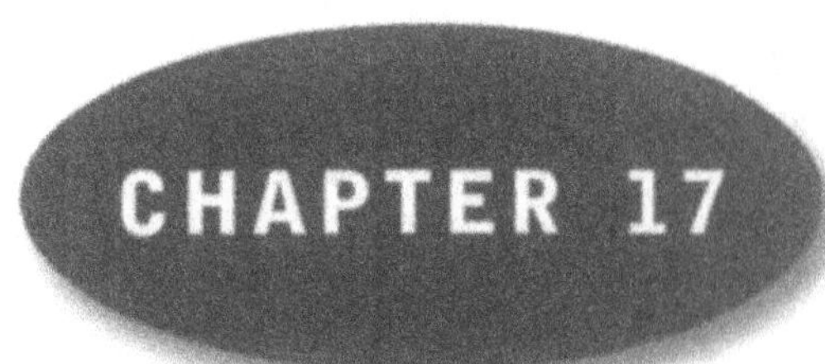

The Endocrine System

Objectives

This chapter introduces the structures that make up the endocrine system and discusses the diseases and disorders that can affect these structures.

Keywords:

Endocrine system
Hormones
Hypothalamus
Antidiuretic hormone (ADH)
Oxytocin (OT)
Anterior pituitary gland
Growth hormone (GH)
Thyroid stimulating hormone (TSH)
Melanocyte stimulating hormone (MSH)

Adrenocorticotropic hormone (ACTH)
Follicle stimulating hormone (FSH)
Luteinizing hormone (LH)
Prolactin (PRL)
Posterior pituitary gland

Thyroid gland
Triiodothyronine (T3)
Thyroxine (T4)
Calcitonin
Parathyroid gland
Parathyroid hormone (PTH)
Pineal gland
Melatonin

Adrenal glands
Aldosterone (ALD)
Cortisol
Cortisone
Epinephrine (adrenaline)

Norepinephrine (noradrenaline)
Pancreas
Islets of Langerhans
Glucagon
Insulin
Ovaries
Estrogen
Progesterone
Testes
Testosterone
Pituitary dwarfism
Gigantism
Acromegaly
Diabetes insipidus
Cretinism
Myxedema
Graves' disease

Thymus gland
Thymosin
Thymopoietin
Goiter
Hypoparathyroidism
Addison's disease
Cushing's syndrome
Diabetes mellitus

17.1 Overview

What Is the Endocrine System?

The ***endocrine system*** consists of glands that secrete chemical messengers called *hormones*.

What Are the Functions of the Endocrine System?

The endocrine system functions in the maintenance of homeostasis by

- Regulating the internal environment
- Regulating metabolism
- Regulating the balance of energy
- Regulating the contraction of muscles
- Regulating glandular secretions
- Helping to regulate the immune response
- Helping in growth
- Helping in development
- Helping in reproduction

What Are Hormones?

Hormones are chemical messengers that affect specific target cells. These cells have special receptor sites that recognize specific hormones. Hormones can be either *water-soluble* or *lipid-soluble*.

Water-soluble hormones include

- Amines
- Proteins
- Eicosanoids

Lipid-soluble hormones include

- Steroids

How Are Hormones Controlled?

Hormones are controlled by

- Electrical signals from the *nervous system*
- Chemical changes that occur in the blood
- Other hormones

17.2 Structures of the Endocrine System

What Are the Structures That Make Up the Endocrine System, and What Are Their Functions?

The principal endocrine glands are shown in Figure 17.1.

- *Hypothalamus.* The ***hypothalamus*** connects the *endocrine system* and the *nervous system* (the two systems that maintain homeostasis).

Where is the hypothalamus located?

  - *Location.* The hypothalamus is located in the diencephalon portion of the brain.

What hormones are associated with the hypothalamus and what are their functions?

- *Hormones.* The hormones that are made in the hypothalamus include
  - *Antidiuretic hormone.* ***Antidiuretic hormone***, or ***ADH***, is stored in and secreted from the *posterior pituitary gland.* This hormone targets the kidneys.
  - *Oxytocin.* ***Oxytocin***, or ***OT***, is also stored in and secreted by the *posterior pituitary gland.* This hormone targets the mammary glands.
- *Anterior pituitary gland.* The ***anterior pituitary gland*** is sometimes referred to as the "master gland." This gland and the hypothalamus are responsible for and govern almost all of the aspects of
  1. Homeostasis
  2. Growth of the body
  3. Development of cells
  4. Metabolism

Where is the pituitary gland located?

  - *Location.* The pituitary gland is located in the sella turcica portion of the sphenoid bone of the skull.

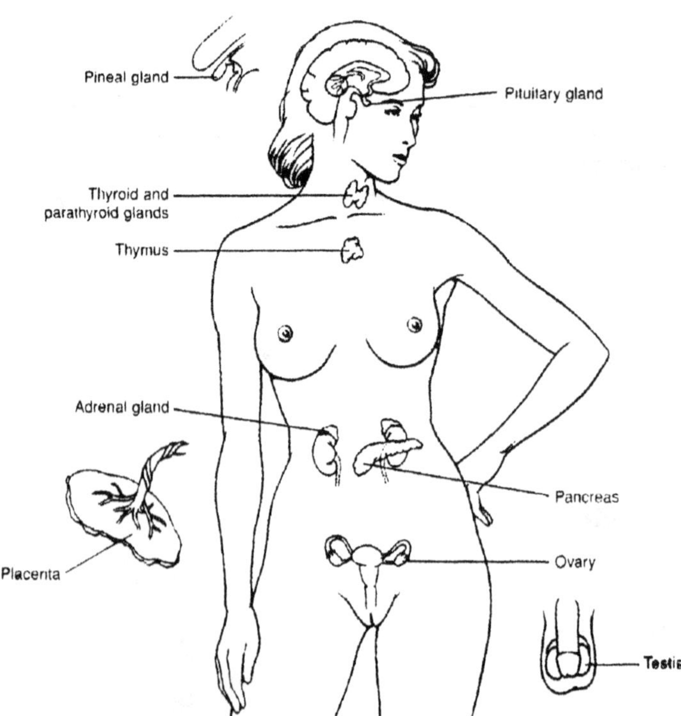

Figure 17.1 The principal endocrine glands.

What hormones are associated with the pituitary gland and what are their functions?

- *Hormones.* The hormones that are associated with the anterior pituitary gland and their functions are
  1. *Growth hormone.* ***Growth hormone***, or ***GH***, is responsible for the maintenance and growth of cells and tissues.
  2. *Thyroid stimulating hormone.* ***Thyroid stimulating hormone***, or ***TSH***, stimulates the thyroid gland to secrete the thyroid hormones T3, T4, and calcitonin. This hormone targets the thyroid gland.
  3. *Melanocyte stimulating hormone.* ***Melanocyte stimulating hormone***, or ***MSH***, stimulates melanocytes located in the epidermis portion of the skin to produce the black/brown pigment melanin. This hormone targets the skin.
  4. *Adrenocorticotropic hormone.* ***Adrenocorticotropic hormone***, or ***ACTH***, stimulates the cortex portion of the adrenal glands (located on top of each kidney), which secretes the hormones *aldosterone* and *cortisol*. This hormone targets the adrenal glands.
  5. *Follicle stimulating hormone.* In males, ***follicle stimulating hormone***, or ***FSH***, will stimulate the production of testosterone and sperm in the testes. In females, it will stimulate the production of the oocyte and estrogen in the ovaries. This hormone targets the gonads.
  6. *Luteinizing hormone.* In males, ***luteinizing hormone***, or ***LH***, is responsible for the production of testosterone. In females, it is responsible for ovulation. This hormone targets the gonads.
  7. *Prolactin.* In males, ***prolactin***, or ***PRL***, works with luteinizing hormone. In females, it stimulates milk production in the mammary glands.
- *Posterior pituitary gland.* The ***posterior pituitary gland*** stores and releases oxytocin and antidiuretic hormone.
  - *Location.* This is the posterior portion of the pituitary gland.
- *Hormones.* The hormones that are associated with the posterior pituitary gland and their functions are
  1. *Oxytocin. Oxytocin*, or *OT*, stimulates the contractions of the uterus during childbirth and is responsible for mammary gland lactation. This hormone targets the uterus and mammary glands.
  2. *Antidiuretic hormone. Antidiuretic hormone*, or *ADH*, stimulates water retention in the kidney, preventing urine production and increasing blood volume. This hormone targets the kidney.
- *Thyroid gland.* The ***thyroid gland*** controls metabolism and affects growth, the development of the nervous system, and the development of the reproductive system.

Where is the thyroid gland located?

  - *Location.* The thyroid gland consists of two lobes and is located inferior and lateral to the larynx.

What hormones are associated with the thyroid gland and what are their functions?

- *Hormones.* The hormones that are associated with the thyroid gland and their functions are
  1. *Triiodothyronine.*
  2. *Thyroxine.*

  Both ***triiodothyronine***, or ***T3***, and ***thyroxine***, or ***T4***, are responsible for growth, development, glucose metabolism, and protein synthesis.

  3. *Calcitonin.* ***Calcitonin*** is responsible for taking calcium out of the blood and putting it into the bone. This hormone targets the bone.
- *Parathyroid gland.* The ***parathyroid gland*** functions in decreasing bone calcium levels and increasing blood calcium levels.

Where is the parathyroid gland located?

  - *Location.* The parathyroid gland is located lateral to the thyroid gland.

What hormones are associated with the parathyroid gland and what are their functions?

- *Hormone.* The hormone that is associated with the parathyroid gland and its functions is
  1. *Parathyroid hormone.* ***Parathyroid hormone***, or ***PTH***, is responsible for the stimulation of osteoclast activity. The matrix of the bone is broken down, and the calcium is released into the

blood. Parathyroid hormone also stimulates the reabsorption of calcium in the kidneys and activates vitamin D. This hormone targets bone, kidneys, and intestines.

- *Pineal gland.* The ***pineal gland*** is responsible for our sleep patterns and for the beginning of puberty.
  - *Location.* The pineal gland is located in the posterior portion of the diencephalon of the brain.
- *Hormone.* The hormone that is associated with the pineal gland and its function is
  1. *Melatonin.* ***Melatonin*** is responsible for our circadian rhythm (internal biological clock) and the onset of puberty. This hormone targets the gonads.
- *Thymus gland.* The ***thymus gland*** is responsible for the maturation of T lymphocytes.

Where is the thymus gland located?

- *Location.* The thymus gland is superficial to the pericardium of the heart and under the sternum.

What hormones are associated with the thymus gland and what are their functions?

- *Hormones.* Two hormones that are associated with the thymus gland and their functions are
  1. Thymosin.
  2. Thymopoietin.

  Both ***thymosin*** and ***thymopoietin*** stimulate the maturation of T cells. These hormones target lymphocytes.
- *Adrenal glands.* The ***adrenal glands*** consist of an outer adrenal cortex and an inner adrenal medulla.

Where are the adrenal glands located?

- *Location.* One of the two adrenal glands is located on top of each kidney.

What hormones are associated with the adrenal glands and what are their functions?

- *Hormones.* Hormones that are associated with the adrenal cortex and their functions are
  1. *Aldosterone.* ***Aldosterone***, or ***ALD***, a mineralocorticoid, stimulates the kidney tubules to retain water and sodium (Na^+) and to excrete potassium (K^+). This will regulate mineral levels in blood. This hormone targets the kidney tubules.
  2. *Cortisol and cortisone.* Both ***cortisol*** and ***cortisone***, which are glucocorticoids, resist stress, have anti-inflammatory properties, and promote cell metabolism.

  The hormones that are associated with the adrenal medulla and their functions are
  1. *Epinephrine.* ***Epinephrine,*** or ***adrenaline***, a catecholamine, increases the heart rate, blood pressure, and metabolic rate; helps us deal with stressful situations; and raises blood sugar. This hormone targets cardiac muscle, blood vessels, and the liver.
  2. *Norepinephrine.* ***Norepinephrine***, or ***noradrenaline***, also a catecholamine, helps us deal with stress and increases the heart rate, respiratory rate, and blood pressure. This hormone also targets cardiac muscle, blood vessels, and the liver.
- *Pancreas.* In the ***pancreas***, the ***islets of Langerhans*** contain two types of cells: alpha cells and beta cells.
  - *Location.* These cells are located in the tail portion of the pancreas.
- *Hormones.* The hormones that are associated with the islets of Langerhans and their functions are
  1. *Glucagon.* Alpha cells secrete ***glucagon***. Glucagon breaks down glycogen into glucose in the liver. This hormone raises blood sugar (glucose) levels. This hormone targets the liver and adipose tissue.
  2. *Insulin.* Beta cells secrete ***insulin***. Insulin lowers blood sugar (glucose) levels by increasing the cell's ability to take in glucose.
- ***Gonads.*** The *gonads* are the organs of reproduction. The female gonads are called the *ovaries*. The male gonads are called the *testes*.

Where are the female and male gonads located?

- *Location.* The ovaries are located in the pelvic cavity. The testes are located in the scrotum.

What hormones are associated with the gonads and what are their functions?

- *Hormones.* The hormones that are associated with the ***ovaries*** and their functions are
   1. *Estrogen*. ***Estrogen*** is a female reproductive hormone. Estrogen maintains the secondary sexual characteristics. It stimulates the development of the lining of the uterus. This hormone targets the mammary glands and female reproductive organs, regulates the female reproductive cycle, and maintains pregnancy.
   2. *Progesterone*. ***Progesterone*** stimulates the development of the mammary glands and the lining of the uterus. This hormone targets the mammary glands and the uterus.

   The hormone that is associated with the ***testes*** and their functions is

   1. *Testosterone*. ***Testosterone*** is responsible for the production of sperm and the development and maintenance of the male secondary characteristics. This hormone targets the male reproductive organs.

17.3 Pathophysiology of the Endocrine System

What Are Some Common Diseases and Disorders of the Anterior Pituitary Gland?

The common diseases and disorders that affect the anterior pituitary gland include the following:

- Pituitary dwarfism
- Gigantism (also called giantism)
- Acromegaly

What Is Pituitary Dwarfism and How Does It Occur?

Pituitary dwarfism occurs when there is hyposecretion of *growth hormone* during childhood. Trauma and tumor growth can also affect pituitary gland secretion.

What are the signs and symptoms associated with pituitary dwarfism?
Pituitary dwarfism will present with a shortness in stature, facial bone abnormalities, frequent headaches (cephalgia), and delayed puberty.

What Is Gigantism and How Does It Occur?

Gigantism occurs when there is hypersecretion of growth hormone during childhood (while the bones are still growing).

What are the signs and symptoms associated with gigantism?
Gigantism presents with a thickening in the bones of the face, growing very tall, and a delay in puberty.

What Is Acromegaly and How Does It Occur?

Acromegaly occurs when there is hypersecretion of growth hormone during adulthood (after the bones have stopped growing) or because of a pituitary gland tumor.

What are the signs and symptoms associated with acromegaly?
Acromegaly presents with an increase in the growth of the hands, feet, and skull bones, and a thickening of the skin. The individual will also experience arm, leg, and head pain; fatigue; weight gain; increase in hair growth; heart disease; and arthritis.

What Is a Common Disease or Disorder of the Posterior Pituitary Gland?

A common disease or disorder of the posterior pituitary gland is diabetes insipidus.

What Is Diabetes Insipidus and How Does It Occur?

Diabetes insipidus occurs when the kidneys lose the ability to reabsorb water. This is caused by the hyposecretion of antidiurectic hormone, or ADH. Hyposecretion of ADH will lead to excessive urine output.

What are the signs and symptoms associated with diabetes insipidus?
The signs and symptoms of diabetes insipidus include increased urination, increased thirst, and cramping of muscles. Cardiac arrhythmias may occur as a result of the electrolyte imbalances that are caused by extreme fluid loss.

What Are Some Common Diseases or Disorders of the Thyroid Gland?

Common disorders and diseases of the thyroid gland include

- Cretinism
- Myxedema
- Graves' disease
- Goiter

What Is Cretinism?

Cretinism occurs when there is hyposecretion of thyroid hormones during fetal development. The fetal skeleton fails to grow, causing dwarfism. Hyposecretion can be the result of decreased stimulation of the thyroid gland by the pituitary gland, absence of the thyroid gland during fetal development, or malformations or abnormalities of the thyroid gland during fetal development.

What are the signs and symptoms associated with cretinism?
The signs and symptoms of cretinism are mental retardation, short stature, and abnormal bone growth.

What Is Myxedema?

Myxedema is *hypothyroidism* in adults, which is caused by inadequate amounts of thyroid hormone being secreted by the thyroid gland. This can be the result of a congenital defect, obesity, or the surgical removal of the thyroid gland.

What are the signs and symptoms associated with myxedema?
The signs and symptoms of myxedema include an increase in metabolic rate, muscle weakness, dry hair and skin, and lethargy.

What Is Graves' Disease?

Graves' disease is *hyperthyroidism* in adults, which is caused by large amounts of thyroid hormones being secreted by the thyroid gland. This oversecretion can be caused by an autoimmune response.

What are signs and symptoms associated with Graves' disease?
The signs and symptoms of Graves' disease include an increase in metabolic rate, a decrease in weight, nervousness, increased sweating, insomnia, and edema behind the eyes, which causes the eyeball to bulge (this condition is called *exophthalmos*).

What Is a Goiter?

A ***goiter*** is an enlargement of the thyroid gland. This can be caused by a decrease in the ingestion of iodine in an individual's diet.

What are the signs and symptoms associated with a goiter?
A goiter presents with a swelling in the anterior portion of the cervical region and thyroid.

What Is a Common Disease of the Parathyroid Gland?

A common disease of the parathyroid gland is hypoparathyroidism.

What Is Hypoparathyroidism?

Hypoparathyroidism is a decrease in parathyroid hormone secretion by the parathyroid glands.

What are the signs and symptoms associated with hypoparathyroidism?
The signs and symptoms of hypoparathyroidism include muscular spasms, tetany (a sustained muscle contraction), and death.

What Are Some Common Diseases of the Adrenal Glands?

Common diseases of the adrenal glands include Addison's disease and Cushing's syndrome.

What Is Addison's Disease?

Addison's disease is the hyposecretion by the adrenal gland of corticosteroid hormones, glucocorticoids, and aldosterone. This hyposecretion is due to a failure in the function of the adrenal cortex.

What are the signs and symptoms associated with Addison's disease?
Addison's disease will present with lethargy and tiredness, nausea, vomiting, fatigue, muscle weakness, muscle pain, loss of appetite, anorexia, weight loss, diarrhea, and dehydration.

What Is Cushing's Syndrome?

Cushing's syndrome is hypersecretion of the glucocorticoids, especially cortisol. Cushing's syndrome is also called *hypercortisolism*. This condition can be caused by a pituitary gland tumor, an adrenal gland tumor, or the chronic use of steroid hormones for many years.

What are the signs and symptoms associated with Cushing's syndrome?
The signs and symptoms that present with Cushing's syndrome include a redistribution of body fat, which includes a "buffalo hump" at the back of the neck, a "moon face" or obese-looking face, and a hanging, obese abdomen that can have stretch marks (striae). This individual will also present with thin, "spindlelike" upper and lower extremities. The individual may also experience fatigue, muscle aches, hypertension, high blood glucose levels, increased urination, and increased thirst.

What Is a Common Disease of the Pancreas?

A common disease of the pancreas is diabetes mellitus.

What Is Diabetes Mellitus?

Diabetes mellitus is a chronic autoimmune disease that affects the beta cells of the pancreas. These beta cells produce insulin. An individual with one form of diabetes mellitus will not produce insulin. This type of diabetes mellitus is commonly referred to as Type 1, early-onset, insulin-dependent, or autoimmune diabetes.

Type 2, late-onset, or non-insulin-dependent diabetes commonly occurs during adolescence to adulthood. Type 2 diabetes can be linked to inactivity, lack of exercise, poor diet, and obesity.

What are the signs and symptoms associated with diabetes mellitus?
The signs and symptoms of diabetes mellitus include high blood glucose levels, increased hunger, decreased weight, increased urination, and increased thirst. Neglectful or poor treatment of the disease can result in blood vessel damage or disease (atherosclerosis), heart disease, kidney disease, eye problems and blindness, poor blood circulation, poor wound healing, fatigue and tiredness, and erectile dysfunction in men.

Chapter 17 Review Questions

Fill In the Blank

1. Chemical messengers that travel through blood are called ______________.
2. Hormones can be water- or ______________-soluble.
3. The structure that is the link between the endocrine system and the nervous system is the _______.
4. The hormone that is stored in the posterior pituitary gland and targets the kidneys is _________.
5. The pituitary gland is located in the ___________ of the sphenoid bone.
6. The gland that is sometimes referred to as the master gland is the ______________.
7. The hormone that is responsible for the maintenance and growth of cells and tissues is ______.
8. The hormone that stimulates the thyroid gland is __________________.
9. The hormone that stimulates the production of melanin is _________________.
10. In males, the hormone that stimulates the production of testosterone and sperm in the testes is ___________.
11. In females, the hormone that will stimulate the production of the oocyte and estrogen in the ovaries is ____________.
12. The hormone that stimulates the production of milk in the mammary glands of the female is _______________.
13. The gland that affects growth, development, and metabolism is the ______________.
14. The thyroid gland consists of two _________________.
15. The hormone that stimulates water retention is ______________.
16. The hormone that is responsible for the stimulation of osteoclast activity is ____________.
17. The gland that is responsible for our sleep patterns is the ________________.
18. The glands that are located on top of the kidneys are the ________________.
19. The gland that is associated with our immune response is the __________________.
20. The cells in the pancreas that secrete glucagon are __________________.
21. The cells in the pancreas that secrete insulin are _________________.
22. The organs of reproduction are the _________________.
23. The hormone that is responsible for male secondary sexual characteristics is ___________.
24. The hormone that is responsible for female secondary sexual characteristics is ___________.
25. Hyposecretion of growth hormone in children can result in __________________.
26. Hypersecretion of growth hormone in children can result in _________________.

27. Hypersecretion of growth hormone in adults can result in ________________.

28. Hyposecretion of thyroid hormones during fetal life can result in ____________.

29. Hyposecretion of parathyroid hormone can result in ________________.

30. Hyposecretion by the adrenal glands can result in ________________.

True/False

31. Thyroxine is classified as a hormone.

32. The nervous system has no effect on hormone secretion.

33. Oxytocin is produced in the posterior pituitary gland.

34. The hypothalamus is located in the brain.

35. Luteinizing hormone is responsible for ovulation.

36. Calcitonin is secreted by the thyroid gland.

37. Melatonin is responsible for circadian rhythms.

38. B lymphocytes mature in the thymus gland.

39. Epinephrine is secreted by the adrenal medulla.

40. Alpha cells are located in the thyroid gland.

Matching

41. Hyposecretion by the anterior pituitary gland

42. Hypersecretion by the posterior pituitary gland

43. Hyposecretion of antidiuretic hormone

44. Hyposecretion of thyroid hormone

45. Hypersecretion of thyroid hormone

46. Hyposecretion by the adrenal glands

47. Hypersecretion by the adrenal glands

48. An inability to secrete insulin

49. Hypersecretion of growth hormone in adults

50. Enlargement of the thyroid gland

    A. Gigantism
    B. Addison's disease
    C. Myxedema
    D. Cushing's syndrome
    E. Graves' disease
    F. Diabetes mellitus
    G. Acromegaly
    H. Pituitary dwarfism
    I. Goiter
    J. Diabetes insipidus

Chapter 17: Review Questions and Answers

Fill In the Blank Answers

1. Hormones
2. Lipid
3. Hypothalamus
4. Antidiuretic hormone
5. Sella turcica
6. Pituitary gland
7. Growth hormone
8. Thyroid stimulating hormone
9. Melanocyte stimulating hormone
10. Follicle stimulating hormone
11. Follicle stimulating hormone
12. Prolactin
13. Thyroid gland
14. Lobes
15. Antidiuretic hormone
16. Parathyroid hormone
17. Pineal gland
18. Adrenal glands
19. Thymus gland
20. Alpha cells
21. Beta cells
22. Gonads
23. Testosterone
24. Estrogen
25. Pituitary dwarfism
26. Gigantism
27. Acromegaly
28. Cretinism
29. Hypoparathyroidism
30. Addison's disease

True/False Answers

31. True
32. False
33. False
34. True
35. True
36. True
37. True
38. False
39. True
40. False

Matching Answers

41. H
42. A
43. J
44. C
45. E
46. B
47. D
48. F
49. G
50. I

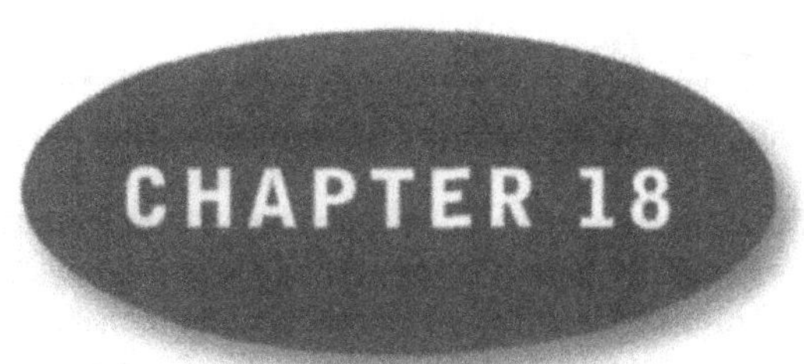

The Nervous System

Objectives

This chapter will discuss the structures and functions of the nervous system. It will also discuss the common disorders of the brain, spinal cord, sensory and motor pathways, and special senses.

Keywords:

Central nervous system
Peripheral nervous system
Somatic nervous system
Autonomic nervous system
Enteric nervous system

Sympathetic nervous system
Parasympathetic nervous system
Neurons
Neuroglia
Ganglion
Neuralgia
Neuritis
Neuropathy
Tay-Sachs disease
Multiple sclerosis
Guillain-Barré syndrome
Meninges
Brain stem
Diencephalon
Cerebellum
Cerebrum
Trigeminal neuralgia (tic douloureux)
Bell's palsy
Alzheimer's disease
Amyotrophic lateral sclerosis (ALS)
Cerebral palsy

Cerebrovascular accident (CVA)
Epilepsy
Encephalitis
Huntington's disease (Huntington's chorea)
Parkinson's disease
Plexuses
Meningitis
Poliomyelitis
Spina bifida
Astigmatism

Myopia
Hyperopia
Nyctalopia
Conjunctivitis
Strabismus
Glaucoma

Cataracts
Tinnitus
Otitis media
Otitis interna
Meniere's disease

18.1 Overview

What Are the Main Functions of the Nervous System?

The nervous system *detects* changes in our internal and external environment, *interprets* these changes, and *responds* to them. The portion of the nervous system that detects changes is considered the *sensory* portion. The portion of the nervous system that interprets these changes is considered the *integrating* portion. The portion of the nervous system that reacts to the changes is considered the *motor* portion.

What Are the Divisions of the Nervous System?

The nervous system is divided into two main parts:

1. The ***central nervous system***, or CNS, includes the *brain* and the *spinal cord.*
2. The ***peripheral nervous system***, or PNS, includes the *cranial nerves* exiting from the brain and the *peripheral nerves* exiting from the spinal cord. There are 12 pairs of cranial nerves and 31 pairs of spinal nerves. The peripheral nervous system consists of the:
   - ***Somatic nervous system***, which controls skeletal muscles
   - ***Autonomic nervous system,*** which controls cardiac and smooth muscles
   - ***Enteric nervous system,*** which controls the glands

   The autonomic and enteric nervous systems consist of the
   - ***Sympathetic nervous system***, which uses energy or speeds up or increases body functions
   - ***Parasympathetic nervous system***, which conserves energy or slows down or decreases body functions, returning them to normal

Remember: The somatic nervous system is under conscious control, and the autonomic nervous system is under unconscious control.

The autonomic nervous system is like our "automatic nervous system."

The sympathetic nervous system is used for "fight or flight" situations.

The parasympathetic nervous system is used for "rest and digest" or "feeding and breeding."

18.2 Histology of the Nervous System

What Types of Cells Form the Nervous System?

There are two main types of cells that make up the nervous tissue:

1. *Neurons*. ***Neurons*** elicit the electrical impulse.
2. *Neuroglia*. ***Neuroglia*** support the neurons.

What Types of Neuroglia Are There?

There are six types of neuroglia cells:

1. *Astrocytes*. The astrocytes are responsible for creating a barrier that prevents infectious organisms from entering the brain from the blood.
2. *Oligodendrocytes*. The oligodendrocytes form the myelin sheath in the central nervous system.
3. *Microglia cells*. Microglia cells engulf foreign materials and organisms in the process called phagocytosis.
4. *Ependymal cells*. Ependymal cells line the ventricles of the brain. These cells have cilia, which circulate the cerebrospinal fluid (CSF).

5. *Neurolemmocytes*. Neurolemmocytes are also called Schwann cells. These cells produce the myelin sheath in the peripheral nervous system.
6. *Satellite cells*. These cells support the cell bodies of neurons in a ganglion.

What Is a Ganglion?

A ***ganglion*** is a group of neuron cell bodies that form what looks like a swelling or lump within the nerve.

What Are the Main Types of Neurons?

There are three main types of neurons:

1. *Multipolar neurons*. These neurons are located mostly in the brain and spinal cord.
2. *Bipolar neurons*. These neurons are associated with special senses, which include sight, hearing, smelling, tasting, and equilibrium.
3. *Unipolar neurons*. These neurons are associated with general senses. These senses include crude touch, vibration, pain, cold/hot temperature, pressure, and soft touch.

Figure 18.1 shows the structure of a neuron.

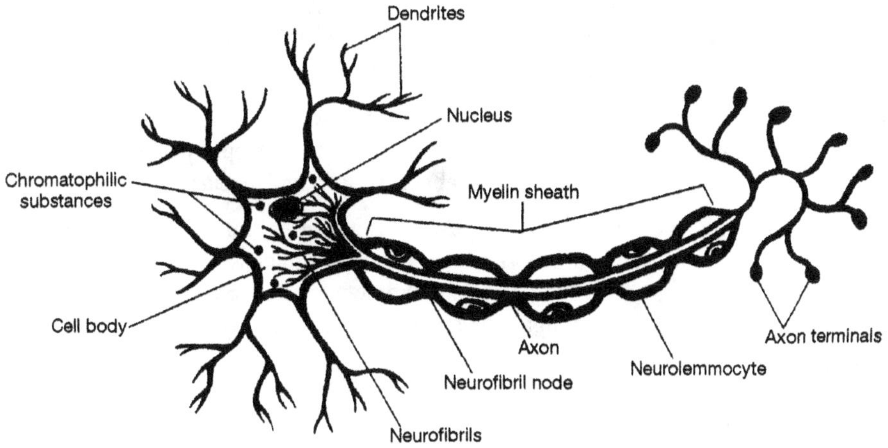

Figure 18.1 The structure of a neuron.

What Is the Difference between a Neuron That Is Myelinated and One That Is Unmyelinated?

Myelin is a lipoprotein insulator that surrounds the neuron. Oligodendrocytes form this insulator in the CNS, and Schwann cells or neurolemmocytes form this insulator in the PNS. Myelinated neurons look white and are said to be white matter, whereas unmyelinated neurons are said to be gray matter. Myelinated neurons have a faster conduction time then those that are unmyelinated.

What Are Some Common Diseases and Disorders That Can Affect Nerves?

1. *Neuralgia*. **Neuralgia** is simply nerve pain.

What are the signs and symptoms associated with neuralgia?
Signs and symptoms associated with nerve pain are

- Numbness or tingling, which is called *paresthesia*
- A hot or burning sensation, which is called *causalgia*
- Shooting or radiating pain

2. *Neuritis*. ***Neuritis*** is the inflammation of a nerve.

What are the signs and symptoms associated with neuritis?
The signs and symptoms of nerve inflammation are neuralgia or loss of function.

3. *Neuropathy*. A ***neuropathy*** is any condition that can cause dysfunction or weakness to peripheral nerves. This dysfunction can be caused by a trauma, degeneration, nerve impingement, or a subluxation.

What Are Examples of Disorders or Diseases That Can Affect the Myelin Sheath?

Some disorders that can affect the myelin sheath are Tay-Sachs disease, multiple sclerosis, and Guillain-Barré syndrome.

- *Tay-Sachs disease*. ***Tay-Sachs disease*** is a progressive genetic disease in which there is an accumulation of lipids (lipidosis) around and within the myelin sheath.

What are the signs and symptoms associated with Tay-Sachs disease?

- Tay-Sachs disease presents with paralysis, blindness, and mental retardation, and death usually occurs by the age of four.
- *Multiple sclerosis*. ***Multiple sclerosis***, or MS, is a progressive disease in which there is a demyelination of neurons in the brain and spinal cord. Plaquing can be seen in the area of demyelination. The causes of MS are unknown, although genetics may be a factor, since a higher incidence within families has been observed. Also, an autoimmune component may play a role because of elevated IgG antibodies and T lymphocytes. Multiple sclerosis can occur in men but is more common in women between the ages of 20 and 40.

What are the signs and symptoms associated with multiple sclerosis?
Multiple sclerosis presents with numbness in the extremities, thorax, and face; optic pain and/or blindness in one eye; hand and leg pain; muscle weakness and joint stiffness; abnormal gait; and dizziness.

- *Guillain-Barré syndrome*. ***Guillain-Barré syndrome*** is a serious, potentially fatal immune disorder in which the body's immune system attacks peripheral nerves and causes inflammation and demyelination of these nerves. Guillain-Barré syndrome can affect both men and women, commonly between the ages of 25 and 50, although it can occur at any age. This disease occurs in three phases:
  1. Acute
  2. Plateau
  3. Recovery

  The recovery phase can last three years as remyelination and axon growth occur. The cause is unknown, although vaccines, viruses, pregnancy, Hodgkin's disease, lupus, and bacterial infections such as *Campylobacter jejuni* may start the disease process.

What are the signs and symptoms associated with Guillain-Barré syndrome?
Guillain-Barré syndrome presents with muscle paresthesia, weakness, paralysis, myalgia, difficulty breathing, and abnormal heart rhythms.

18.3 The Brain

What Is the Main Function of the Brain?

The main function of the brain is to take sensory information from the periphery, interpret and process the information, then react to that information with motor commands in order to maintain homeostasis of the body.

How Much Does the Brain Weigh?

The brain weighs only about three pounds, although it uses around 20 percent of our oxygen intake.

What Protects the Brain?

The brain is protected by the ***meninges***.

What Are the Meninges?

The meninges are three layers of connective tissue that protect the brain and spinal cord. These three layers, from superficial to deep, are

1. Dura mater
2. Arachnoid mater
3. Pia mater

The cerebrospinal fluid is located in the space between the arachnoid mater and the pia mater. This region is called the *subarachnoid space*. The brain has what are called four ventricles through which cerebrospinal fluid circulates. There are two lateral ventricles, a third ventricle, and a fourth ventricle.

An area called the *choroid plexus* forms the cerebrospinal fluid from blood plasma.

What Are the Parts of the Brain?

The parts of the brain include the

1. Brain stem
2. Diencephalon
3. Cerebellum
4. Cerebrum

What Is the Brain Stem?

The ***brain stem*** is the most inferior portion of the brain and is attached to the spinal cord. It has four parts:

1. Medulla oblongata
2. Pons
3. Midbrain
4. Red nucleus

1. *Medulla oblongata*. The medulla oblongata is the most inferior portion of the brain stem and extends from the pons to the spinal cord.

What is the function of the medulla oblongata?

- *Functions*. The medulla oblongata is a relay station between sensory and motor impulses. It regulates our *vital reflexes*, such as heart rate, respiratory rate, and blood vessel diameter. The medulla oblongata also controls our *nonvital reflexes*, such as swallowing, sneezing, coughing, hiccupping, and regurgitation. The motor tracts located in the medulla oblongata carry impulses to skeletal muscles.

2. *Pons*. The pons bridges many parts of the brain. The pons contains two respiratory centers. The *apneustic* and *pneumotaxic centers*, together with the medulla oblongata, help control breathing.

What is the function of the pons?

- *Function*. The apneustic center increases the inflow of air by prolonging inhalation. The pneumotaxic center increases the amount of air that is exhaled.

3. *Midbrain*. The midbrain extends from the hypothalamus to the diencephalon to the pons. It connects the third and fourth ventricles and relays sensory impulses from the spinal cord to the thalamus and motor impulses from the cerebral cortex to the pons.

What is the function of the midbrain?

- *Function*. The midbrain is responsible for the visual and auditory reflexes. It contains the
    - *Superior colliculi*, which coordinate the movements of the eyeballs and head in response to visual stimuli
    - *Inferior colliculi*, which coordinate the movement of the head and trunk in response to visual stimuli
    - *Substantia nigra*, which produces and secretes dopamine for subconscious fine motor control

4. *Red nucleus*. The red nucleus works with the basal ganglion and the cerebellum to coordinate muscle movement. The red nucleus is an extrapyramidal tract.
    - Extrapyramidal tracts coordinate nondominant movement.
    - Pyramidal tracts coordinate controlled movement.

What Is the Diencephalon?

The ***diencephalon*** contains these parts:

1. Epithalamus
2. Thalamus
3. Hypothalamus

1. *Epithalamus*. The epithalamus contains the pineal gland. The pineal gland promotes sleepiness when it secretes the hormone melatonin in response to darkness at night.
2. *Thalamus*. The thalamus is the main region of the brain for relaying sensory impulses that reach the cerebrum from the spinal cord, brain stem, and cerebellum. The thalamus is also the location for the *reticular activating system*, which controls our levels of consciousness. This system is also located in the midbrain and helps control our sleep and wake cycles (circadian rhythms).
3. *Hypothalamus*. The hypothalamus is the link between the endocrine system and the nervous system. It is located inferior to the thalamus. The hypothalamus monitors and regulates our thirst centers, hunger centers, satiety centers (the feeling that your stomach is full), thermostat center, and pleasure centers. The hypothalamus also regulates behavioral and emotional patterns and contributes to the maintenance of our sleep and wake patterns.

What Is the Cerebellum?

The ***cerebellum*** makes up the posterior portion of the brain. It is located in back of the cerebrum. It contains an outer cortex composed of gray matter and an inner portion of white matter called the ***arbor vitae*** (tree of life).

The cerebellum is responsible for our equilibrium, or balance, and our proprioception, or our sense of our body's position in relation to space. The cerebellum is also responsible for motor information that maintains muscle tone and coordination. These tasks are involuntary.

What Is the Cerebrum?

The ***cerebrum*** is the largest portion of the brain. It has left and right hemispheres that are divided by a *longitudinal fissure*. These two hemispheres communicate with each other by a structure made up of around 200 million neurons called the *corpus callosum*. The cerebrum contains an outer cerebral cortex made up of gray matter. Inferior to the gray matter is white matter, which connects all parts of the brain.

What Are the Basal Ganglia?

The ***basal ganglia*** are gray matter that contain nuclei that are deep in the cerebrum.

The basal ganglia control emotion, memory, muscle tone, and learned reflexes, such as writing, tying shoes, or brushing teeth.

What Are the Lobes of the Cerebrum?

The lobes of the cerebrum are named for the skull bones that protect them. The lobes of the cerebrum are

1. *Frontal lobes*. The frontal lobes contain the premotor area for voluntary muscle action. The left frontal lobe controls the right side of the body, and the right frontal lobe controls the left side of the body.
2. *Parietal lobes*. The parietal lobes are the area for general sensory perception. The right lobe is sensitive to the left side of the body, and the left lobe is sensitive to the right side of the body.
3. *Temporal lobes*. The temporal lobes have an auditory area and an olfactory area.
   - *Auditory area*. The auditory area receives sensory impulses from the inner ear and interprets the sound for hearing.
   - *Olfactory area*. The olfactory area receives sensory impulses from the nasal cavity and interprets the information as smell.
4. *Occipital lobes*. The occipital lobes contain the visual areas. The visual areas receive sensory information from the eye (retina) and interpret the information as sight.

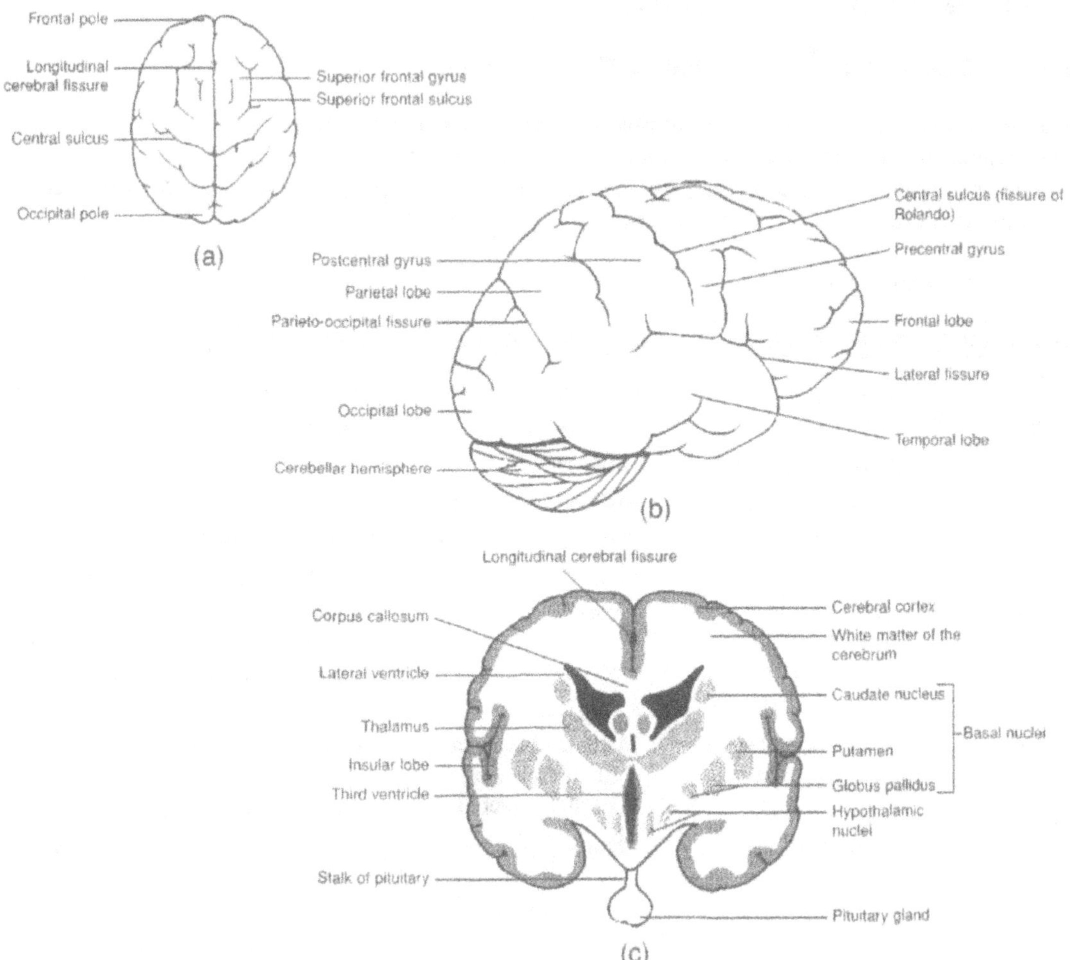

Figure 18.2 The cerebrum. (*a*) A superior view, (*b*) a lateral view, and (*c*) a coronal view.

What Is Broca's Area?

Broca's area is a region of the brain that is found in the left frontal lobe and is responsible for *speech*.

What Is the Primary Somesthetic Area?

The primary somesthetic area is located in the postcentral gyrus (a gyrus is a fold in the brain). This area is responsible for tactile sensation.

What Is the Primary Gustatory Area?

The primary gustatory area receives and interprets sensations of taste.

What Is the Hippocampus?

The *hippocampus* is the region of the brain that is responsible for our memory.

What Are the Left and Right Hemispheres of the Brain Responsible For?

- *Left hemisphere*. The left hemisphere is responsible for logic, language, intellectual skills, math skills, scientific skills, and reasoning.
- *Right hemisphere*. The right hemisphere is responsible for artistic ability, musical ability, creative thinking, imagination, and pattern perception.

What Are Cranial Nerves, and What Is Their Function?

Cranial nerves exit the brain and are responsible for sensory function, motor function, or both. Cranial nerves that are responsible for both sensory and motor information are said to be mixed.

There are 12 pairs of cranial nerves, and they are part of the peripheral nervous system. For each cranial nerve, Table 18.1 shows the cranial nerve number, its name, and its function.

TABLE 18.1 Cranial Nerves

NERVE NUMBER	NERVE NAME	ORIGIN IN BRAIN	NERVE FUNCTION
C.N. I	Olfactory nerve	Cerebral cortex	Sensory for smell
C.N. II	Optic nerve	Cerebral cortex	Sensory for sight
C.N. III	Oculomotor nerve	Midbrain	Motor to eyeball
C.N. IV	Trochlear nerve	Midbrain	Motor to eyeball
C.N. VI	Abducens nerve	Pons	Motor to eyeball
C.N. V	Trigeminal nerve	Pons	Motor to muscles of chewing
C.N. VII	Facial nerve	Pons	Sensory to face, motor to muscles of face expression, sensory taste to anterior 2/3 of tongue (sweet, sour, salty taste)
C.N. VII	Vestibulocochlear nerve	Medulla oblongata and cerebrum	Sensory for hearing
		Pons and cerebellum	Sensory for equilibrium
C.N. IX	Glossopharyngeal nerve	Medulla oblongata	Motor to pharynx (uvula), sensory to posterior 2/3 of tongue (bitter taste)
C.N. X	Vagus nerve	Medulla oblongata	Motor to larynx, sensory to pharynx
C.N. XI	Spiral accessory nerve	Medulla oblongata	Motor to sternocleidomastoid and trapezius muscles
C.N. XII	Hypoglossal nerve	Medulla oblongata	Motor to tongue

What Are Some Examples of Diseases or Disorders of Cranial Nerves?

Two examples of diseases that can affect cranial nerves are trigeminal neuralgia and Bell's palsy.

1. *Trigeminal neuralgia*. ***Trigeminal neuralgia*** is also called ***tic douloureux***. Trigeminal neuralgia can be caused by degenerative changes or by a compression or impingement of the trigeminal nerve (C.N. V) as a result of trauma to the nerve.

What are the signs and symptoms associated with trigeminal neuralgia?
Trigeminal neuralgia presents with deep, sharp, stabbing pain along the nerve distribution. This pain can be extremely severe.

2. *Bell's palsy*. ***Bell's palsy*** is the inflammation of C.N. XII. This neuritis will cause temporary paralysis of one side of the face. The causes of Bell's palsy include trauma to the nerve and an infection caused by a virus or bacterium.

What are the signs and symptoms associated with Bell's palsy?
The signs and symptoms of Bell's palsy present with a loss of function of the muscles of facial expression, tearing of the eye on the affected side, and drooling from the side of the mouth on the affected side. The individual may also experience headaches.

18.4 Pathophysiology of the Brain

What Are Some Diseases and Disorders That Can Affect the Brain?

Diseases that can affect the brain include

- Alzheimer's disease
- Amyotrophic lateral sclerosis
- Cerebral palsy
- Cerebrovascular accident (stroke)
- Epilepsy (seizures)
- Encephalitis
- Huntington's disease
- Parkinson's disease

What Is Alzheimer's Disease?

Alzheimer's disease is a progressive degenerative disease that can occur in the cerebral cortex of the brain.

The direct cause of Alzheimer's disease is unknown, although the lack of certain neurotransmitters, such as acetylcholine, somatostatin, and norepinephrine, may be a factor. Also, tangled fibers in the neurons, degeneration of neurons, trauma, family history, and genetic defects contribute to the development of Alzheimer's disease.

What are the signs and symptoms associated with Alzheimer's disease?
The signs and symptoms of Alzheimer's disease include loss of memory, dementia, disorientation, confusion, irritability and restlessness, personality changes (mood swings, depression, anger, hostility), and deterioration of speech.

What Is Amyotrophic Lateral Sclerosis?

Amyotrophic lateral sclerosis, or ***ALS***, is commonly called *Lou Gehrig's disease* after the New York Yankees first baseman who died from the disease. This is a progressive degenerative disease that affects the motor neurons of the cranial and spinal nerves.

The direct cause of ALS is unknown, although hereditary and environmental factors (such as viruses, metabolic imbalances, and immune disorders) may contribute to it. ALS occurs more commonly in men between the ages of 40 and 75. As the neurons deteriorate and eventually die, the skeletal muscles that they innervate weaken and eventually atrophy. This disease commonly results in death within six years of onset.

What are the signs and symptoms associated with amyotrophic lateral sclerosis?
The signs and symptoms associated with ALS include muscle spasms and cramps, fatigue, muscle weakness, slurred speech, difficulty chewing, difficulty swallowing, and, in the later stages, choking, muscle paralysis, and difficulty breathing.

What Is Cerebral Palsy?

Cerebral palsy is a nonprogressive disorder that affects the motor portion of the brain. This disease, although nonprogressive, is permanent.

Cerebral palsy is caused by an infection, trauma, or other toxic conditions that damage the brain during or before birth.

What are the signs and symptoms associated with cerebral palsy?
The signs and symptoms of cerebral palsy will present with an impairment of motor function (speech, walking), muscle spasms, and spastic paralysis.

What Is a Cerebrovascular Accident?

A ***cerebrovascular accident***, or ***CVA***, is commonly referred to as a *stroke*. A CVA results when the blood flow from one or more blood vessels in the brain is impaired, interrupted, or stopped. This lack of blood supply (ischemia) results in brain cell and tissue necrosis (cell death) and brain damage.

The cause of a CVA can be either an occlusion or blockage in an artery, called an *embolism*; clotting in an unbroken blood vessel, called a *thrombosis*; or a rupture in an artery, causing a *hemorrhage* (bleeding). Contributing factors that can increase the risk of a CVA include a family history, hypertension, atherosclerosis, diabetes mellitus, cardiovascular disease, high cholesterol, poor diet, and smoking.

What are the signs and symptoms associated with a cerebrovascular accident?
The signs and symptoms associated with a CVA include numbness, paralysis of one side of the face and/or one side of the body (hemiparesis), slurred speech (dysphasia), lack of ability or inability to speak (aphasia), muscle weakness, loss of time or memory, mental confusion, impairments of sight, coma, and even death.

What Is Epilepsy?

Epilepsy is an abnormal brain condition that causes seizures. These seizures occur as a result of an abnormal increase in electrical impulses of neurons in the brain.

Most epileptic cases and seizures are of unknown cause. Causes and contributing factors can include brain injuries, brain tumors or lesions, diabetes mellitus, chemical toxins, CVA, fevers, infections (meningitis, encephalitis), problems with normal metabolism, phenylketonuria, hypocalcemia, hyponatremia, hypoglycemia, and withdrawals from drug and alcohol addiction.

What are the signs and symptoms associated with epilepsy?
Signs and symptoms associated with epilepsy include nausea; visual disturbances; bad, abnormal, or unusual tastes and smells; abnormal levels or loss of consciousness; muscle tremors or convulsions; and loss of sensation.

What Is Encephalitis?

Encephalitis is an inflammation of the brain. This inflammation can cause seizures, delirium, cephalgia, damage to the brain, coma, and death as a result of the degenerative changes that occur within the brain.

Encephalitis is caused by an infection. Viral infections are most common.

What are the signs and symptoms associated with encephalitis?
Signs and symptoms associated with encephalitis include fever, cephalgia, lethargy, delirium, and seizures.

What Is Huntington's Disease?

Huntington's disease, or ***Huntington's chorea***, is a progressive, hereditary disorder in which signs and symptoms commonly begin between 35 and 50 years of age. This disorder will eventually lead to death. Before death, the individual becomes totally incapacitated, with severe choreiform movements (rapid contortions and rigidity of muscles).

Huntington's chorea is an autosomal dominant disorder affecting the front lobe of the cerebral cortex of the brain. It causes a decrease in the levels of the neurotransmitter GABA, resulting in severe nerve damage to the cortex.

What are the signs and symptoms of Huntington's disease?
The signs and symptoms of Huntington's chorea present with rigidity in the muscles of the face, trunk, and upper extremities; mental changes; depression; dystonia; ataxia; muscular writhing; choreic movement of muscles; difficulty swallowing; and dementia.

What Is Parkinson's Disease?

Parkinson's disease, or shaking palsy, is a slow, progressive degenerative disease that affects motor neurons. Parkinson's disease tends to be more common in men between the ages of 40 and 65, although women and younger people can also have this disease.

The cause of Parkinson's disease is unknown, although the cells of the substantia nigra portion of the midbrain fail to produce adequate amounts of the neurotransmitter dopamine. This may be the result of a brain tumor, carbon monoxide poisoning, drugs, or repeated chronic head trauma.

What are the signs and symptoms associated with Parkinson's disease?
Signs and symptoms associated with Parkinson's disease include resting tremors, slow movements, slowed speech, lack of coordination and balance, a shuffling gait, and a freezing, masklike facial expression.

18.5 The Spinal Cord

What Is the Spinal Cord?

The *spinal cord* is part of the central nervous system. It extends inferiorly from the medulla oblongata of the brain stem to L1 (the first lumbar vertebra).

At L1, the spinal cord narrows to a "V" shape. This is called the *conus medullaris*. From the conus medullaris, the spinal cord fans out like a horse's tail. This is called the *cauda equina*.

The *filum terminale* anchors the spinal cord to the coccyx bone.

A cross section of the spinal cord is shown in Figure 18.3.

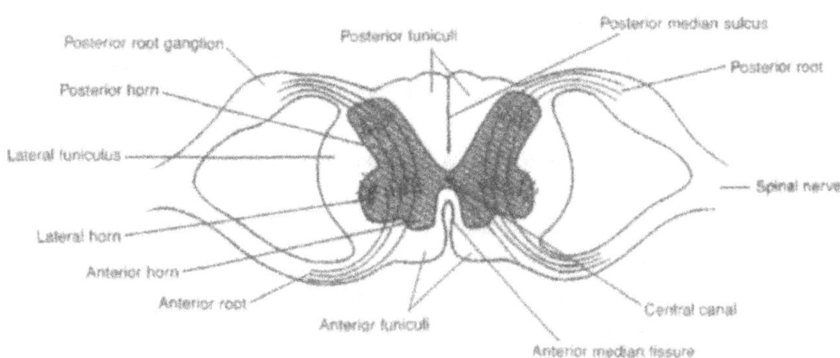

Figure 18.3 A cross section of the spinal cord and the roots of a paired spinal nerve.

What Protects the Spinal Cord?

The spinal cord is protected by the *meninges*.

What Are Spinal Nerves?

Spinal nerves are part of the peripheral nervous system.

How Many Spinal Nerves Are There, and Where Do They Exit the Spinal Cord?

There are 31 pairs of spinal nerves:

- 8 cervical
- 12 thoracic
- 5 lumbar
- 5 sacral
- 1 coccyx

These spinal nerves consist of spinal nerve roots. Each spinal nerve contains a dorsal root for sensory information and a ventral root for motor information.

Remember: Sensory information enters the posterior portion of the spinal cord. Motor information exits from the anterior portion of the spinal cord.

The cervical, lumbar, and sacral spinal nerves come together to form ***plexuses.*** These plexuses, the cervical, brachial, lumbar, and sacral plexuses, become the peripheral nerves that provide nervous innervation (supply) to the skin and muscles of the neck, upper extremities, buttocks, and lower extremities.

Figure 18.4 shows the spinal nerves and plexuses.

What Are the Sensory Pathways, and What Are They Responsible For?

The sensory pathways of the spinal cord are called *ascending tracts*. The ascending pathways to the cerebral cortex of the brain include the following:

- The *anterior spinothalamic tract* is responsible for the sensation of crude touch, itch, tickle, pressure, and light touch.
- The *lateral spinothalamic tract* is responsible for the sensation of temperature and pain.

These two tracts are located on the anterior and lateral portions of the spinal cord.

- The *fasciculus gracilis* is responsible for fine touch, vibration, two-point discrimination, weight discrimination, proprioception, and stereognosis (the ability to recognize familiar objects by sense or touch) sensations from the lower portion of the body.
- The *fasciculus cuneatus* is responsible for fine touch, vibration, two-point discrimination, weight discrimination, proprioception, and stereognosis sensations from the upper portion of the body.

The ascending pathways to the cerebellum of the brain are as follows:

- The *posterior spinocerebellar tract* is responsible for the sensations associated with equilibrium, posture, unconscious proprioception, and balance.
- The *anterior spinocerebellar tract* is responsible for the sensations associated with posture and coordination of fine skilled movement.

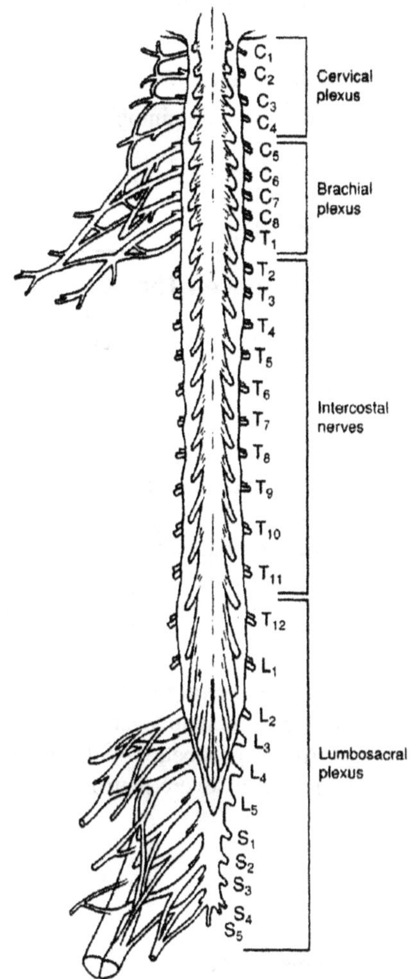

Figure 18.4 The spinal cord, spinal nerves, and plexuses.

What Are the Motor Pathways, and What Are They Responsible For?

The motor pathways of the spinal cord are called *descending tracts*. The descending pathways take either a direct route (which is called a pyramidal pathway) or a complex or indirect route (which is called an extrapyramidal pathway).

The direct routes include the

- *Lateral corticospinal tract*. This is responsible for conscious voluntary, skilled movements of the hands and feet.
- *Anterior corticospinal tract*. This is responsible for conscious voluntary, coordinated movement of the axial skeleton.
- *Corticobulbar tract*. This is responsible for conscious voluntary movement of muscles innervated by cranial nerves.

The indirect routes include the

- *Lateral reticulospinal tract*. This flexes the flexor muscles and inhibits the extensor muscles.
- *Medial reticulospinal tract*. This extends the extensor muscles and inhibits the flexor muscles.

- *Rubrospinal tract.* This is responsible for precise fine movements of hands and feet on the opposite side of the body.
- *Tectospinal tract.* This turns the head, neck, and eyes in response to visual stimuli.
- *Vestibulospinal tract.* This is responsible for maintaining same side of the body balance.

18.6 Pathophysiology of the Spinal Cord

What Are Examples of Disorders and Diseases That Can Affect the Spinal Cord?

Examples of diseases and disorders that can affect the spinal cord are meningitis, poliomyelitis, and spina bifida.

What Is Meningitis?

Meningitis is the inflammation of the protective covering of the brain and spinal cord. This protective covering is called the *meninges.*

Meningitis can be caused by either a virus or a bacterium, such as *Staphylococcus aureus, Streptococcus pneumoniae*, or *Neisseria meningitides*, that is transmitted through droplets from the respiratory system by coughing, sneezing, and exhaling. The organisms can enter the blood through the nasopharynx, then make their way to the cerebrospinal fluid.

What are the signs and symptoms associated with meningitis?
The signs and symptoms associated with meningitis include fever, sleepiness, headache, neck ache and stiffness, confusion, and vomiting. Viral meningitis normally gets better on its own in about two weeks. Bacterial meningitis, on the other hand, if not treated, can result in severe neurological malfunctions, such as paralysis and death.

What Is Poliomyelitis?

Poliomyelitis is a disease that causes inflammation of the gray matter of the spinal cord. This inflammation destroys motor neurons in the brain and spinal cord.

Poliomyelitis is caused by infection with the polio virus.

What are the signs and symptoms associated with poliomyelitis?
The signs and symptoms associated with poliomyelitis include paralysis, flaccid paralysis, muscle atrophy, respiratory failure, and infections of the digestive system and respiratory system. Death can occur as a result of respiratory failure.

What is Spina Bifida?

Spina bifida is a congenital defect in which the posterior arches of the vertebrae (L5 and/or LS1) fail to fuse. The posterior arch includes the spinous process and laminae. There are two different types of spina bifida:

1. *Spina bifida occulta.* Spina bifida occulta presents with no protrusion; just a small impression or dimple may be present in the region of the defect. No symptoms are present.
2. *Spina bifida cystica.* Spina bifida cystica presents with a sac or cystlike protrusion at the level of L5-S1. There are two types:
    - *Spina bifida cystica meningocele.* In this condition, the meninges and cerebrospinal fluid protrude into the saclike protrusion.
    - *Spina bifida cystica meningomyelocele.* In this condition, the spinal cord and/or the spinal nerves protrude into the saclike protrusion.

Spina bifida is a congenital abnormality and can be linked to low levels of folic acid (B vitamin) during pregnancy.

What are the signs and symptoms associated with spina bifida cystica meningomyelocele?
Spina bifida cystica meningomyelocele is the most serious and presents with severe neurological dysfunction, which includes partial or complete paralysis and loss of bowel and urinary bladder control.

18.7 The Special Senses

The special senses include smell, taste, vision, and hearing. This section will review vision and hearing.

What Are the Structures of the Eye?

The eyeball is about one inch in diameter and is covered by a thin mucous membrane called the *conjunctiva*. The eyeball can be divided into three layers:

1. *Fibrous tunic*. The fibrous tunic makes up the outer portion of the eyeball. It consists of the
   - *Cornea*. The cornea lets light into the eye and also bends the light. The cornea is the clear portion of the eye.
   - *Sclera*. The sclera provides protection and shape. The sclera is the white portion of the eye.
2. *Vascular tunic*. The vascular tunic contains the
   - *Choroid*. The choroid provides the blood supply to the eye and also absorbs scattered light rays.
   - *Iris*. The iris contains an opening in the anterior portion of the eye called the *pupil*. The iris regulates the amount of light entering the eyeball.
   - *Ciliary body*. The ciliary body contains the ciliary processes, ciliary muscle, and suspensory ligaments, which are attached to and change the shape of the lens.
   - *Lens*. The lens is made of proteins called *crystallins*. The lens refracts (bends) the light that enters the eye. As the lens becomes more rounded or convex (the curve becomes greater), the focusing power increases. For example, the lens becomes *more* curved when viewing objects that are up close. The lens becomes *less* curved when the objects being viewed are far away.
3. *Nervous tunic*. The nervous tunic contains the *retina*. The retina contains photoreceptors that receive the light that enters the eye and convert that light into receptor potentials or electrical impulses. These electrical impulses enter the brain (sensory input) through bipolar neurons that form the optic nerve (cranial nerve II).

   There are two types of photoreceptors:

1. *Rods*. Rods are used during dim light. We see shades of gray (black and white) with rods.
2. *Cones*. Cones are used during bright light for seeing color.

Remember: You can see orange safety *cones* in the street because of your *cones*.

What Are Some Common Diseases Associated with the Eye?

Diseases that can affect the eye include

- Astigmatism
- Myopia
- Hyperopia
- Nyctalopia
- Conjunctivitis
- Strabismus
- Glaucoma
- Cataracts

What Is Astigmatism?

Astigmatism is the abnormal bending of the light that enters the eye. It is caused by an abnormal curve in the lens of the eye. This causes the light entering the eye to bend irregularly.

What Is Myopia?

Myopia is a condition in which an individual can see objects that are close but cannot see objects that are far away clearly. Myopia occurs when the eyeball has an elongated shape.

What Is Hyperopia?

Hyperopia is a condition in which an individual can see objects that are far away but cannot see objects that are close clearly. Hyperopia occurs when the eyeball has a shortened shape.

What Is Nyctalopia?

Nyctalopia is commonly referred to as night blindness. The individual is unable to see objects in the darkness of night. Nyctalopia can occur when there is a retinol or vitamin A deficiency or if there is a degeneration of the retina. (Nyctamblyopia is a decrease in vision at night with no visible structural changes in the eye.)

What Is Conjunctivitis?

Conjunctivitis is commonly called "pinkeye" and occurs when the protective mucous membrane that covers the eyeball, the conjunctiva, is inflamed. Conjunctivitis is very contagious and can be caused by bacterial infections or viral infections.

What Is Strabismus?

Strabismus is the deviation of one or both eyes. This deviation can be medial or lateral, and can converge or diverge. When one eye deviates medially, it is called *convergent strabismus*. When one eye deviates laterally, it is called *divergent strabismus*. Strabismus can be caused by a traumatic injury to the eye and/or brain, or it can be inherited.

What Is Glaucoma?

Glaucoma occurs when there is an increase in intraocular pressure. This is a potentially dangerous disorder. If left untreated, it can result in damage to the optic nerves, and blindness can occur. Glaucoma is caused by an excessive buildup of aqueous humor in the anterior chamber of the eye. This buildup can be the result of an obstruction or trauma.

What Is a Cataract?

A ***cataract*** is a cloudiness or fogginess in vision caused by a buildup of calcium within the lens or cornea of the eye. A cataract can be caused by degeneration of aging, trauma, exposure to sunlight, and certain medications.

What Are the Structures of the Ear?

The ear is composed of three regions:

1. *Outer ear.* The outer ear consists of three parts:
    - Auricle or earlobe
    - External auditory canal
    - Eardrum or tympanic membrane

2. *Middle ear.* The middle ear contains the auditory ossicles (malleus, incus, and stapes) and the auditory or eustachian tubes, which connect to the nasopharynx.
3. *Inner ear.* The inner ear, also called the *labyrinth*, contains the *cochlea* and the *vestibular apparatus*. The cochlea portion of the inner ear is responsible for *hearing*. The vestibular portion of the inner ear is responsible for *equilibrium*. Sensory information for both hearing and equilibrium travel to the brain by the vestibulocochlear nerve, or cranial nerve VIII.

What Are Some Common Diseases Associated with the Ear?

Some common diseases that are associated with the ear include

- Tinnitis
- Otitis media
- Otitis interna
- Meniere's disease

What Is Tinnitus?

Tinnitus is the term used to describe "ringing" in the ears. Tinnitus can be caused by an injury, an infection, otosclerosis (which is a type of conductive hearing loss resulting from a stapes that is immobile), and presbyacusis (which is caused by the deterioration of the auditory system that can occur during the normal aging process).

What Is Otitis Media?

Otitis media is a middle ear infection that causes pain, inflammation, and fever. It is more common in children and occurs as a result of an upper respiratory infection that has spread up the eustachian tubes into the middle ear.

What Is Otitis Interna?

Otitis interna is also called labyrinthitis and is an inner ear infection that results in inflammation, dizziness (vertigo), and nausea. Otitis interna occurs when there is an infection of the inner ear.

What Is Meniere's disease?

Meniere's disease most commonly occurs in males and affects the inner ear. The individual will experience dizziness (vertigo), a ringing sound in the ears (tinnitus), and nausea. This condition progresses to a loss of hearing. Meniere's disease occurs when the endolymph (the fluid found in the inner ear) accumulates in the inner ear.

Chapter 18 Review Questions

Fill In the Blank

1. The portion of the nervous system that responds to changes is called the ____________ portion.
2. The portion of the nervous system that reacts to these changes is called the ____________ portion.
3. The division of the nervous system that includes the brain and the spinal cord is referred to as the ________________.
4. The division of the nervous system that includes the cranial nerves and the peripheral nerves is referred to as the ________________.
5. There are ____________ of cranial nerves.

6. There are ______________ of spinal nerves.
7. The subdivision of the peripheral nervous system that controls skeletal muscle activity is the ____________.
8. The subdivision of the peripheral nervous system that controls cardiac and smooth muscle activity is the ________________.
9. The subdivision of the peripheral nervous system that controls glands is the ______________.
10. The subdivision of the autonomic nervous system that is referred to as "fight or flight" is the ______________.
11. The subdivision of the autonomic nervous system that is referred to as "rest and digest" is the ________________.
12. The nerve cells that elicit electrical impulses are the __________________.
13. The nerve cells that have a supporting role are the __________________
14. Neurons that are found mostly in the brain and spinal cord are the __________________.
15. Neurons that are associated with special senses are the ________________.
16. Neurons that are associated with general senses are the __________________.
17. If a neuron is myelinated, it is said to be ____________________.
18. If a neuron is unmyelinated, it is said to be ____________________
19. A word that means "nerve pain" is __________________.
20. A word that means "nerve inflammation" is ____________________.
21. Dysfunction of the peripheral nerves is called ____________________.
22. The most superficial layer of the meninges is the ___________________.
23. The middle layer of the meninges is the ____________________.
24. The innermost layer of the meninges is the ____________________.
25. The cerebrospinal fluid is located in the ____________________.

Matching

26. Microglia cells
27. Ependymal cells
28. Neurolemmocytes
29. Astrocytes
30. Oligodendrocytes
31. Satellite cells
32. Ganglion
33. MS
34. Guillain-Barré syndrome
35. Tay-Sachs disease
    - A. Blood-brain barrier
    - B. Responsible for phagocytosis
    - C. Circulate cerebrospinal fluid

D. Also called Schwann cells
E. Form myelin sheath in the CNS
F. Support cell bodies in the ganglion
G. "Swelling" or "lump"
H. Causes an accumulation of lipids around the myelin sheath
I. Demyelination and plaquing occur within the myelin sheath
J. The immune system attacks peripheral nerves

True/False

36. The medulla oblongata regulates vital reflexes.

37. Sneezing would be considered a vital reflex.

38. The pons is part of the midbrain.

39. Pons means "bridge."

40. The substantia nigra secretes the neurotransmitter dopamine.

41. The thalamus is located in the diencephalon portion of the brain.

42. Tic douloureux is caused by an impingement or degeneration of cranial nerve V.

43. Bell's palsy is neuritis of cranial nerve X.

44. ALS is a progressive degenerative disease in which neurons deteriorate. It is more common in males.

45. Cerebral palsy is a progressive disorder.

Matching

46. CVA

47. Slurred speech

48. Epilepsy

49. Thrombosis

50. Cerebral palsy

A. Caused by an infection or trauma during birth
B. Referred to as a stroke
C. A clot in an unbroken blood vessel
D. Dysphasia
E. Causes seizures

Chapter 18: Review Questions and Answers

Fill In the Blank Answers

1. Sensory

2. Motor

3. Central nervous system

4. Peripheral nervous system

5. 12 pairs

6. 31 pairs

7. Somatic nervous system

8. Autonomic nervous system

9. Enteric nervous system
10. Sympathetic
11. Parasympathetic
12. Neurons
13. Neuroglia cells
14. Multipolar neurons
15. Bipolar neurons
16. Unipolar neurons
17. White matter
18. Gray matter
19. Neuralgia
20. Neuritis
21. Neuropathy
22. Dura mater
23. Arachnoid mater
24. Pia mater
25. Subarachnoid space

Matching Answers

26. B
27. C
28. D
29. A
30. E
31. F
32. G
33. I
34. J
35. H

True/False Answers

36. True
37. False
38. False
39. True
40. True
41. True
42. True
43. False
44. True
45. False

Matching Answers

46. B
47. D
48. E
49. C
50. A

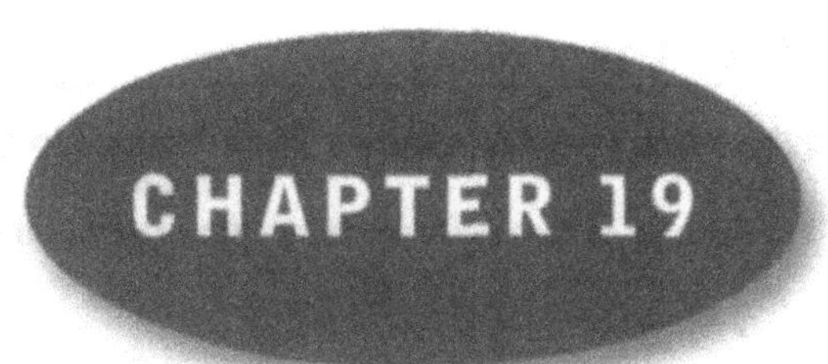

The Gastrointestinal System

Objectives

This chapter will review the structures that make up the gastrointestinal tract, review the functions of these structures, and discuss the diseases and disorders that can affect these structures.

Keywords:

Mouth
Pharynx
Esophagus
Hiatal hernia
Gastroesophageal reflux disease (GERD)
Stomach
Gastritis
Stomach ulcers
Stomach cancer
Small intestine
Crohn's disease
Ulcerative colitis
Large intestine
Rectum
Anus
Appendicitis
Colorectal cancer
Diverticulosis
Diverticulitis
Hemorrhoids
Liver
Hepatitis
Gallbladder
Cholecystitis
Gallstones
Pancreas
Pancreatitis
Pancreatic cancer
Ductal adenocarcinoma

19.1 Overview

What Are the Structures That Make Up the Gastrointestinal Tract?

The structures that make up the gastrointestinal tract include the

- Mouth
- Pharynx
- Esophagus
- Stomach
- Small intestine
- Large intestine
- Rectum
- Anus

Figure 19.1 shows the structures of the digestive system.

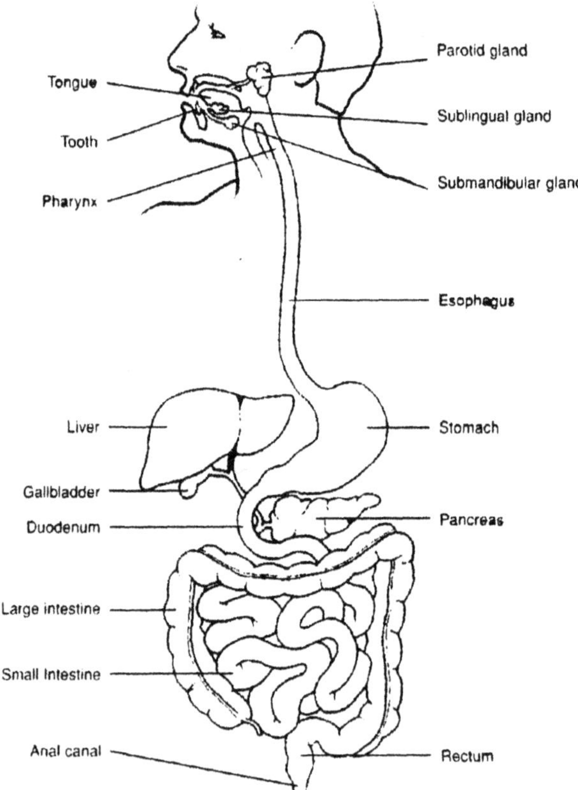

Figure 19.1 The digestive system.

What Structures Make Up the Mouth?

The *mouth* contains the teeth, which include the

- Incisors
- Cuspids

- Bicuspids (premolars)
- Molars

The mouth also contains the tongue, which contains papillae.

What Are Papillae?

Papillae are projections of the lamina propria. There are three types:

1. *Filiform papillae.* Filiform papillae have no taste buds but create friction to move food around your mouth.
2. *Fungiform papillae.* These taste buds resemble mushrooms and are scattered all over the surface of the tongue.
3. *Circumvallate papillae.* These taste buds form an inverted "V" on the posterior portion of the tongue.

What Part of the Tongue Senses Taste?

The anterior two-thirds of the tongue senses sweet, sour, and salty tastes. The posterior one-third of the tongue senses bitter tastes.

What Is Saliva?

Saliva contains water, mucin, and salivary amylase. The pH of saliva is 6.35 to 6.85. There are three glands that secrete saliva into the mouth:

1. Parotid gland
2. Submandible gland
3. Sublingual gland

What Is the Pharynx and Where Is It Located?

The ***pharynx*** is the throat. The pharynx has three regions:

1. *Nasopharynx.* The nasopharynx is located posterior to the nasal cavity.
2. *Oropharynx.* The oropharynx is located posterior to the oral cavity.
3. *Laryngopharynx.* The laryngopharynx is located posterior to the larynx and connects the mouth to the esophagus.

What Is the Esophagus?

The ***esophagus*** is a collapsible muscular tube that connects the pharynx to the stomach.

What Diseases or Disorders Can Affect the Esophagus?

Two diseases that can affect the esophagus are hiatal hernia and gastroesophageal reflux disease.

- *Hiatal hernia.* A ***hiatal hernia*** occurs when a portion of the stomach gets pushed up through the opening of the diaphragm (called the esophageal hiatus).

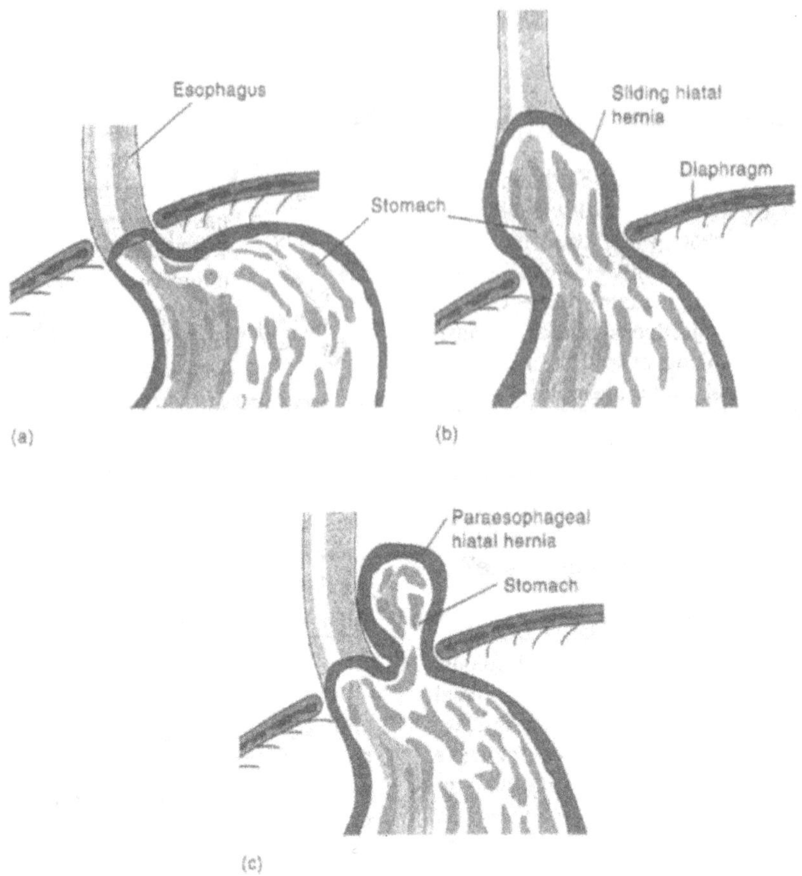

Figure 19.2 Hiatal hernia.

- *Gastroesophageal reflux disease.* ***Gastroesophageal reflux disease***, or ***GERD***, is also referred to as "heartburn." Gastroesophageal reflux disease occurs when the hydrochloric acid that is maintained in the stomach gets pushed into the esophagus.

Causes of GERD include hiatal hernia, pregnancy, a malfunction of the esophageal sphincter, foods such as chocolate or fatty foods, and smoking.

What are the signs and symptoms associated with gastroesophageal reflux disease?
The signs and symptoms associated with gastroesophageal reflux disease include burning sensations in the epigastric region and/or throat, especially after meals and in the supine position. Nausea and vomiting with blood can also occur.

What Is the Stomach, Where Is It Located, and What Is Its Function?

The ***stomach*** is located in the right upper quadrant of the abdominopelvic cavity. The stomach mixes ingested food, saliva, and gastric juices (secretions) to form *chyme*, and also holds food until the small intestine is ready to accept this food.

What Is Gastric Juice Made Up Of?

Gastric juice consists of hydrochloric acid, intrinsic factor, gastric lipase, and pepsinogen.

Which Stomach Cells Secrete Gastric Juice?

1. *Surface mucous cells* and *mucous neck cells* secrete mucus, which acts as a protective barrier that prevents damage to the stomach.
2. *Parietal cells* secrete
   - *Hydrochloric acid*, which kills most microorganisms and denatures proteins.
   - *Intrinsic factor*, which is needed to absorb vitamin B_{12}. (Vitamin B_{12} is needed to make red blood cells.)
3. *Chief cells* secrete:
   - *Gastric lipase*, which breaks down fats.
   - *Pepsinogen*, which is converted to pepsin (the active form) when it makes contact with the hydrochloric acid. Pepsin breaks down protein.

What Are Examples of Diseases and Disorders That Affect the Stomach?

Some examples of stomach diseases are gastritis, stomach ulcers, and stomach cancer.

What Is Gastritis?

Gastritis occurs when the lining of the stomach becomes inflamed. Gastritis can be caused by bacterial or viral infections, medicines, alcohol, stress, and certain foods, such as foods that are hot and spicy.

What are the signs and symptoms associated with gastritis?
Gastritis presents with an upset stomach, nausea and vomiting, and heartburn.

What Are Stomach Ulcers?

Stomach ulcers are erosions of the stomach lining. If they are severe enough, these ulcerations can bleed.

These ulcers can be caused by a bacterial infection, *Helicobacter pylori*. Increased amounts of stomach hydrochloric acid, cigarette smoking, drinking alcoholic beverages, and chronic aspirin use can contribute to stomach ulcers.

What are the signs and symptoms associated with stomach ulcers?
Stomach ulcers commonly present with severe abdominal pain and nausea associated with vomiting and loss of weight. The vomit can have a coffee grounds appearance, representing digested blood, or the blood can be red.

What Is Stomach Cancer?

The cause of ***stomach cancer*** is unknown, although stomach ulcers may be a factor.

What are the signs and symptoms associated with stomach cancer?
Stomach cancer commonly presents with a bloating sensation, gas, abdominal pain and cramping, bloody stool, nausea, and vomiting.

What Is the Small Intestine?

The ***small intestine*** is a muscular tube that extends from the stomach to the cecum of the large intestine. Most of the digested food is absorbed into the blood through the small intestine. The small intestine has three sections:

1. Duodenum
2. Jejunum
3. Ileum

The cells that make up the endothelial lining of the small intestine contain microvilli that increase the surface area for the absorption of digested food. The small intestine contains glands that secrete an alkaline mucus that protects the lining from digestive enzymes and stomach acid, called *Brunner's glands*, and glands that secrete digestive enzymes, called *crypts of Licherkühn*.

What Are Examples of Disorders That Affect the Small Intestine?

A condition that affects the small intestines is Crohn's disease.

Crohn's disease. ***Crohn's disease***, or ***CD***, is also known as *regional enteritis* and is a chronic inflammatory disease that affects the mucosa layer, resulting in inflammation and ulceration. Intestinal stenosis can occur as a result of fibrosis in the submucosa layer and the hypertrophic muscular layer. Crohn's disease typically affects both the small and large intestines, but it can occur anywhere in the gastrointestinal tract, from the mouth to the anus.

This is regional enteritis because tissue changes can occur at any given section without adjacent regions being involved.

The causes of Crohn's disease are unknown, although there tends to be a familial pattern as well as an autoimmune component. Infectious agents, such as enteric bacteria, mycobacteria, viruses, and chlamydiae, have also been suspected.

What are the signs and symptoms associated with Crohn's disease?

Crohn's disease presents with abdominal pain and cramping, fever and diarrhea, decreased weight, and decrease in red blood cell production (caused by malabsorption).

What Is the Large Intestine?

The ***large intestine*** extends from the small intestine to the anus. The large intestine is also called the *large bowel* or *colon* and consists of five sections or parts.

The large intestine begins as the *cecum*, which is attached to the ileum of the small intestine. Off the cecum is a wormlike projection called the *vermiform appendix* or *appendix*. The appendix has no purpose in humans. The *ascending colon* travels superiorly to the *transverse colon*, which travels transversely across the abdomen to hook up with the *descending colon*. The descending colon travels inferiorly to the *sigmoid colon*, an S-shaped structure connected to the rectum. The ***rectum*** stores feces. The feces empty along the *anal canal* and exit the body through a muscular opening called the ***anus***.

What Is the Function of the Large Intestine?

The large intestine functions in the absorption of water, ions, and vitamins and the formation of feces. Water, inorganic salts, epithelial cells, undigested food (such as fiber), and bacteria are expelled from the body as feces.

What Are Examples of Diseases or Disorders That Can Affect the Large Intestine, Rectum, and Anus?

Examples of diseases or disorders that can affect the large intestine, rectum, and anus include appendicitis, colorectal cancer, diverticulosis, hemorrhoids, and **ulcerative colitis.**

What Is Appendicitis?

Appendicitis is inflammation of the appendix. Appendicitis can be caused by an obstruction of hard fecal matter in the lumen, resulting in bacterial growth. The fecal matter is called a *fecalith* and starts the inflammatory process. Inflammation can also be caused by the compression from a mass, such as a tumor, an abscess, or even a gallstone. Parasites can also cause blockages. An example of such a parasite would be pinworms.

What are the signs and symptoms associated with appendicitis?
The signs and symptoms of appendicitis initially present as mild epigastric or umbilical pain. As the appendix continues to swell, it pushes against the abdominal wall and parietal peritoneum, causing severe localized pain in the lower right quadrant.

What Is Colorectal Cancer?

Colorectal cancer is cancer that affects the mucosal lining of the rectum and colon. Most tumors that grow in the gastrointestinal tract tend to be carcinomas. These carcinomas can be found in the colon, stomach, esophagus, and small intestine. Cancer of the colon is the most common, and cancer of the small intestine is the least common.

The cause of colon cancer is unknown, although high-fat, low-fiber diets may contribute, and polyps in the colon and/or rectum can become cancerous.

What are the signs and symptoms associated with colorectal cancer?
Colorectal cancer presents with abdominal pain, especially at night; blood in the feces; "pencil thin" feces; bowel obstruction; weight loss; and anemia.

What Is Diverticulosis?

Diverticulosis is a condition of the colon (most common in the sigmoid colon) in which pouchlike sacs called *diverticula* protrude through the mucosa wall of the colon. When these sacs become inflamed or swell, the condition is called ***diverticulitis***.

The cause of diverticulosis is unknown, although infections of the diverticula and a poor diet lacking fiber have been known to cause the condition. Eating peanuts and seeds has been known to exacerbate the condition.

What are the signs and symptoms associated with diverticulosis?
Diverticulosis is often asymptomatic (having no symptoms). If the condition is becoming exacerbated, the individual may experience abdominal pain, constipation, diarrhea, blood in the feces, nausea, and fever.

What Are Hemorrhoids?

Varices in the veins of the rectum and anus are referred to as ***hemorrhoids***. Hemorrhoids can be caused by an increased or elevated pressure in veins, pregnancy and labor, obesity, and chronic constipation that causes the individual to strain while moving his or her bowels.

What are the signs and symptoms associated with hemorrhoids?
Hemorrhoids present as bulges in the anal region. Bright red blood can be found in the feces, and there is pain during defecation and itching in the anal region.

What Is Ulcerative Colitis?

Ulcerative colitis, also known as ***UC***, can be chronic or acute and is also an inflammatory and ulcerative process. This disease process is restricted to the large intestine, beginning at the rectosigmoid region and extending upward, until it eventually affects the entire colon. The cause of ulcerative colitis is unknown.

What are the signs and symptoms associated with ulcerative colitis?
The signs and symptoms of ulcerative colitis include watery diarrhea that contains blood and mucus. This diarrhea can be sudden and urgent. The individual can also present with a high fever, weight loss, anemia (decrease in red blood cells), malaise, and toxemia. There is also a risk of hemorrhage, which is a common complication of ulcerative colitis.

19.2 Accessory Structures of the Gastrointestinal Tract

What Are the Accessory Structures of the Gastrointestinal Tract?

The accessory structures of the gastrointestinal tract include the liver, gallbladder, and pancreas.

What Is the Liver and Where Is It Located?

The ***liver*** is composed of a right and a left lobe and is located in the right upper quadrant of the abdominopelvic cavity. The lobes of the liver are connected to each other and to the common bile duct (coming off the gallbladder) by the common hepatic duct.

What Is the Function of the Liver?

The liver functions in the metabolism of carbohydrates, lipids, and proteins; processes hormones and drugs; stores vitamins; and excretes bilirubin.

What Is a Disease That Can Affect the Liver?

A disease that can affect the liver is ***hepatitis***. Hepatitis is the inflammation of the liver. Hepatitis can be caused by a bacterial infection; a viral infection, such as hepatitis B virus (HBV); a parasitic infection; alcohol abuse and drug abuse, including overuse of acetaminophen; and undercooked or contaminated food.

What are the signs and symptoms associated with hepatitis?
Hepatitis commonly presents with an enlarged liver, jaundice (yellow color to the skin and sclera of the eyes), abdominal pain, nausea and vomiting, weakness, and urine that is very dark.

What Is the Gallbladder and Where Is It Located?

The ***gallbladder*** lies between the lobes of the liver in the right upper quadrant.

What Is the Function of the Gallbladder?

The gallbladder stores *bile*. Under the influence of the hormone cholecystokinin, the gallbladder contracts, ejecting bile through the cystic duct into the common bile duct and into the duodenum of the small intestine, where it emulsifies fats.

What Is a Disease of the Gallbladder?

A common disease of the gallbladder is ***cholecystitis***, which is the inflammation of the gallbladder as a result of the blockage of a cystic duct by a gallstone.

What are the signs and symptoms associated with cholecystitis?
Cholecystitis commonly presents as recurring colicky pain in the right upper quadrant that refers pain to the inferior angle of the right scapula.

What Are Gallstones?

Gallstones are made up of solidified bile salts, phospholipids, and cholesterol.

What Is the Pancreas?

The ***pancreas*** is located posterior to the stomach and is both an endocrine gland and an exocrine gland. About 99 percent of pancreatic cells are *acini cells* and function in exocrine secretion of pancreatic digestion. The other 1 percent are endocrine cells and are called the *islets of Langerhans*.

What Do the Acini Cells Secrete?

The acini cells secrete:

- *Pancreatic lipase.* Pancreatic lipase breaks down fats (triglycerides).
- *Pancreatic amylase.* Pancreatic amylase breaks down starches (polysaccharides).
- *Pancreatic nucleases.* Pancreatic nucleases include *ribonuclease* and *deoxyribonuclease*, which break down nucleic acids.
- *Trypsinogen.* Trypsinogen is converted to its active form *trypsin* (in the intestines by enterokinase), which breaks down protein.

What Are Diseases That Can Affect the Pancreas?

Two disorders of the pancreas are pancreatitis and pancreatic cancer.

What Is Pancreatitis?

Pancreatitis is inflammation of the pancreas. There are two forms:

1. *Acute pancreatitis.* This form of pancreatitis resolves and is commonly the result of a biliary obstruction, usually calculi (stone).
2. *Chronic pancreatitis.* This form of pancreatitis involves tissue changes that are not reversible and that result in progressive loss of both endocrine and exocrine function. The most common cause of chronic pancreatitis is chronic alcohol consumption. Pancreatitis presents as severe abdominal pain that is referred to the midthoracic region of the back and is described as a steady, deep, boring pain accompanied by nausea and vomiting.

What Is Pancreatic Cancer?

Pancreatic cancers that are exocrine tumors are called ***ductal adenocarcinomas***. The majority of these tumors occur in the head of the pancreas and cause obstructions that result in jaundice. Pancreatic cancer is twice as common in men at an average age of 55 years.

The cause of pancreatic cancer is unknown, although alcohol consumption and smoking are risk factors. Pancreatic cancer commonly presents with severe abdominal pain that radiates to the thoracic region of the vertebral column, accompanied by weight loss, jaundice, nausea, vomiting, and fatigue.

Chapter 19 Review Questions

Fill In the Blank

1. Projections of the lamina propria of the tongue are called ____________________.
2. Papillae that have no taste buds are called __________________.
3. Papillae that resemble mushrooms are called ____________________.
4. The throat is called the ____________________.
5. The collapsible muscular tube that connects the pharynx to the stomach is called the _____________.
6. When a portion of the stomach gets pushed up through the opening of the diaphragm, it is called a(n) _____________________.
7. The disorder that is also known as "heartburn" is _________________.
8. A mixture of food, saliva, and gastric juice in the stomach is called ________________.
9. The cells that are located in the stomach and secrete hydrochloric acid and intrinsic factor are called __________________.

10. The cells that are located in the stomach and secrete gastric lipase and pepsinogen are called ____________.
11. Inflammation of the lining of the stomach is called ____________.
12. Erosions in the stomach lining are called ____________.
13. The bacteria that are known to cause ulcerations of the stomach lining are ____________.
14. The jejunum is part of the ____________.
15. The glands that secrete an alkaline mucus that protects the lining of the small intestine are ____________.
16. An inflammatory condition that affects the mucosa layer, resulting in ulcerations, is called ____________.
17. Ulcerative colitis is an inflammatory and ulcerative process that begins at the ____________ region.
18. A "wormlike" projection off the cecum is called the ____________.
19. An S-shaped structure connected to the rectum is the ____________.
20. Feces are stored in the ____________.
21. An obstruction or fecalith can cause ____________.
22. A condition of the colon in which "pouchlike" sacs called diverticula protrude through the mucosa wall of the colon is called ____________.
23. When diverticula become inflamed, the condition is called ____________.
24. Varicose veins that occur in the rectum and anus are called ____________.
25. Inflammation of the liver is called ____________.
26. A common inflammation of the gallbladder is called ____________.
27. Cholecystitis occurs as a result of a blocked ____________.
28. Blockage of the cystic duct is commonly caused by ____________.
29. Gallstones are made up of ____________, ____________, and ____________.
30. Inflammation of the pancreas is called ____________.

True/False

31. A burning sensation in the epigastric region and/or throat is a symptom of GERD.
32. Pepsinogen breaks down fats.
33. Bacterial infections can cause stomach ulcers.
34. Crohn's disease is also referred to as regional enteritis.
35. Crohn's disease has *no* relationship to malabsorption.
36. Ulcerative colitis is an inflammatory disorder.
37. Appendicitis presents only as lower right quadrant pain.
38. Colorectal cancer can cause "pencil-thin" feces.
39. The gallbladder produces bile.
40. Hepatitis can be caused by undercooked or contaminated seafood.

Matching

41. GERD
42. Stomach ulcer
43. Crohn's disease
44. Ulcerative colitis
45. Appendicitis
46. Colorectal cancer
47. Diverticulitis
48. Hemorrhoids
49. Hepatitis
50. Pancreatitis

   A. Fever, cramping, decreased weight, decrease in red blood cell production
   B. Severe localized lower right quadrant pain
   C. Pain after meals or in the supine position
   D. Sudden, violent, watery diarrhea containing blood and mucus
   E. History of polyps in the colon
   F. Abdominal pain after eating peanuts
   G. Pain during defecation and itching in the anal region
   H. Yellow appearance to the skin and sclera
   I. Severe abdominal pain that radiates to the thoracic region
   J. Vomit that looks like coffee grounds

Chapter 19: Review Questions and Answers

Fill In the Blank Answers

1. Papillae
2. Filiform papillae
3. Fungiform papillae
4. Pharynx
5. Esophagus
6. Hiatal hernia
7. Gastroesophygeal reflux disease
8. Chyme
9. Parietal cells
10. Chief cells
11. Gastritis
12. Stomach ulcers
13. *Helicobacter pylori*
14. Small intestine
15. Brunner's glands
16. Crohn's disease
17. Rectosigmoid
18. Appendix
19. Sigmoid colon
20. Rectum
21. Appendicitis
22. Diverticulosis
23. Diverticulitis
24. Hemorrhoids
25. Hepatitis
26. Cholecystitis
27. Cystic duct
28. Gallstones
29. Solidified bile salts; phospholipids; cholesterol
30. Pancreatitis

True/False Answers

31. True
32. False
33. True
34. True
35. False
36. True
37. False
38. True
39. False
40. True

Matching Answers

41. C
42. J
43. A
44. D
45. B
46. E
47. F
48. G
49. H
50. I

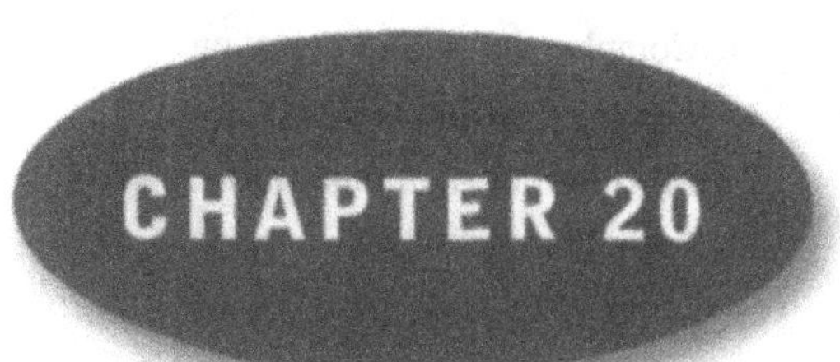

The Diagnosis and Treatment of Disease

Objectives

This chapter will introduce and explain some of the tools that physicians and scientists use to diagnose various diseases and also will give examples of ways of treating these diseases.

Keywords:

Precipitation reaction
Agglutination reaction
Hemagglutination reaction
Neutralization reaction
Complement-fixation reaction
Fluorescent-antibody reaction
Enzyme-linked immunosorbent assay (ELISA)
Radioimmunoassay (RIA)
Antibiotic
Broad-spectrum antibiotic
Narrow-spectrum antibiotic
Bactericidal antimicrobial drugs
Bacteriostatic antimicrobial drugs
Cell wall inhibitors
Protein inhibitors
Plasma membrane inhibitors
Nucleic acid inhibitors
Antimetabolites
Antifungal drugs
Antiviral drugs
Antiprotozoan drugs
Antihelminthic drugs

20.1 Overview

What Are Some of the Reactions That Scientists Use in Determining the Causes of a Disease?

Scientists use eight principal types of reactions to diagnose a disease process:

1. Precipitation reaction
2. Agglutination reaction
3. Hemagglutination reaction
4. Neutralization reaction

5. Complement-fixation reaction
6. Fluorescent-antibody reaction
7. Enzyme-linked immunosorbent assay
8. Radioimmunoassay

What Is a Precipitation Reaction?

A ***precipitation reaction*** combines the antibodies IgG or IgM with soluble antigens. This mixture forms an antigen-antibody complex called a *lattice.* This lattice contains the best possible ratio of antigen and antibody, forming an insoluble precipitate. The antibody that is responsible for creating a precipitating reaction is called a *precipitin*.

Precipitation reactions are commonly used in the following tests:

1. *Precipitation ring test.* In a precipitation ring test, a ring will appear when there is an optimal ratio between antibodies and antigens. This ring is called the *zone of equivalence* and indicates a positive finding.
2. *Immunodiffuse test.* An immunodiffuse test is a type of precipitation reaction that takes place in an agar gel. A visible line will appear in the optimal ratio area, indicating a positive test.
3. *Immunoelectrophoresis test.* Some antigen-antibody mixtures are too complex to be separated by simple diffusion or precipitation. This test uses electrophoresis, which speeds up the separation of these antigens. These tests are commonly used to identify the different proteins in human blood serum for certain diagnostic tests.

What Are Agglutination Reactions?

Agglutination reactions are reactions that add particulate or soluble antigens to antibodies, forming an aggregate (clumping) reaction called *agglutination*. These aggregates can be seen with the naked eye. Agglutination tests are used to determine antibody titer.

There are two types of agglutination reactions:

1. *Direct agglutination test.* This test detects huge cellular antigens. The direct agglutination test uses a microtiter plate containing a series of pits or indentations. Each indentation contains antigen and serum antibody. This measures the concentration of antibody in the serum.
2. *Indirect agglutination test.* In the indirect agglutination test, antigens that are soluble are absorbed in latex spheres and react to the antibodies in around 10 minutes. This test is normally used in diagnosing strep throat.

What Is a Hemagglutination Reaction?

A ***hemagglutination reaction*** is used in blood typing and in diagnosing mononucleosis. In hemagglutination, the antigens that are found on the plasma membrane of the red blood cell react with the antibodies and clump together. The clumping is considered a positive reaction.

What Is a Neutralization Reaction?

A ***neutralization reaction*** takes the antibody of a certain antigen and puts it in a culture that consists of cells and the antigen. If the antigen does not destroy the cells, the toxin of the bacteria or virus is neutralized. This reaction uses antibodies as an "antitoxin" to block the exotoxins and toxoids of bacteria and viruses.

What Tests Use a Neutralization Reaction, and What Are They Used to Diagnose?

The *hemagglutination inhibitor test* is a neutralizing reaction and is used to diagnose influenza, measles, and mumps.

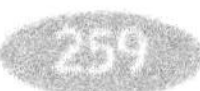

What Is a Complement-Fixation Reaction?

A ***complement-fixation*** reaction uses a group of serum proteins to bond with antigen-antibody complexes. The serum proteins are "fixed" when they completely bind to the antigen-antibody complex. Complement-fixation tests are used to identify very small amounts of antibody in serum. They are used to diagnose certain viral infections, protozoan infections, fungal infections, and bacterial infections, such as those caused by *Chlamydia* and *Rickettsia*.

What Is a Fluorescent-Antibody Reaction?

A ***fluorescent-antibody*** reaction, or RA reaction, uses fluorescent dyes to make the antibodies fluorescent when they are exposed to ultraviolet light. This test is used to diagnose rabies.

What Is an Enzyme-Linked Immunosorbent Assay Test?

An ***enzyme-linked immunosorbent assay*** test, or ***ELISA*** test, uses reagents to identify antigens or antibodies. There are two types of ELISA tests:

1. A *direct ELISA test* identifies antibodies for a specific antigen.
2. An *indirect ELISA test* identifies antigens for specific antibodies.

What Is Radioimmunoassay?

Radioimmunoassay, or ***RIA***, uses tag markers that are radioactive to mark the antibodies and the antigens. The samples are scanned for the presence of these tags.

20.2 Drugs

Chemical agents that are used to treat and cure diseases are called *drugs*.

What Is an Antibiotic?

An ***antibiotic*** is a chemical that inhibits the growth of a microorganism.

What Are Examples of Organisms That Produce Antibiotic Compounds?

Examples of organisms that produce antibiotic compounds are *Streptomyces* (bacteria that live in soil) and *Cephalosporium* and *Penicillium*, which are molds.

What Is a Broad-Spectrum Antibiotic?

A ***broad-spectrum antibiotic*** is one that will destroy a wide variety of infectious organisms.

What Is a Narrow-Spectrum Antibiotic?

A ***narrow-spectrum antibiotic*** is one that will kill only a few different kinds of bacteria.

What Are Bactericidal Antimicrobial Drugs?

Bactericidal antimicrobial drugs are drugs that kill the pathogen and prevent it from spreading.

What Are Bacteriostatic Antimicrobial Drugs?

Bacteriostatic antimicrobial drugs prevent the growth of the pathogen, but allow the immune system of the host to fight the organism.

20.3 Antimicrobial Drugs

How Are Antimicrobial Drugs Classified?

Antimicrobial drugs are classified by their activity. These activities include cell wall inhibitors, protein inhibitors, plasma membrane inhibitors, nucleic acid inhibitors, antimetabolites, antifungal drugs, antiviral drugs, antiprotozoan drugs, and antihelminthic drugs.

What Are Cell Wall Inhibitors?

Cell wall inhibitors are antimicrobial drugs that inhibit the functions and growth of the cell walls of pathogenic organisms.

Some examples of cell wall inhibitors are penicillin antibiotics, which are used in fighting against infections involving staphylococci, streptococci, and several forms of spirochetes. Some examples of penicillin drugs would include ampicillin, amoxicillin, and carbenicillin.

What Are Protein Inhibitors?

Protein inhibitors are drugs that interfere with the pathogenic organism's ability to make proteins. Protein inhibitor drugs include the following:

1. *Aminoglycosides* are antibiotics that were once commonly used in treating gram-negative bacteria. The downside of using these types of antibiotics is their toxic side effects. Examples of aminoglycosides include *streptomycin,* which is used as a secondary treatment against tuberculosis, and *neomycin*, a topical antibiotic used for superficial infections.
2. *Tetracyclines* are broad-spectrum antibiotics that are used to treat urinary tract infections, rickettsial infections, and chlamydial infections. They are also used as a secondary treatment for gonorrhea and syphilis. Examples of tetracycline drugs include oxytetracycline, chlorotetracycline, and minocycline.

What Are Plasma Membrane Inhibitors?

Plasma membrane inhibitors interfere with the structure and function of the microorganism's plasma membrane. An example of a plasma membrane inhibitor would be polymyxin B, which is used to treat *Pseudomonas* infections.

What Are Nucleic Acid Inhibitors?

Nucleic acid inhibitors are drugs that interfere with the formation of nucleic acids. Examples of nucleic acid inhibitors include

1. *Rifamycins.* Rifamycins inhibit the production of mRNA. Rifamycins are used against tuberculosis and leprosy.
2. *Quinolones.* Quinolones interfere with the enzyme DNA gyrase, which is needed for the replication of DNA. These drugs are used to treat urinary tract infections.
3. *Fluoroquinolones.* Fluoroquinolones enter the cell to attack the organism. Examples of these types of drugs are norfloxacin and ciprofloxacin.

What Are Antimetabolites?

Antimetabolites interfere with the cell's normal metabolism (the chemical reactions that take place within a cell that are needed for proper cell function).

What Are Antifungal Drugs?

Antifungal drugs are drugs that stop the growth of fungi. Examples of commonly used antifungal drugs include

1. *Clotrimazole.* Clotrimazole is used to treat athlete's foot and vaginal yeast infections.
2. *Griseofulvin.* Griseofulvin is used to treat fungal infections of the hair and nails.

What Are Antiviral Drugs?

Antiviral drugs stop viruses from replicating.

Nucleoside analogs are drugs that inhibit the synthesis of viral DNA and RNA. Examples of some commonly used nucleoside analogs are

1. *Acyclovir.* Acyclovir is used in treating herpes.
2. *Ganciclovir.* Ganciclovir is used in treating cytomegalovirus.
3. *Zidovudine.* Zidovudine, or AZT, is used in treating HIV.

What Are Antiprotozoan Drugs?

Antiprotozoan drugs are used to treat parasite infections. Commonly used antiprotozoan drugs include

1. *Chloroquine.* Chloroquine is used in treating malaria.
2. *Quinacrine.* Quinacrine is used in treating giardiasis.
3. *Diiodohydroxyquin.* Diiodohydroxyquin is used to treat amoebic infection of the intestine.
4. *Nifurtimox.* Nifurtimox is used to treat Chagas' disease.

What Are Antihelminthic Drugs?

Antihelminthic drugs are used to treat infections by parasitic flatworms called helminths. Some commonly used antihelminthic drugs include

1. *Niclosamide.* Niclosamide is used in treating tapeworm infections.
2. *Praziquantel.* Praziquantel is used to treat fluke infections.
3. *Mebendazole.* Mebendazole is used to treat whipworm and pinworm infections.

Chapter 20 Review Questions

Fill In the Blank

1. A reaction that combines the antibodies IgG and IgM with antigens is called a(n) _______.
2. In this test, a "ring" will appear when there is an optimal ratio between antibodies and enzymes: _____________.
3. In this test, a visible line will appear, indicating a positive test: _____________.

4. The test that uses electrophoresis to identify the different proteins in human serum is ________.

5. A test that adds soluble antigens to antibodies to form an agglutination is called a(n) ______.

6. The two types of agglutination reactions are called ______________ and __________.

7. The test that is used in blood typing and in diagnosing mononucleosis is called ________.

8. In this test, antibodies from a certain antigen are placed in a culture with cells and the antigen. If the antigen does not destroy the cells, the toxin produced by the pathogen is neutralized. This is a(n) ________________.

9. In this test, a group of serum proteins bind with antigen-antibody complexes. When the proteins completely bind to the antigen-antibody complex, it is called a(n) _____________.

10. The type of test that is used to diagnose rabies is ________________.

11. The type of test that uses reagents to identify antigens or antibodies is a(n) _______________.

12. The form of the ELISA test that identifies antibodies for a specific antigen is a(n) ___________.

13. The form of the ELISA test that identifies antigens for specific antibodies is a(n) _______________.

14. The type of test that uses radioactive tag markers is ________________.

15. Chemical agents that are used to treat and cure diseases are called ______________.

16. Drugs that inhibit the growth of microorganisms are called _________________.

17. Antibiotics that destroy a wide variety of bacteria are _________.

18. Types of antibiotics that kill only specific types of bacteria are called ______________.

19. Drugs that kill pathogens are _________________.

20. Drugs that prevent the growth of pathogens are _____________.

21. Antimicrobial drugs that inhibit the growth and function of an organism's cell wall are called ____________.

22. Antimicrobial drugs that interfere with the organism's ability to make protein are called ____________.

23. Antimicrobial drugs that interfere with the structure and function of the organism's plasma membrane are called __________________.

24. Antimicrobial drugs that interfere with the formation of nucleic acids are called ___________.

25. Antimicrobial drugs that interfere with the normal chemical reactions that take place within the pathogenic cell are called __________________.

Matching

26. Ampicillin

27. Streptomycin

28. Penicillin

29. Neomycin

30. Minocycline

31. Rifamycin

32. Quinolones

33. Fluoroquinolone

34. Clotrimazole

35. Griseofulvin

36. *Pseudomonas*

37. Tetracyclines

38. Nucleoside analogs

39. Acyclovir

40. Ganciclovir

41. Zidovudine

42. Chloroquine

43. Quinacrine

44. Diiodohydroxyquin

45. Nifurtimox

46. Niclosamide

47. Praziquantel

48. Mebendazole

49. ELISA

50. Polymyxin

A. Cell wall inhibitor drugs used to fight staph and strep infections
B. An example of a tetracycline drug
C. A plasma membrane inhibitor
D. Polymyxin B is used to treat
E. Inhibits mRNA production
F. Broad-based antibiotics used to treat rickettsial and chlamydial infections
G. Inhibit DNA gyrase
H. Ciprofloxacin is of this type
I. Drugs used to inhibit the synthesis of viral RNA and DNA
J. Used to treat herpes
K. Used to treat cytomegalovirus
L. Also known as AZT
M. Used to treat malaria
N. Used to treat giardiasis
O. An example of a penicillin drug
P. Used to treat amoebic infections
Q. Used to treat Chagas' disease
R. Used to treat tapeworm infections
S. Used to treat fluke infections
T. Used to treat whipworm and pinworm infections
U. Enzyme-linked immunosorbent assay test
V. This drug is used to treat fungal infections of nails
W. This drug is used to treat athlete's foot
X. A topical antibiotic used for superficial infections
Y. An example of an aminoglycoside

Chapter 20: Review Questions and Answers

Fill In the Blank Answers

1. Precipitation reaction
2. Precipitation ring test
3. Immunodiffuse test
4. Immunoelectrophoresis test
5. Agglutination reaction
6. Direct agglutination; indirect agglutination
7. Hemagglutination reaction
8. Neutralization reaction
9. Complement-fixation reaction
10. Fluorescent-antibody test
11. ELISA test
12. Direct ELISA test
13. Indirect ELISA test
14. Radioimmunoassay test
15. Drugs
16. Antibiotics
17. Broad-spectrum antibiotics
18. Narrow-spectrum antibiotics
19. Bactericidal drugs
20. Bacteriostatic drugs
21. Cell wall inhibitors
22. Protein inhibitors
23. Plasma membrane inhibitors
24. Nucleic acid inhibitors
25. Antimetabolites

Matching Answers

26. O
27. Y
28. A
29. X
30. B
31. E
32. G
33. H
34. W
35. V
36. D
37. F
38. I
39. J
40. K
41. L
42. M
43. N
44. P
45. Q
46. R
47. S
48. T
49. U
50. C

INDEX

About the Author

TOM BETSY is a Professor of Biology at Bergen Community College where he teaches anatomy and physiology, biology, and human biology courses. He also teaches anatomy and physiology at the Academy of Massage Therapy in Hackensack, NJ and is a chiropractic doctor. He is the author of *Microbiology Demystified* and has reviewed several health-related science books.

CPSIA information can be obtained
at www.ICGtesting.com
Printed in the USA
FSHW021814110920
73403FS

9 780071 623698